DIVERSITY AND CULTURAL

COMPETENCE IN

HEALTH CARE

DIVERSITY AND CULTURAL

COMPETENCE IN

HEALTH CARE

A Systems Approach

JANICE L. DREACHSLIN

M. JEAN GILBERT

BEVERLY MALONE

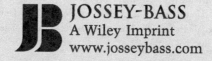

JOSSEY-BASS
A Wiley Imprint
www.josseybass.com

Cover design by Michael Rutkowski
Cover image © 501room/iStock

Published by Jossey-Bass
A Wiley Imprint
One Montgomery Street, Suite 1200, San Francisco, CA 94104-4594—www.josseybass.com

Jossey-Bass books and products are available through most bookstores. To contact Jossey-Bass directly call our Customer Care Department within the U.S. at 800-956-7739, outside the U.S. at 317-572-3986, or fax 317-572-4002.

Wiley publishes in a variety of print and electronic formats and by print-on-demand. Some material included with standard print versions of this book may not be included in e-books or in print-on-demand. If this book refers to media such as a CD or DVD that is not included in the version you purchased, you may download this material at http://booksupport.wiley.com. For more information about Wiley products, visit www.wiley.com.

Library of Congress Cataloging-in-Publication Data
Dreachslin, Janice L.
     Diversity and cultural competence in health care : a systems approach / Janice L. Dreachslin, M. Jean Gilbert, Beverly Malone.—1st ed.
       p. cm.
     Includes bibliographical references and index.
     ISBN 978-1-118-06560-0 (pbk.); ISBN 978-1-118-28216-8 (ebk.);
     ISBN 978-1-118-28385-1 (ebk.); ISBN 978-1-118-28428-5 (ebk.)
       I. Gilbert, M. Jean. II. Malone, Beverly. III. Title.
[DNLM: 1. Cultural Diversity—United States. 2. Delivery of Health Care—United States.
3. Cultural Competency—United States. 4. Healthcare Disparities—United States.
5. Systems Analysis—United States. WA 31]
362.1—dc23
                                                                          2012030239

Printed in the United States of America

FIRST EDITION
PB Printing   V10005474_101918

CONTENTS

FIGURES AND TABLES

LIST OF FIGURES

LIST OF TABLES

PREFACE

Major changes are occurring in the US population and the nation's health care institutions and delivery systems. The population is aging rapidly, with the proportion of senior citizens to youthful workers becoming larger than it has ever been. The population is increasingly ethnically and racially diverse, and groups that were long ignored in health care, such as the LGBT community, are being recognized as having specific health needs that are not being met. The health care enterprise, with all its integrated and disparate parts, has been slow to respond to the needs of our rapidly diversifying population. Millions are uninsured in a system in which insurance is critical to receiving health care, and enormous disparities in health status are visible across diverse groups in the nation's population. Legislation, such as the Affordable Care Act of 2010, is driving change in the way health care services are delivered. Health care institutions, public and private, are seeing the need to recognize and respond to the needs of discrete population groups.

This book was written as an argument for the incorporation of cultural competence and diversity management as important components of the current and emerging systems of health care in the United States. In this argument, we recognize that health care in this country is actually the integration of three systems: a prevention and curative treatment system, a workforce system, and a business system. The book identifies cultural competence and diversity management as integral to all three systems.

All three authors have worked intimately for more than twenty-five years with health care systems at all levels: national, state and local governments, professional associations, and public and private health care delivery organizations. We see cultural competence and diversity management as essential elements of any workable system organized to meet the needs of all Americans.

WHO SHOULD READ THIS BOOK?

This book was designed to be read by students in health sciences and health administration as well as current and future professionals in nursing, medicine, and other clinical and allied health fields. The essentials of cultural competence and diversity management covered in this book will be helpful to a wide variety of students because they encompass principles and practices that can be realistically incorporated into the ongoing work of any health care field or organization.

HOW THIS BOOK IS ORGANIZED

This book is divided into four parts. Part One, "The Diversity Imperative," provides a rationale for incorporating diversity understandings and cultural competence as key components of the US health care system. Chapter One describes the seven dimensions of diversity considered throughout the book. It defines cultural competence and introduces health care disparities across US population groups as a critical issue facing the nation. The role of diversity management as a key component of culturally competent health care is discussed. The second chapter in this section examines the breadth of disparities and differences in health care status across major population groups. It documents sources of these disparities and outlines past and current responses to this issue by the health care establishment, including the slowness with which the nation has come to grips with the problem. Legislation, advocacy, and accreditation policy are described as drivers of cultural competence strategies to address disparities. Chapter Three addresses changing workforce demographics and their impact on the health care workforce. Most particular, the effects of an aging workforce and an ethnically and racially diverse workforce are described. The authors point out how social factors work to narrow the pipeline of minority students entering health care professions. The management of diverse workforces in terms of philosophy and practice are examined, as is the business case for a diverse workforce.

The chapters in Part Two describe the development of cultural competence. Chapter Four discusses how cultural competence in health care is practically defined and integrated into more recent care philosophy and service delivery. An emphasis is placed on understanding the meaning of culture in the lives of all persons and on what constitutes a cultural group. The growth of cultural competence as an important strategy of health care is reviewed as are guides and models for culturally competent care.

Chapter Five describes the complex processes underlying personal biases toward others, both implicit and explicit. It discusses the nature of professional resistance to training in cultural competence. A framework for transforming the role of the health care professional to explicitly include the perspectives of cultural competence is presented. Chapter Six emphasizes training modalities that include general and specific kinds of knowledge and skills needed by health care managers, clinicians, and frontline workers in order to be culturally competent in the work they do.

The chapters in Part Three, "Cultural Competence and Health Care Delivery," address specific issues in cultural competence as they relate to interactions between health care providers and diverse patients. Chapter Seven focuses our attention on the most fundamental element in health care: the patient-provider interaction. The chapter describes several conceptual models that can assist clinicians in preparing for crosscultural transactions. Chapter Eight introduces the critical issue of language access in the United States, where 8 percent of the population has no or limited proficiency in English. It examines the severity of issues that can arise in a health care setting when interpretation and translation are not available, the legislation and regulation that have developed around the provisions of language services, as well as several model programs and practices that health care organizations have devised to reduce language barriers. Chapter Nine examines the process of group identity development and the role that group identity plays in the delivery of health care services. The operation of in-group–out-group behavior and relationships are described and their effect on health care delivery is explored.

Part Four, the last section of the book, is devoted to cultural competence as it relates to and is expressed in diversity management, organizational behavior, and policy. Chapter Ten explains why organizational behavior is essential to a systems approach to cultural competence. It describes the practices that create a culture of inclusion in which people can perform to their highest potential, providing a motivating context for culturally competent health care. Chapter Eleven makes the business case for culturally competent health care organizations by pointing to improvements in productivity, patient satisfaction, health outcomes, and market expansion that accrue to diversity management of the workforce and the provision of culturally competent health care. Chapter Twelve explores the future of diversity and cultural competence in health care with emphasis on the continuing diversification of the US population, legislation such as the Affordable Care Act, which not only will bring into the health system millions of minority patients but also mandates examination of how health care practices affect those populations, making public and private systems of care accountable for health care outcomes and health status across diverse groups. The chapter predicts that the systems approach to diversity and cultural competence will increasingly be the norm, not the exception, in health care organizations and identifies trends that support and trends that work against this prediction.

Following the text of each chapter are questions and suggested activities designed to allow students to explore and examine concepts and practices identified in the chapter, helping to foster group discussion.

CHALLENGES TO THE STUDENTS

Health care in the United States is receiving intense scrutiny as the nation attempts to control escalating costs and at the same time improve health care quality and reduce problematic disparities. Developing culturally competent care and capable diversity management are important but challenging approaches to resolving these issues. Students are encouraged to consider these strategies in the context of their other studies that deal with health care organization and service delivery and be inventive in applying and integrating them. The authors also strongly suggest that students follow up on the websites and many online publications that are listed throughout the chapters because they will greatly amplify the information in this book.

The ultimate goal of cultural competence and diversity management is to create and maintain a cost-effective and efficient health care system that produces good health care outcomes for all the nation's citizens. Although many cultural competence and diversity management strategies are intuitively appropriate to this goal, many remain to be tested in order to develop a strong evidence base for their use in health care. It is appropriate, then, for students to challenge these concepts, improve them, and test their effectiveness in the health care work that they do.

ACKNOWLEDGMENTS

When a book is the product of three people each spending over twenty years working in complementary fields such as diversity management and cultural competence, there are many, many people who have provided important insights, education, counsel, and support along the way. We are particularly grateful for the long-term, pioneering inspiration and collaborative support of Julia Puebla-Fortier of Diversity Rx; Robert C. Like, MD, of the Center for Healthy Families and Cultural Diversity; Tawara Goode of the National Center for Cultural Competence; Guadalupe Pacheco of the Office of Minority Health; Joseph Betancourt, MD, of the Disparities Solutions Center; Beatriz Solis of L.A. Care; Fred Hobby of the Institute for Diversity in Health Management; and Rob Weech-Maldonado of the University of Alabama. Without their innovation, collegial spirit, and, yes, dogged persistence, the fields of cultural competence and diversity management would not have developed as fully as they have!

Jan Dreachslin owes special thanks to Portia Hunt of Temple University, her treasured mentor, colleague, and friend, whose love, guidance, and encouragement were key to her development in the field of diversity management over the last thirty-plus years. She is grateful to the American College of Healthcare Executives for the 1999 Health Management Research Award that was instrumental in launching her exploration of the role that leadership behavior and organizational practices play in the delivery of culturally and linguistically appropriate care. Subsequent and ongoing support from the National Center for Health Care Leadership and Sodexo ensured that her work in the field would continue to evolve.

Jean Gilbert owes special thanks to the many doctors and managers of Kaiser Permanente who willingly embraced the concepts of cultural competence and taught her much about patient care and the structuring of health care delivery.

She benefitted from learning about medical interpretation and translation from colleagues Gayle Tang and Cindy Roat and is thankful for the insights they shared. The California Endowment is also gratefully acknowledged for the strong support they provide for culturally and linguistically appropriate health care services in general and also for the specific support they provided for Gilbert's research on medical interpretation in clinical settings and the development of the *Principles and Standards for the Cultural Competence Education of Health Care Professionals*.

Bev Malone is indebted to Drs. Hattie B. Bessent and Gloria Smith, who lived a commitment to diversity and inclusion in their clinical and organizational work. Dr. Bessent, with the wisdom of those over eighty years old, is still developing creative strategies to include minority professionals as leaders in the care of others. Bev also wants to extend a special thank-you to Dr. David Satcher, former surgeon general and assistant secretary for health during the Clinton administration, who provided supervision, mentoring, and inspiration to her as she took up the role of deputy assistant secretary for health. Finally she wishes to extend kudos to her British colleagues, Bruce Irvine, Jean Reed, and John Bazalgette, who believe in co-creation when working with organizations, differences, and others honoring the person in their role in the system.

We are all indebted to the health care managers, clinicians, and consultants who work every day to ensure that diverse patients receive culturally and linguistically appropriate care and that health care organizations and their leaders engage in best practices in diversity management.

Janice L. Dreachslin, PhD, is a professor of health policy and administration at the Penn State Great Valley School of Graduate Professional Studies in Malvern, Pennsylvania, and co-professor-in-charge of the MBA program. With over thirty years' experience, Dr. Dreachslin has consulted with health care organizations in the United States, Canada, Great Britain, and Australia. She is the author of numerous publications and presentations in diversity leadership and maintains an active consulting practice in the field. Dr. Dreachslin is author of the first academic book on strategic diversity management in health care, *Diversity Leadership*, published in June 1996 by the American College of Healthcare Executive's Health Administration Press. Dr. Dreachslin and her collaborators received the 1999 ACHE Health Management Research Award for their Survey of Diversity Practices in Pennsylvania Hospitals. As chair of the Association of University Programs in Health Administration's (AUPHA) Diversity Forum (2000–2004), Dr. Dreachslin led an initiative to define domains and core competencies for diversity leadership in health services management nationwide. She served as an invited member of the Institute for Diversity in Health Care Management's benchmarking project advisory council. She was the lead investigator for a study of factors that affect career advancement for women and people of color in health services management, commissioned by the National Center for Healthcare Leadership (NCHL). Dr. Dreachslin is principal investigator for a Sodexo-funded NCHL diversity demonstration project. The project employs pre- and postintervention assessment of systemwide diversity change initiatives and involves two major hospital systems. Dr. Dreachslin was inducted into the NCHL Innovator's Circle in 2010 in recognition for her work in diversity leadership.

M. Jean Gilbert, PhD, an applied medical anthropologist, received her PhD from the University of California, Santa Barbara. She has conducted crosscultural research in childbirth, health services use, and substance use and abuse in the United States and Mexico. She was National Institute of Alcohol Abuse and Alcoholism Research Scholar in Latino alcohol studies at UCLA for six years, then joined Kaiser Permanente in 1990 to help initiate its cultural competence programs as consultant to its national diversity council and director of cultural competence for its California Regions. In this role, she collaborated in the design of cultural competence curricula for a wide variety of health care professionals and consulted in the delivery of services to diverse populations. Dr. Gilbert was on the advisory team that created the original Department of Health and Human Services' CLAS standards and a member of the California Health Services' Cultural and Linguistic Task Force that developed mandatory cultural and linguistic requirements for MediCal. She was an organizing charter member of the California Healthcare Interpreters Association (CHIA) and has conducted research into the impact of interpreter training on dual role interpreters. In 2003, she led the national team of health care professionals that developed the Principles and Standards for the Cultural Competence Education of Health Care Professionals under a grant from The California Endowment. Dr. Gilbert was project director for the national and international award winning Multicultural Health Series video modules created in collaboration with Kaiser Permanente's MultiMedia Communications Department to train health care professionals in cultural competence. Currently, she consults on cultural competence and diversity issues to foundations, governmental agencies, and professional schools. She is a Fellow of the Society for Applied Anthropology.

Beverly Malone, PhD, RN, FAAN, is the chief executive officer of the National League for Nursing (NLN). Dr. Malone's tenure at the NLN has been marked by a retooling of the League's mission to reflect the core values of caring, diversity, integrity, and excellence and an ongoing focus on advancing the nation's health.

In 2010, the year she was ranked number twenty-nine among the one hundred most powerful people in health care by *Modern Healthcare* magazine, Dr. Malone served on the Institute of Medicine's Forum on the Future of Nursing Education, contributing to the IOM's groundbreaking report, "The Future of Nursing: Leading Change, Advancing Health," and on the Advisory

Committee on Minority Health, a federal panel established to advise the US Secretary of Health and Human Services.

Her distinguished career has mixed policy, education, administration, and clinical practice. Dr. Malone has worked as a surgical staff nurse, clinical nurse specialist, director of nursing, and assistant administrator of nursing. During the 1980s she was dean of the School of Nursing at North Carolina Agricultural and Technical State University. In 1996, she was elected to two terms as president of the American Nurses Association, representing 180,000 nurses in the United States. In 2000, she became deputy assistant secretary for health within the US Department of Health and Human Services. Just prior to joining the NLN, Dr. Malone was general secretary of the Royal College of Nursing, the United Kingdom's largest professional union of nurses, from June 2001 to January 2007. Dr. Malone was also a member of the Higher Education Funding Council for England.

To Elaine Smith with love and appreciation

—JLD

To Lisa Gilbert with love and respect

—MJG

To Addie Blanche Olden and Dorothy Black with admiration and love

—BJM

DIVERSITY AND CULTURAL

COMPETENCE IN

HEALTH CARE

THE DIVERSITY

IMPERATIVE

The chapters in Part One provide background and context for the systems approach to cultural competence and diversity management in health care. They supply a rationale for health care services designed to meet the needs of a diverse population. In Chapter One, "Systems Approach to Cultural Competence," we explain the unifying systems concept as it is applied to health care. The authors see cultural competence and diversity management, integrated into a systems approach, as critical to meeting the health care challenges of the nation's diverse population. Although the United States rightly considers itself one people, there is significant diversity within the population, and this diversity has implications that affect the way health care is structured and delivered. We discuss several important dimensions of diversity and address the unfortunate reality that there are serious disparities in health care access and status that divide the nation's diverse groups. Major changes in how health care services are conceptualized and delivered are taking place, and we briefly point out how cultural competence and diversity management integrate these changes.

In Chapter Two, "Systematic Attention to Health Care Disparities," the term *disparities* is clarified. In-depth attention is then given to the kinds and degrees of health care disparities that are visible throughout segments of the nation's population. After a long period of inattention to the nature of these disparities and their consequences, the health care establishment, private philanthropy, and government agencies are gearing up to address them with data, legislation, and new strategies of care. We discuss how collecting data on the characteristics and health of patient populations is important for all health care organizations and emphasize its use as a driver for changing health care approaches. Organizations that are implementing data-driven strategies are described, as are some of the tools that have been developed for collecting and using data about diverse groups.

A diversifying population means a diversifying labor force, and Chapter Three, "Workforce Demographics," addresses significant changes in the nation's workforce as minorities become majorities in many parts of the country. The health care workforce is a major sector of the US labor force, and its complex structure of many different kinds of professionals, support, and service staff is reviewed in this chapter. Majority and minority groups are integrated differently in health care's hierarchical workforce structure, and the reasons for and implications of this are significant when it comes to the nation's being able to provide culturally appropriate care and reduce health disparities. Additionally, we point out that such a diverse workforce, with its many occupational specialties and levels as well as its racial, ethnic, age, and gender composition, offers many performance challenges to management. Group identity has important social meaning for persons inside and outside groups, and these meanings are reflected in constructive and destructive workplace behavior. We make clear that the need for informed diversity management, with its emphasis on inclusion, opportunity, and equity, is critical.

Chapter 1

SYSTEMS APPROACH TO CULTURAL COMPETENCE

LEARNING OBJECTIVES

- To clarify what is meant by a systems approach
- To define key terms including *diversity*, *cultural competence*, *disparities*, and *strategic diversity management*
- To describe the dimensions of diversity that will be discussed throughout this text
- To gain an understanding of health care disparities in the United States
- To become familiar with essential systems approaches to cultural competence and reducing disparities
- To characterize the relationship between strategic diversity management and culturally competent health care delivery

Fundamentally, a **system** is a structure of interconnected people, policies, and practices designed to work in concert to achieve a common goal. The **systems approach** is the process of considering how different parts of the whole structure influence and integrate with each other and viewing problems in a system as affecting the system overall. Component parts of a system can best be understood in the context of their relationships with each other. In a well-integrated, smoothly functioning system, each part contributes to the achievement of the goals for which the system was put into place. In the case of the health care system in the United States, the goal is a high level of health within the nation's population. Thus, this system can be said to be a preventive and curative system. It is also, most important, a major employment system and a key business system. The health care system is an "open system"; that is, elements from outside the system in its environment are constantly affecting and being admitted to the system. In other words, there are transactions across the external and internal boundaries of the system. As this occurs, a well-designed system includes feedback mechanisms so that those operating the system can assess, evaluate, and readjust its structure and processes, enabling it to continue to meet its goals. In this book, we view **diversity** within the population and **disparities** in health care access and treatment as factors with which the US health care system must successfully adjust in order to meet its goal of good health for the overall population rather than just segments of the population.

Cultural competence is a major strategy for helping the system successfully meet the challenges of diversity and disparities. From its initial conceptualization in health care, cultural competence was seen as an essential systems component. Cross, Barzon, Dennis, and Issacs (1989) defined it as "a set of congruent behaviors, attitudes and policies that come together in a system, agency, or amongst professionals and enables that system, agency, or those professionals to work effectively in cross-cultural situations" (p. 2). Another excellent definition of cultural competence put forth by the National Quality Forum (2008) is "the ongoing capacity of healthcare systems, organizations, and professionals to provide for diverse patient populations high-quality care that is safe, patient and family centered, evidence based and equitable" (p. 3). Cultural competence incorporates all of the strategies and practices needed to work effectively with patients from diverse groups based on an understanding of their beliefs, values, and social milieu. We take the position in this book that by systematically integrating the philosophy and practices of cultural competence and diversity management into the processes, transactions, and structures of the health care system, appropriate care for diverse groups and the elimination of disparities could better be accomplished and the goal of good health care across the nation more completely realized.

Figure 1.1 is a visual representation of the authors' overall conceptualization of a systematic approach to the development of cultural competence and diversity in health care, moving from a rationale for the development of cultural competence in health care, to the adoptions of appropriate attitudes, skills, and knowledge, then to an application of those capabilities in service delivery, and finally to the use of organizational leadership and **strategic diversity management** to create well-functioning, diverse organizations able to provide appropriate health care to all populations.

This first chapter provides an overview of the seven key dimensions of diversity that will be considered in this book as well as the roots of diversity in the United States. In this text, the term *diversity* refers to differences that make each person or group unique when compared with other persons or groups. Our individual uniqueness is driven by the groups we are identified with, such as race and ethnicity, socioeconomic status, gender, age and generation, sexual orientation,

FIGURE 1.1 Systematic Approach to Development of Cultural Competence

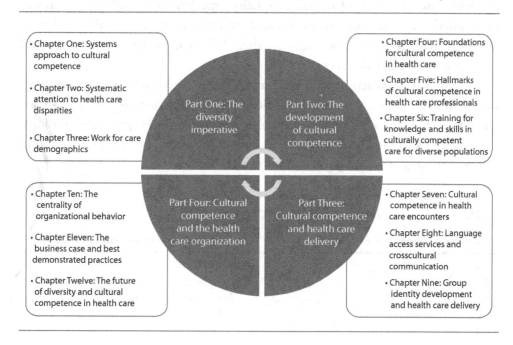

and religious preference, and also by what our **identity groups** mean to others and ourselves. Diversity is important in health care because what patients, caregivers, families, and health care organizations believe about key diversity dimensions affects how patient care is structured and delivered and how the health care work force is managed. And the United States is changing: not only are we becoming more diverse across multiple dimensions of diversity but our attitudes toward diversity are also evolving. In this chapter we review the diversity demographic trends for the seven key dimensions of diversity that have special implications for health care and are referenced throughout this text: race and ethnicity, gender, sexual orientation, age, language, socioeconomic status, and religion (see Table 1.1). The first three dimensions of diversity are personal, almost **immutable**, qualities of personhood; the last four are important social variables that create diversity among people, **crosscutting** the immutable dimensions and contributing to diversity within them. A moment's reflection also will tell us that these dimensions of diversity frequently overlap and interact with each other and intersect with the health care system in many complex ways. This complexity will be addressed in this book many times over.

This chapter next introduces the critical issue of health care disparities across diverse population groups in the United States. The glaring disparities in access to health care and levels of treatment quality experienced by different groups in the United States is a significant societal problem that can be addressed only through careful assessment of diverse needs and the structuring of appropriate and systematic health care delivery.

Several new approaches to the creation of health care delivery systems that require culturally competent care will be briefly introduced, including evidence-based care, medical homes, person-centered health care, and interdisciplinary professional teams. Cultural competence is seen as an important factor in needs assessment and the creation of appropriate **personalized care**.

TABLE 1.1   The Seven Dimensions of Diversity

Immutable Dimensions of Diversity	Crosscutting Dimensions of Diversity
Race and ethnicity	Age
Gender	Language
Sexual orientation	Socioeconomic status
	Religion

Finally, it is clear that the changes needed to create and implement more systematic and culturally competent health care policies and practices will not take place without the informed management and leadership of health care professionals and policy makers. The chapter ends by urging students to take up the challenge of leadership in the creation of health care systems and organizations that truly meet the needs of all the nation's residents.

DIMENSIONS OF DIVERSITY

The following section examines each of the dimensions of diversity in depth so that when the terms are used throughout the book, the reader will understand exactly what is meant by each term.

Ethnicity and Race

The growing attention to diversity and cultural competence in health care has been in great part driven by the United States' increasing racial and ethnic diversity and by the fact that health care access and quality of care differ substantially across diverse groups, resulting in critical differences in health status (Smedley, Stith, & Nelson, 2002). The 2010 Census confirmed that, by the middle of this century, the United States will be a majority minority nation; less than half of the population will be non-Hispanic white (Mather, Pollard, & Jacobsen, 2011). *Cultural* or *ethnic groups* are not the same as *racial groups*, though culture and race are both aspects of human diversity. An ethnic group is defined by its **culture**; it is a group of people whose members identify with each other through a common language, behavioral norms, **worldview**, history, and ancestry. Culture, like language, is learned, not biologically inherited. An ethnic group is also generally recognized as a discrete group by persons outside the group. **Ethnicity** is often associated with national origin, but there are usually many ethnic groups within a single nation, and there are ethnic groups that cross national boundaries. Examples of ethnic groups are Mexican-Americans, Navajo, Hmong, Berber, and Zulu.

Race is a term used by scientists and the general public to identify groups of people by physiological characteristics such as skin color, hair texture, facial features, bone structure, and the like. As pointed out by Byrd and Clayton (2002) in *Unequal Treatment*, "Scientists who study race consider it a socially determined category based on shared physical characteristics . . . most commonly dividing the human family into three to five major racial groups" (p. 474). Very recently, population geneticists studying the genetic constitution of populations around the world through genomewide studies have been able to link genetic heritage with the ancient continental, geographic distribution of populations that correspond closely with commonly used racial designations such a Caucasian (Europe and Middle East), African, Asian, Pacific Islander (for example, New Guinean and Melanesian), and Native American (Li et al., 2008; Risch et al., 2002). However, it is clear that virtually none of the authorities contend there are "pure" races because many groups overlap the racial classification systems that have been used and are blurred due to migration, contact, and intermarriage. It should be noted as well that there are almost always many ethnic groups falling within a racial category (Collins, 2004). Research has been able to link disease resistance, risk, and response to pharmaceuticals to these different racial heritage groups as well as to some ethnic groups whose gene pools have been isolated for extended periods of time. This is just one of the several reasons why epidemio-logical studies usually consider race and ethnicity as important variables in determining health care disparities across population groups. To take note of the genetic aspects of race, however, is not to deny the importance of historical and current social constructions around the meaning of race and ethnicity because these are critical to understanding the environmental, economic, and societal factors that are associated with disparities in health status, health care access, and treatment. Our understanding of the complex relationship between self-reported race and ethnicity, genetics, and health continues to evolve and will be discussed in the context of disparities in Chapter Two.

As a result of the immigration history of the United States, it has also been common to describe segments of the US population by nation of origin. Clearly, most nations are made up of several ethnic and racial groups. An individual, for example might be a British national but ethnically Pakistani and racially Asian. Sometimes persons from a particular nation are thought to subscribe to a national culture that adds to and overlies the cultures of various groups making up its population. In contemporary society, the historic connection between ethnicity and nationality is growing weaker. In the United States, national identity or citizenship is by design and values distinct from ethnic or racial identity, a topic that we will discuss in greater detail later in this book.

The ethnic, racial, and national background characteristics of the US popu-lation are mostly the result of US policy regulating immigration to the country during the country's history. Although the United States prides itself on being a nation of immigrants, not all races, ethnicities, and nationalities were accepted with equally open arms. To a great extent, immigration policies have been driven by the nation's need for specific types of labor over the years. Black Americans were enslaved and forcibly brought to the United States to meet the labor needs of the agricultural South. The need for unskilled labor during the building of the transnational railroads in the latter part of the 1800s allowed the immigration of many workers from China, and, later, Mexico. When that need was over, very restrictive policies such as the Chinese Exclusion Act of 1882 were enacted. The country's need for Mexican labor has waxed and waned, and immigration policies have restricted or encouraged immigration from that nation accordingly. In the late 1800s and early 1900s, the huge waves of immigrants from southern and eastern Europe who found employment in the burgeoning industries of America as well as the fewer immigrants from northern and western Europe came to work in mainly low-skilled factory work. By 1921, however, the Emergency Quota Act was passed; in it, the incoming immigrant population was limited to 198,082 from northern and western Europe, and 158,367 from southern and eastern Europe. A few years later, the National Origins Act strictly limited the number of persons who could emigrate from *any* eastern hemisphere country. During the Depression and before and after World War II, immigration was severely curtailed. The Immigration and Nationality Act of 1952 continued restrictions based on nationality quotas with an emphasis on allowing European immigration more than from other parts of the world. The outcome of these various policies through the generations was a very homogeneous, primarily white US population in the two decades just following World War II. This apparent homogeneity enabled little appreciation of diverse health care needs. At the same time, the health care of black Americans was relegated to black institutions or segregated facilities (Skloot, 2010).

Radical policy change came with the Hart-Celler Immigration Act of 1965, which removed quotas based on national origins and labor needs. The major source countries of immigration shifted from Europe to Latin America and Asia. Thousands of undocumented persons also entered the country from Mexico and Central America, many of whom were granted amnesty in 1986 through the Immigration Reform and Control Act. Following the Vietnam War in 1975, large numbers of southeast Asians, such as Hmong, Mien, and Vietnamese, were granted admission. Refugees from Afghanistan, Pakistan, Iran, Somalia, and other war-torn nations sought asylum and settled in the country. After the first terrorist attack on the World Trade Center occurred in 1992, public support for restricted immigration and curtailment of undocumented entry began to grow again. Nevertheless, as a result of the push-pull policies of the prior three decades (Orchowski, 2008), the nation's population had become more ethnically, racially, and linguistically diverse than it ever had been in its history.

This cultural and linguistic diversity was making itself felt in the patient populations of the country's hospitals and clinics. Health care organizations and personnel, surprised and unprepared to respond to diversity of this magnitude, were often reluctant to make changes that would enable them to better serve diverse patients. Further, assessment of the health status of the different races and ethnic groups revealed very significant disparities in health status across several of the country's population groups, which included but were not restricted to black-white differences. These circumstances gave rise in the early to mid-1990s to the beginnings of the cultural competence movement in health care and to national policies that were directed to the reduction of serious disparities in health care access and treatment. Whereas the differing racial and ethnic health statuses first prompted these directions within health care, proponents soon realized that the women's health movement, issues related to sexual orientation made more explicit by the HIV epidemic, and the aging of the population made a broader understanding of diversity and health disparities necessary.

Gender

Although more boys than girls are born each year, the US population overall is about 51 percent female and 49 percent male. Researchers attribute this to differences in mortality that favor women over men, and, due to their longer life expectancy, women predominate in the oldest age cohorts that consume relatively more health care services. Interestingly, prior to the 1950 Census, the male-to-female ratio was over 100, indicating that there were more males than females in the United States. From 1950 through 1990, the male-to-female ratio dipped below 100 but began a gradual rise from 94.5 in 1980 to 96.3 in 2000, which researchers attribute to the combined effects of immigration, which has brought in more men than women, and a decline in the male death rate that exceeded the decline for women during the same time period (Smith & Spraggins, 2001).

Prior to the 1970s, women's health needs were rarely differentiated from those of men. Research examining medical, health-related, and pharmaceutical agents infrequently included women, and, if women were included, results were seldom broken out by gender. It was assumed the women's bodies differed from men's only by their reproductive organs. However, the feminist movement had a women's health thrust, the women's health movement. At first, the major concerns centered on birth control, abortion, and reproductive health but the focus soon expanded as it became clear that there was widespread dissatisfaction among women regarding their health care and the attitudes about women prevalent in the medical community. The publication of *Our Bodies, Ourselves* (Boston Women's Health Collective, 1973) was a milestone in women's early articulation of their special health needs. In 1985 a United States Public Health Service task force concluded that exclusion of women from clinical research was detrimental to their health, in 1986 the National Institutes of Health (NIH) adopted guidelines urging the inclusion of women in clinical studies, and in 1993 NIH mandated that women and members of minority groups be included in all government-sponsored research (Society for Women's Health Research, nd). The research literature now robustly shows that differences between the genders exist in the prevalence and severity of a broad range of diseases and conditions and at every stage of life. The National Institute of Medicine summarized much of what is known so far about gender differences in health in the book, *Exploring the Biological Contributions to Human Health: Does Sex Matter?* (Wizemann & Pardue, 2001) and more recently have updated the progress of women's health research in Committee on Women's Health Research, *Women's Health Research: Progress, Pitfalls, and Promise* (2010).

As Owens (2008) observes, women consume more health care services overall than do men: "Research spanning several decades shows that in comparison with men, women use more physician services, have more episodes of acute illness, require reproductive care, and need more long-term care over their longer life span. An analysis of Express Scripts' integrated database of medical and pharmacy claims revealed that women contribute to 60% of medical spending and consume 59% of the prescription volume. In addition, women represent the majority of Medicare beneficiaries" (p. S2).

Health care insurance premium prices and the proportion of the uninsured also vary by gender. Historically, insurers have employed gender rating, that is, routinely charged women more than men for individual health care insurance policies. Effective in 2014, the Affordable Care Act of 2010 will prohibit this practice.

Biology most certainly plays a role in the significance of gender to health care. However, as with the other dimensions of diversity discussed previously, what we believe about gender is driven by our cultures' values and behavioral norms. These beliefs in turn shape gender roles and relationships in society, such as spousal and parenting behaviors. They influence career choices, patient-clinician interactions, and treatment seeking as well as health care decisions.

Sexual Orientation

Estimating the proportion of the US population that self-identifies as lesbian, gay, bisexual, or transgender (LGBT) is challenging for researchers, producing figures ranging from less than 2 percent to about 5½ percent. Estimates will vary depending on how sexual orientation is defined and how questions about sexual orientation are posed. The Williams Institute at UCLA Law puts the percentage of lesbian, gay, or bisexual US adults at 3½ percent and transgender at .3 percent (Gates, 2011). Lofquest (2011), using data from the 2010 American Community Survey (ACS), estimates that 1 percent of couples sharing a household in the United States are same-sex domestic partners. ACS data reveal that the percentage of same-sex couple households ranged from .29 percent in Wyoming to 4.01 percent in the District of Columbia, and nearly 20 percent of same-sex couple households in the United States have children. Dade (2011) notes an 80 percent increase in the percentage of households consisting of same-sex domestic partners from Census 2000 to Census 2010. Dade (2011) attributes this to growing acceptance of LGBT relationships in the United States and a concomitant willingness to disclose sexual identity on government surveys such as the census. Based on 2010 census data, Gates (2011) observes that the percentage of same-sex couples that are interracial or interethnic (20.6 percent) is higher than for either different-sex unmarried couples (18.3 percent) or different-sex married couples (9.5 percent).

Because of the social stigma attached to any sexual orientation other than heterosexual, prior to the 1980s and the AIDS epidemic, the LGBT population was a hidden population as far as health data were concerned. Societal adjustment in perspectives has occurred during the last three decades, and there is greater acceptance of and attention to the health needs of people of different sexual orientations in many of the nation's health care organizations. The LGBT community has itself worked to build an infrastructure to address its health needs and has lobbied successfully to obtain recognition of these needs from scientific bodies and the government (Committee on Lesbian, Gay, Bisexual and Transgender Health Issues, 2011).

Sexual orientation is relevant to health in myriad ways that will be discussed throughout this book. Although LGBT people share with the rest of society the full range of health risks, they also face a set of additional risks due to social stigma. One of these risks is their "invisibility" to health care providers because of their reluctance to come out to health care professionals and the failure of providers and health care institutions to foster an accepting environment. Domestic partner health benefits for the workforce of health care organizations, hospital visitation rights, the health care decision-making role and space for a patient's domestic partner, and establishing trust to encourage disclosure of sexual orientation are among the issues relevant to patients and employees who self-identify as LGBT.

There are still challenges to obtaining clear, generalizable data on the health risks of the LGBT population that are related to appropriately defining inclusion criteria for studies, reluctant self-identification of research subjects, and the costs of obtaining and analyzing data from small or hidden populations (Dean et al., 2000; Gilbert & Sabin, 2008;). Nevertheless, an actionable picture of the needs of the LGBT population throughout the life course is emerging (Committee on Lesbian, Gay, Bisexual and Transgender Health Issues, 2011) and there are indications that some health systems are responding to the needs of the LGBT community in positive ways. In considering culturally competent approaches to the LGBT group, it is important to realize that different racial and ethnic and religious groups perceive sexual orientation issues differently and that LGBT persons need to be understood in terms of the larger group in which they are culturally embedded.

Age and Generation

The US population as a whole is growing older. The US Census Bureau (2008) predicts that by 2030, 20 percent of the population will be sixty-five and older, which is more than double the 2008 proportion. Whereas the eighty-five and older population will triple by 2050, the working age population will decline from 63 percent in 2008 to 57 percent. There is perhaps is no greater challenge to the health care institutions of the United States than that posed by its aging population. Much has been made recently of the leading front of the baby boomer age wave passing into retirement and into the embrace of Medicare. Another issue that has not been as widely discussed is the fact that the aging population is predominantly white and the younger working age population is increasingly made up of people of color, a large proportion of whom have lower levels of education and have difficulty entering a health care workforce that is increasingly technical, specialized, and cybernetic in nature. As will be noted in Chapter Three, the black and Latino pipeline for future professional level jobs in health care is very narrow. This situation is exacerbated by the fact that the health care workforce is itself highly stratified and hierarchical, with most professional and high-level administrative positions requiring postgraduate educations. This age, race, and ethnic workforce gap is a critical diversity issue facing the US health care system.

The health care issues surrounding the aging of the population aren't just those of changes in the ratio of age cohorts. People in the United States are living much longer than they used to. For example, under current mortality conditions, people who survive to age 65 can expect to live an average of 18.5 more years, about 4 years longer than people aged 65 in 1960 (Federal Interagency Forum on Age-Related Statistics, 2010). Along with extended life spans come much more chronic disease and multiproblem illness that lower functioning levels and require more intensive and ongoing health care. And, whereas chronic diseases such as type 2 diabetes can be modified with behavioral changes, such interventions need to be culturally sensitive to diverse populations in order to be effective. Differing cultural groups also have long-held beliefs about aging and caretaking of the elderly that are important to consider in planning for elder care. For example, cultural concepts around death and dying are important issues in end-of-life decision making that are critical to elders and their families.

Related to and yet distinct from age is the concept of generational diversity. With its origins in consumer marketing, this body of research studies cultural differences among generational cohorts in the United States: veterans (1922–1943); baby boomers (1943–1960); generation X (1960–1980), and generation Y (1980–2000). Due to shared social, political, economic, and technological events during their formative years, each generation has developed a set of beliefs and core values that undergird their work style and choices, including career decisions as well as health care expectations and preferences (Howe, 2009; Zemke, Raines, & Filipczak, 2000). These generational shifts in expectations and preferences will require change in health care delivery organizations. Issues as diverse as the replacement of paper with electronic medical records, expanding modes of communication between patient and provider, and addressing shortages of personnel in key clinical roles including registered nurses and primary care physicians are among those that health care organizations must address.

Additionally, another common use of the word *generation* in health care literature and epidemiology refers to whether an individual is first generation in the United States, that is, immigrated from another country; second generation, the child of an immigrant; and so on. An understanding of a patient's generational remove from immigrant status is useful in evaluating his or her knowledge of the US health care system, perceptions around disease etiology, and the like, all necessary to operating within a culturally competent framework.

Socioeconomic Status

Although people in the United States like to think of themselves as a highly socially mobile, almost classless society, the facts belie this belief. The country is highly stratified by every measure of social class. A measure that is often used, socioeconomic status (SES), is an economic and sociological composite measure that is based on a combination of three highly related factors: income (and sometimes wealth or accumulated assets), education, and occupation. Typically, socioeconomic status is broken into three levels called *classes*: low, middle, and high. Some analyses use finer breakdowns, for example, lower-middle, middle-middle, and upper-middle as indicated by SES of individual and family of origin. Often, as in the US Census, individuals, families, and households are categorized separately by each of the three indicators, income, education, and occupation. Recently, much has been written about the economic decline of the middle class and a growing wealth disparity between the very wealthy and the remainder of the US population. These changes in wealth distribution cannot help but affect access to and delivery of health care in important ways.

Socioeconomic status is a diversity factor that crosscuts all of the other diversity indicators in critical ways. For example, SES is associated with race and ethnicity. In 2009, the median family income for whites was $54,461; for Asians, $65,469; for Hispanics, $38,039; and for blacks, $32,584. With the official poverty level for a family of four set at $22,128, more than 24 percent of black and Hispanic families fell at or below that level, and just slightly more than 10 percent of white and Asian families did (DeNavas-Walt, Proctor, & Smith, 2010). Because SES differs so dramatically across racial and ethnic groups, many measures of health status and access are linked to racial and ethnic identification through SES. Blacks, for example, are disproportionately represented among the uninsured and lower SES (Williams, 1999). SES is a strong predictor of health behavior, health status, and mortality (Marmot, 2004). SES is of course linked to the ability to buy good health insurance and concomitant access to the most recent advances in care. Asians, as a whole, because of their higher incomes and educations, fare better, healthwise, than many other population groups, although this is not the case with all Asian groups. Education levels, also racially and ethnically linked, also affect health literacy, a growing issue as health care becomes more technologically and genetically driven.

Because race and ethnicity are so closely associated with SES, it is often difficult to determine whether health behavior is influenced by cultural or economic factors; in many cases, both need to be considered as skilled professionals, trained in considering all aspects of a patient's diversity, are able to do. Low SES often interacts with gender, compounding health access problems because of the growing number of female-headed, single-income families in all racial and ethnic groups.

Language

The variety of languages spoken in the United States creates significant problems in health care settings, where good communication between patients and health care providers is critical. The report *Language Use in the U.S.: 2007*, produced by the US Census in 2010 with data from the American Community Survey, showed that of 281 million people over age five, 55,444,485 million, or 20 percent, spoke a language other than English at home. This didn't mean that all these millions of Americans couldn't speak any English, but many reported that they didn't speak English well. For example, 29 percent of Spanish speakers and 22 percent of Asian and Pacific Island language speakers reported limited proficiency in English. Spanish was by far the most predominant language other than English spoken in the home, followed by Chinese, Tagalog, Vietnamese, French, German, and Korean. Language is, of course, a learned diversity factor, but a native language is learned rapidly in childhood and quickly embeds the culture from which it springs.

Clearly, the languages spoken in the United States reflect the immigration patterns of the last fifty years. Although these major languages are associated with nations of origin, there are also many languages such as Hmong, Mien, and Mixteco that are associated with ethnic groups within donor nations. The Census Bureau codes for 381 languages spoken in the United States including Native American languages! However, and fortunately for most health care institutions, speakers of languages other than English are not distributed evenly across the nation. For example, just 2 percent of West Virginians over the age of five spoke a language other than English at home and 43 percent of people in California, a state that is home to many Chinese, Vietnamese, Hmong, and Spanish speakers, reported speaking a language other than English in the home. Even within states certain metropolitan areas have concentrated clusters of foreign languages speakers such as Khmer (Cambodian) in Long Beach, California, Somali in Minneapolis, and Hmong in Fresno, California. Thus, health care institutions can often concentrate their language-access services on specific languages spoken within their catchment areas. Because communication is so critical in health care, providers and health care organizations often make attention to language-access needs their first step in integrating cultural competence into their systems of care. As they accomplish this, it opens wide the door to greater cultural understanding and appreciation. Later in this book we will look at how language access is being provided in many health care institutions and the growth of a new medical profession: the medical interpreter.

Religion

Because illness, injury, and death are critical issues in peoples' lives, they have, from time immemorial, been linked to religious beliefs and practices. Concepts about birth, the vital functioning of the body, the association between body and spirit, belief in the efficacy of prayer and personal agency, dietary practices, illness and punishment, and death and dying are very frequently religion based and dramatically affect the acceptance and compliance with health care prevention and treatment practices. Recognizing this, health care professionals have grown to accept that patient's religious and spiritual lives need to be considered as part of their diversity, and that health care systems should accommodate patients' varying religious practices when at all possible. This is no easy task when the complexity of the religious landscape in the United States is appreciated and its changing nature is considered.

Religion is one of the crosscutting diversity dimensions. One's religious beliefs, like language, are usually learned (or not) through socialization. The Pew Forum on Religion and Public Life released its most recent US Religious Landscape

Survey (2008) and concluded that "religion in the United States is often described as a vibrant marketplace where individuals pick and choose religions that meet their needs and religious groups are compelled to compete for members" (p. 22). Although religious and ethnic identities continue to be strongly related, the survey reports that 28 percent of US residents have changed their religious affiliation from the one in which they were raised; this percentage would be even higher (44 percent) if changes between denominations within a religious tradition, for example, Protestantism, were included as well. Rates of change in religious affiliation vary by racial and ethnic group, with lower rates for Hispanics and Asian ethnicities and higher rates for African Americans and whites.

Based on current trends, the Landscape Survey projects that the United States will become less Protestant, that an ever-growing proportion of Catholics will be Latino, and that immigration patterns will continue to add to America's religious diversity with a small but growing proportion of the population, mostly people of Middle Eastern background, affiliating with the Muslim faiths and persons of Asian or South Asian heritage remaining Buddhist or Hindu. The percentage of US residents who report no religious affiliation is also growing but varies with race, ethnicity, and age. African Americans, for example, are the least likely racial ethnic group to report having no religious affiliation. One quarter of all adults under age thirty are not affiliated with any religion, which is three times the percentage of people seventy and above.

The American Religious Identity Survey (ARIS) (Kosmin & Keysar, 2009) reveals related trends. Although in 1990, 86 percent of US adults identified as Christian, that number declined to 76 percent in 2008. The decline is attributed to an increasing percentage of Americans reporting no religious preference or self-identifying as atheist or agnostic, from 8.2 percent in 1990 to 15 percent in 2008.

ARIS also saw growth in religions other than Christianity from 3.3 percent of the US population in 1990 to 3.9 percent in 2008. Those reporting a Jewish religious identity declined from 1.8 to 1.2 percent of the population whereas respondents reporting a Muslim religious affiliation doubled from .3 percent of the population to .6 percent in 2008. ARIS reported that affiliations with Eastern religions as a group, including Buddhism, Hinduism, Taoism, Baha'i, Shinto, Zorastrian, and Sikh, more than doubled during this same time frame.

As these trends demonstrate, religion is truly a diversity dimension that is not immutable. However, ethnicity and religious identities are still closely associated and immigration patterns will continue to drive increasing religious diversity in the United States. As the US Religious Landscape Survey (2008) reported, "immigration is adding even more diversity to the American religious quilt. For example, Muslims, roughly two-thirds of whom are immigrants, now account for roughly 0.6 percent of the U.S. adult population; and Hindus, more than eight in ten of whom are foreign born, now account for approximately 0.4 percent of the population" (p. 11).

HEALTH CARE DIVERSITY CHALLENGES

The seven dimensions of diversity discussed in the previous section present health care with a number of challenges. A major goal of this book is to clarify these challenges in detail and point out ways in which integrating cultural competence into the health care system equips the reader with the necessary knowledge and skills to respond effectively.

Research confirms that we develop a sense of community not through our differences but through our similarities. Differences in fact generate conflict unless they are managed appropriately. Health care providers will need to hone the diversity management and cultural competencies needed to create **inclusion** and deliver patient-centered care in the context of diversity (Dreachslin, 2007).

Following are just a few of the many implications of the changing demographic and cultural landscapes discussed in the previous section:

- An aging population increases the demand for health care services.

- Generational differences in work style preferences may exacerbate the shortage of nurses and other professionals unless addressed by role and work redesign.

- The gap between the levels of technical and scientific education required of health care workers and the levels of education currently achieved by blacks and Hispanics may perpetuate the concentration of Asians and non-Hispanic whites in professional, administrative, and policy-making positions.

- Provider bias and lack of cultural awareness can contribute to disparities in health care, as can poorly structured service delivery.

- The issue of language access caused by the high number of limited English speakers will call for innovative and cost-effective solutions.

- The association of low SES with racial and ethnic groups that are under-represented among physicians, nurses, and the allied health professions can make concordance difficult; that is, it may be difficult to provide patients with clinicians who share their racial or ethnic identity.

- Growing religious diversity will require health care organizations to review and adapt their human resource policies and patient care practices, for example, holiday leave and accommodations for religious observances, hospital diets, and family involvement in care.

- Learning to understand and value diversity's multiple dimensions will help health care providers adhere to the many new standards, accreditation measures, and legislation calling for patient-centered communication. For example, the Joint Commission's (2010) accreditation standards for culturally competent, patient-centered care prohibit "discrimination based on age, race, ethnicity, religion, culture, language, physical or mental disability, socioeconomic status, sex, sexual orientation, and gender identity or expression" (p. 61).

HEALTH CARE DISPARITIES IN THE UNITED STATES

A critical diversity issue confronting health care institutions throughout the United States is that of seemingly intractable disparities in health access and status across population groups

Disparities in health status across different population groups have become an important topic in the ongoing dialogue about the cost, quality, and cultural competence of health care in the United States. This has not always been the case, so it is important to understand just what is meant when the term *disparities* is used. The National Institutes of Health (2000) defines health care disparities as "differences in the incidence, prevalence, mortality, and burden of diseases and other health conditions that exist among several populations in the United States" (p. 4). Put simply this means that groups living in this country, when compared with each other, do not enjoy the same life expectancies or levels of good health. Disparities in health status across population groups in the United States are so significant that they may in part be responsible for the unfavorable comparison of the United States to other industrialized nations with respect to key health indicators.

The study of disparities is a special issue in the overall science of epidemiology, that is, the study of risk for and occurrence of disease and disorders in population groups. The great preponderance of attention focused on health care equity has centered on racial and ethnic disparities that are so large as to affect the nation's overall health landscape and significant enough to erode trust in health institutions among minority groups. These racial and ethnic disparities will be explored in detail in Chapter Two, as will disparities related to gender, age, and sexual orientation.

Little notice of disparities in health status across racial and ethnic groups was taken before the 1980s. A pivotal research report, published by the NIH in 1986, the *Secretary's Task Force Report on Black and Minority Health*, and subsequent research done on Hispanics (Mexican Americans, Cubans, and Puerto Ricans) as an adjunct to the *National Health and Nutrition Survey* conducted from 1982 to 1985 by the National Center for Health Statistics (1985) and referred to as the HHANES, made the existence of racial and ethnic health disparities across populations very clear. However, it wasn't until the mid-nineties, when the US population began to diversify even further through immigration, asylum, and natural increase and the disparities noted in the earlier reports appeared intractable, that disparities began to be associated with the cultural and linguistic competence of health care providers and organizations as well as the structuring of health care delivery. The disparities in health status revealed in early and current studies are consistently reflected in research that shows disparities across the entire health care system: access, prevention, treatment, health care literacy, and health outcomes. Health care disparities across racial and ethnic groups are strongly linked to socioeconomic differences and tend to be reduced when these factors are controlled but many disparities have been shown to remain after these factors are accounted for. Therefore, the causes of disparities in health status across population groups are as multiple and complex as the disparities themselves, and will be covered in Chapter Two. Reduction of disparities will ultimately depend on the cultural and linguistic competencies of health care policies, delivery systems, organizations, and practitioners systematically organized.

CHANGING THE US HEALTH CARE SYSTEM

No one who is familiar with topics of current interest can fail to be aware that the structure of health care delivery in all its aspects has been a major subject of focus and debate in US public policy for at least four decades. There is significant agreement across all sectors of the health care establishment that reform is needed and that culturally competent care will play a role in that reform.

Starting with the creation of Medicaid and Medicare by the Social Security Act of 1965 through the recent passage of the Patient Protection and Affordable Care Act of 2010, the structure, cost, and outcomes of the national health care system have been constantly under discussion and reorganization. As the costs of US health care have mounted and the nation's health profile has declined in comparison with those of other developed nations, the government, health care providers, health care institutions, evaluators and accreditors, as well as private philanthropic organizations have sought solutions to the costly disarray and lack of systematic approaches that characterize much of US health care (Shea, Shih, & Davis, 2008). Important critiques, for example, can be found in three of the publications of the national Institute of Medicine (IOM). *To Err Is Human: Building a Safer Health System* (Kohn, Corrigan, & Donaldson, 1999) caused national dismay over its revelation of the massive number of medical errors that harmed tens of thousands of patients as a result of uncoordinated and fragmented medical care. *Crossing the Quality Chasm: A New Health System for the 21st Century* (Committee on Quality of Healthcare in America, 2001) stated unequivocally, "Indeed, between the health care that we now have and the health care we could have lies not just a gap, but a chasm" (p. 1). This chasm was seen to be, in great part, a failure to translate the new learnings of medical science and rapid technological development into safe and integrated systems of practice. The report states that the delivery of care is often overly complex and uncoordinated, requiring steps and patient "handoffs" that slow down care and decrease patient safety, wasting resources. Finally, in *Unequal Treatment: Confronting Racial and Ethnic Disparities in Healthcare* (Snedley, Stith, & Nelson, 2002), the IOM documents the differences in medical treatment experienced by different population groups in the United States that are "not due to access-related factors or clinical needs, preferences, and appropriateness of care" (p. 3) but asserted that these differences are the result of the way health care systems operate within their regulatory contexts as well as discrimination at the individual patient-provider level. These differences in treatment, coupled with socioeconomic and environmental factors, underlie the enormous disparities in health status across different population groups.

Overall, the picture that has emerged from the many analyses of health care delivery in the United States is that there is little that is actually systematic at all in health care. Health care organizations, hospitals, and provider groups typically operate in silos with imperfect communication among them. In a delivery structure with lacunae in shared information, extreme specialization, and, often, dispersed treatment locales, it is often left up to patients low in health literacy to make connections and attempt to create order out of a seemingly impenetrable "un-system." These access and delivery problems are exacerbated when class, language, cultural, and discriminatory barriers are also present.

Recommendations about how to reform the health care industry so that it is a truly equitable enterprise whose parts work smoothly and effectively with each other center on several broad courses of action. First, there is general agreement that practices within the health care system need to be based on **data-driven** and **evidence-based strategies** that are patient centered. Each of these recommendations carries implications for incorporating cultural competence approaches that will support and strengthen them.

In terms of reducing disparities and addressing the needs of diverse groups, a culturally competent approach to building an evidence base means that the health needs and risks of various segments of the population need to be consistently assessed, locally and nationally, and then treatment modalities used to address these needs implemented and evaluated for their efficacy, with the results of these assessments fed back into the system so that upgrades and modifications can be made. Chapter Two includes a discussion of this data-driven strategy.

Second, to reduce fragmentation and discontinuities in care, the interrelated concepts of **medical homes, patient-centered care**, and **interprofessional or multidisciplinary teams** have been proposed and are being put into practice. Together, these three elements enhance continuity of care and improve patient outcomes through a systems approach. In each of these formulations for practice, the individual patient or health care professional is seen in the context of his or her multiple and interrelated connections to all the components involved in the delivery of services. Aspects of the patient's cultural environment and the social determinants affecting the care process are emphasized.

The patient-centered medical home is a model of care in which each patient has an ongoing relationship with a personal health care provider who leads a team that takes collective responsibility for patient care over extended periods of time. Care is coordinated and actively managed across specialists, allied health staff, hospitals, home health agencies, and nursing homes. Key to the success of the medical home is centralized care management. Communication is facilitated by integrated data systems and electronic medical records accessible to all members of the care team. Emphasis is given to preventive care as well as curative care (Abrams, Davis, & Harran, 2009). Medical homes set into various communities need to be sensitive to the dimensions of diversity within those communities; the perspectives and practices of cultural competence are critical in achieving this sensitivity.

Patient-centered care emphasizes that the specific characteristics of each patient, such as gender, age, sexual orientation, ethnicity, and race as well as the patient's social environment, are considered as equally important as medical status or diagnosis. Of great importance, patients and their families are involved with health care decision making facilitated by transparent processes and information sharing. Culturally and linguistically sensitive communication is critical to accurate information sharing and trust building in this context. Here again we see the importance of cultural competence in the system.

According to at least one assessment, *Closing the Divide: How Medical Homes Promote Equity in Health Care: Results from The Commonwealth Fund 2006 Health Quality Survey* (Beal et al., 2007), racial and ethnic disparities in access and quality are reduced or eliminated when patients have a medical home that provides continuity of care. With the implementation of centralized care, access to routine preventive screenings and management of chronic conditions are also greatly improved. Although the medical home model of care is just one example of a coordinated system, it points the way to how institutional policy makers and managers can work with frontline care-giving professionals and managers in the integration of overall philosophies and specific practices that are responsive to the needs of diverse patient populations. For an excellent review of case studies of coordinated care systems, large and small, see The Commonwealth Fund's report, *Organizing for Higher Performance: Case Studies of Organized Delivery Systems— Series Overview, Findings, and Methods* (McCarthy & Mueller, 2009). This report documents the characteristics of health plans, clinics, independent practice associations, safety net providers, and multispecialty group practices, demonstrating that systematic care models can be successfully integrated into a variety of health care delivery structures.

The interprofessional or multidisciplinary team is now considered critical to all models of systematically organized health care. The creation of a synergistic team made up of health care professionals with different areas of specialized expertise works against the fragmentation of care that the proliferation of areas of expertise has tended to produce. Leadership by providers and shared responsibility for the care of patients creates a system of accountability to patients and members of the team. Distribution of patient-related data and information sharing across different areas of expertise gives rise to innovative approaches to patient care. Care teams often include physicians, nurses, pharmacists, social workers, and behavioral health specialists, physical therapists, medical interpreters, and other allied health professionals. Interprofessional teams are particularly useful in managing the care of patients with chronic or multiple illnesses such as diabetes or metabolic syndrome. Given the current cultural and racial diversity of the health care workforce as well as its very hierarchical nature, retraining in areas of cultural competence and skills in working in diverse teams is gaining in importance. A report by the IOM, *Health Professions Education: A Bridge to Quality* (Greiner & Knebel, 2003), recommends that skills development for interprofessional teams should include the following:

- Learning about other disciplines' areas of expertise, background, and values

- Identifying individual roles and processes

- Acquiring basic group collaboration skills including communication, negotiation, delegation, and time management

- Managing transitions and hand-offs

- Acquiring conflict-resolution techniques

- Learning to communicate in a common language

- Creating and adhering to shared guidelines.

In an industry in which professions and positions have typically been extremely hierarchical and partitioned, acquiring and practicing these skills requires mind-set and philosophical changes. When the care is patient centered, the leadership of the interprofessional team is situationally, not traditionally, determined. Additionally, the health care workforce brings together persons of many backgrounds and cultures whose perspectives on work relations and patient-provider relations may differ significantly. Multidisciplinary teams are usually diverse beyond occupational specialization. Cultural competency training around workforce issues is useful for revealing and dealing with different perspectives on leadership and workgroup interactions as well as attending sensitively to the needs of diverse patients.

SYSTEMS APPROACH IN THE HEALTH CARE DELIVERY ORGANIZATION

Coordinated, patient-centered, and culturally competent systems of care need to begin at the policy-making and planning levels of management within health care delivery organizations. Because communities are very different from each other in terms of their diversity, much planning needs to be done at the local level, where policy makers need to be knowledgeable about and consider the diversity characteristics of the community or communities served.

Strategic diversity management includes a careful evaluation of the health care delivery system and its personnel to ensure that it is actually able to meet the needs of the community or communities that make up its catchment area. Information about the populations in the service area and their specific health, cultural, and language needs should be part of ongoing training for staff and health professionals. Goal setting and quality-improvement efforts intended to reduce disparities in access, treatment, and health outcomes need to be focused on evidence-based measures broken down by populations groups whenever feasible. Opportunities for management, staff, patient, and data feedback loops into the system should be built. These policy-making, planning, and quality improvement processes and their importance for the care of diverse patients and the elimination of disparities will be discussed throughout this book.

Again, a system is a structure of interconnected people, policies, and practices designed to work in concert to achieve a common goal. Despite the fragmentation of the US health care system in general, health care organizations themselves can independently follow a systems approach to strategic diversity management and culturally and linguistically appropriate health care delivery. In fact, even if recommended changes to the US health care system overall were in place, individual health care organizations would still need to follow a systems approach within their own organization. Figure 1.2 is a visual representation of the systems approach to diversity and cultural competence at the health care organization level. Fundamental to the systems approach is executive leadership's diversity-sensitive orientation. The organization's top administrators, who are sometimes referred to as C-suite level administrators because their titles often begin with the letter *C* (CEO, CFO, COO, CNO, CMO, etc.), must believe that workforce and patient diversity are important drivers of strategy or the systems approach will not even get out of the gate. With diversity-sensitive orientation at the C-suite level, the

FIGURE 1.2   Systems Approach to Diversity and Cultural Competence

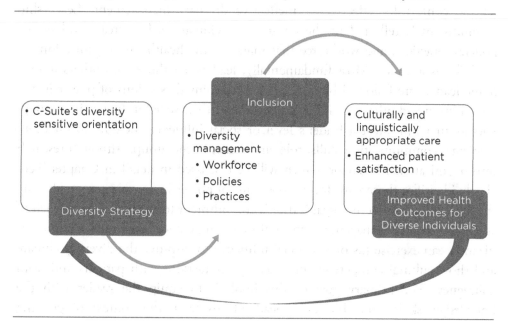

organization will have a diversity strategic plan that is data driven and evidence based and a commitment to continuous improvement, as indicated by the feedback loop at the bottom of Figure 1.2. Diversity management practices, with a focus on the workforce, policies, and practices, are the building blocks of strategic diversity management, which in turn creates a culture of inclusion, in which diverse individuals, families, and communities can perform to their highest potential. A culture of inclusion provides a context in which culturally and linguistically appropriate care is the norm and patient satisfaction is paramount. The result: improved health outcomes for diverse individuals. The role of the systems approach in ameliorating disparities in the process and outcome of health care delivery at the health care organization level will be emphasized throughout this book.

THE IMPORTANCE OF LEADERSHIP

Leadership commitment is essential to the systems approach, to the well-functioning multidisciplinary health care team, and ultimately to the amelioration of disparities in health care and to career accomplishment and satisfaction in health care organizations. Leaders at every level from the C-suite to the patient's bedside set the context for effective or ineffective diversity management. Leadership commitment is reflected in the culture and climate leaders create and in the policies, practices, and workforce that make up the health care organization.

Who is a leader? Most fundamentally, leaders are those who others follow. Some leaders are followed because of their appointed positions of power in the organization and others are followed because of their social influence in a group. Factors that can affect a leader's level of social influence include information, charisma, communication skills, role, and status in the group. Although research into organizational behavior, which will be discussed in detail in Chapter Ten, clearly identifies those with formal positions of power in organizations as having the most influence on the organization's commitment to the systems approach to strategic diversity management and cultural competence, everyone in the organization can exercise his or her social influence to improve the diversity climate and show cultural competence in everyday interactions with patients and team colleagues. The primary goal of this book is to equip the reader with the knowledge, skills, and abilities to lead effectively in the context of growing workforce and patient diversity.

SUMMARY

The United States is made up of many groups. Some are ethnic and defined by their culture. Some are racial and defined loosely by genetic characteristics and ancestry. Within these groups there are men and women, persons of various sexual orientation and age, persons of different social class and religions, as well as persons who speak a variety of languages. Historically, the US healthcare system has tended to reflect the view that health care issues were basically the same for everyone even though the US population has changed significantly in the last few decades. However, a growing body of research refutes this view and shows that each of these groups has distinct health needs and that there are significant disparities in health status across groups. Many of the health disparities are long standing, though a few have developed from the immigration of new groups. Some disparities are certainly the result of personal or institutional discrimination or, at the very least, indifference. Health care in the United States has been fragmented and lacking systematic approaches; the consequence of this is that many people do not enjoy good health, having fallen through the cracks of a disjointed system. Since about 2000, efforts to right the delivery of health care services and eliminate disparities have focused on a systems approach that is based on evidence, personalized care, and continuity of care. Cultural competence conforms well with the new directions in health care and can inform and strengthen them. However, incorporating the philosophy and practices of cultural competence as a vital element of this evolving health care system is, as can be seen in this initial chapter, complex because health care systems are made up of many interlocking and interacting elements: the people served; the people doing the serving; the processes, practices, and environment involved; and the policy and planning that unites all the pieces. The goal of this book is to help students examine these pieces and understand the roles played by cultural competence and diversity management in the health care system so that they can assume leadership in meeting the health needs of all this nation's peoples.

KEY TERMS

crosscutting	inclusion
cultural competence	interprofessional or multidisciplinary teams
culture	medical homes
data-driven strategies	patient-centered care
disparities	personalized care
diversity	race
ethnicity	strategic diversity management
evidence-based strategies	system
identity groups	systems approach
immutable	worldview

REVIEW QUESTIONS AND ACTIVITIES

1. What are your own ethnic, racial, and national backgrounds? How many generations are you from immigrant status? Which of these identities dominates in your concept of self? Why do you think this is? Are there other dimensions

of diversity that play an important role in your life? Compare and share your thoughts about your identity with your classmates.

2. Go to www.census.gov. Look up the racial and ethnic, age, and gender demographics of your city or state. List at least three implications of these demographics for diversity management and culturally competent health care. Support your list with logical argument and factual information.

3. Why is there a strong association among race, ethnicity, and socioeconomic status? Why is lower SES associated with lower health status? Justify your answer.

4. Go to https://www.thinkculturalhealth.hhs.gov/ and join the Center for Linguistic and Cultural Competence in Health Care (CLCCHC). Then, complete one of the free continuing education programs available on the site and list three things you learned from the program.

5. Go to http://www.culturecareconnection.org/index.html and read two of the ethnic group–specific fact sheets accessible through the home page. Identify an area of difference between the two groups and describe how a culturally competent health care provider might address the difference.

6. Imagine you are the primary care physician for three diverse patients diagnosed with type 2 diabetes. Explain how a systems approach that incorporates patient-centered care and cultural competence could be tailored to produce the best outcome for each patient. Assume differences in one or more immutable and crosscutting diversity dimensions among your three patients.

7. Identity three ways in which the systems approach to diversity and cultural competence in an individual health care organization contributes to improved outcomes (see Figure 1.2).

REFERENCES

Abrams, M. K., Davis, K., & Haran, C. (2009). *Can patient-centered medical homes transform health care delivery?* The Commonwealth Fund. Retrieved from http://www.commonwealthfund .org/Content/From-the-President/2009/Can-Patient-Centered-Medical-Homes-Transform-Health-Care-Delivery?

Beal, A. C., et al. (2007). *Closing the divide: How medical homes promote equity in health care: Results from The Commonwealth Fund 2006 health quality survey.* The Commonwealth Fund. Retrieved from http://www.commonwealthfund.org/usr_doc/1035_Beal_closing_divide_medical_homes.pdf

Boston Women's Health Collective. (1973). *Our bodies, ourselves.* Boston: Boston Women's Health Collective.

Byrd, W. M., & Clayton, E. A. (2002). Racial and ethnic disparities in health: A background and history. In B. D. Smedley, A. Y. Stith, & A. R. Nelson (Eds.), *Unequal treatment: Confronting racial and ethnic disparities in healthcare.* Washington, DC: The National Academies Press.

Collins, F. S. (2004). What we do and don't know about "race," "ethnicity," genetics and health at the dawn of the genome era. *Nature Genetics Supplement, 36*(11), S13–S15.

Committee on Lesbian, Gay, Bisexual, and Transgender Health Issues and Research Gaps and Opportunities. (2011). *The health of lesbian, gay, bisexual, and transgender people: Building a foundation for better understanding.* Washington, DC: The National Academy Press.

Committee on Quality of Health Care in America. (2001). *Crossing the quality chasm: A new health system for the 21st century.* National Institute of Medicine. Washington, DC: National Academies Press.

Committee on Women's Health Research (2010). *Women's health research: Progress, pitfalls, and promise.* Washington, DC: National Academies Press.

Cross, T., Bazron, B., Dennis, K., & Issacs, M. (1989). *Towards a culturally competent system of care: A monograph on effective services for minority children who are severely disturbed* (Vol. 1). Washington, DC: Georgetown University.

Dade, C. (2011). *Data on same-sex couples reveal changing attitudes.* Retrieved from http://www.npr.org/2011/09/30/140950989/data-on-same-sex-couples-reveal-changing-attitudes

Dean, L., Meyer, I. H., Robinson, K., Sell, R. L., Sembe, R., Silenzio, V.M.B., et al. (2000). Lesbian, gay, bisexual, and transgender health: Findings and concerns. *Journal of the Gay and Lesbian Medical Association, 4*(3), 101–151.

DeNavas-Walt, C., Proctor, B. D., & Smith, J. C. (2010). *Current population reports, P60–238: Income, poverty, and health insurance coverage in the United States: 2009.* Washington, DC: US Government Printing Office.

Dreachslin, J. L. (2007). Diversity management and cultural competence: Research, practice, and the business case. *Journal of Healthcare Management, 52*(2), 79–96.

Federal Interagency Forum on Age-Related Statistics. (2010). *Older Americans 2010: Key indicators of well-being.* Washington, DC: US Government Printing Office. Retrieved from http://www.agingstats.gov/Main_Site/Data/2010_Documents/docs/Introduction.pdf

Gates, G. (2011). *How many people are lesbian, gay, bisexual, and transgender?* Los Angeles: The Williams Institute.

Gates, G. (2012). *Same-sex couples in Census 2010: Race and ethnicity.* Los Angeles: Williams Institute. Retrieved from http://williamsinstitute.law.ucla.edu/research/census-lgbt-demographics-studies/same-sex-couples-census-2010-race-ethnicity/

Gilbert P., & Sabin, D. (2008). *The importance of sexual orientation and gender identity in health research.* San Francisco: UCSF Lesbian Health and Research Center.

Greiner, A. C., & Knebel, E. (Eds.). (2003). *Health professions education: A bridge to quality.* Washington, DC: National Academies Press.

Howe, M. (2009). *Customer experience: A generational experience.* Washington, DC: Beryl Institute.

The Joint Commission. (2010). *Advancing effective communication, cultural competence, and patient- and family-centered care: A roadmap for hospitals.* Oakbrook Terrace, IL: Author.

Kaiser Family Foundation. (nd). *State health facts.* Retrieved from http://www.statehealthfacts.org

Kohn, L.T., Corrigan, J. M., & Donaldson, M. S. (Eds.). (1999). *To err is human: Building a safer health system.* Washington, DC: National Academies Press.

Kosmin, B. A., & Keysar, A. (2009). *American religious identification survey (ARIS 2008) summary report.* Hartford, CT: Trinity College.

Li, J. Z., Absher, D. M., Tang, H., Southwick, A. M., Casto, A. M., Raachandran, S., Cann, H. M., Barsh, G. S., Feldman, M., Carvilli-Sforza, L. L., & Meyers, R. M. (2008). Worldwide relations inferred from genome-wide patterns of variation. *Science Magazine, 319* (5866), 1100–1104.

Lofquist, D. (2011). *Same sex couple households American community survey briefs.* Washington, DC: US Census Bureau.

Marmot, M. (2004). *The status syndrome: How social standing affects our health and longevity.* New York: Owl Books.

Mather, M., Pollard, K., & Jacobsen, L. A. (2011). *First results from the 2010 census.* Washington, DC: Population Reference Bureau.

McCarthy, D., & Mueller, K. (2009). *Organizing for higher performance: Case studies of organized delivery systems.* The Commonwealth Fund. Retrieved from http://www.commonwealthfund.org/Publications/Case-Studies/2009/Jul/Organizing-for-Higher-Performance-Case-Studies-of-Organized-Delivery-Systems.aspx

National Center for Health Statistics. (1985). *Plan and orientation of the Hispanic health and nutrition survey, 1984–1985.* Vital Health Statistics, Series 1, No. 19. DHHS Publication No. (PHS) 85–1321. Washington, DC: US Government Printing Office.

National Institutes of Health. (1986). *Secretary's task force report on black and minority health, 1982–1984.* Hyattsville, MD: National Center for Health Statistics. Retrieved from http://minorityhealth.hhs.gov/assets/pdf/checked/1/ANDERSON.pdf.

National Institutes of Health. (2000). *Strategic research plan to reduce and ultimately eliminate health disparities* (Vol. 1). Retrieved from http://www.nimhd.nih.gov/our_programs/strategic/pubs/volumei_031003edrev.pdf

National Quality Forum. (2008). *Endorsing a framework and preferred practices for measuring and reporting culturally competent care quality.* Washington, DC: Author.

Orchowski, M. S. (2008). *Immigration and the American dream: Battling the political hype and hysteria.* Lantham, MD: Rowman & Littlefield.

Owens, G. M. (2008). Gender differences in health care expenditures, resource utilization, and quality of care. *Managed Care Pharmacy, 14*(3)(supplement S), S2–S6.

Pew Forum on Religion and Public Life. (2008) *U.S. religious landscape survey religious affiliation: Diverse and dynamic.* Washington, DC: Pew Research Center.

Risch, N., Burchard, E., Ziv, E., & Tang, H. (2002). Categorization of humans in biomedical research: Genes, race and disease. *Genome Biology, 3*(7), 1–12. Retrieved from http://genomebiology.com/2002/3/7/comment/2007

Shea, K. K, Shih, A., & Davis, K. (2008). *Commonwealth commission on a high performance health system data brief: Health care opinion leaders' views on health care system delivery reform.* The Commonwealth Fund. Retrieved from http://www.commonwealthfund.org/Publications/Data-Briefs/2008/Apr/Health-Care-Opinion-Leaders-Views-on-Health-Care-Delivery-System-Reform.aspx

Skloot, R. (2010). *The immortal life of Henrietta Lacks.* New York: Crown Publishers.

Smedley, B. D., Stith, A.Y., & Nelson, A. R. (Eds.). (2002). *Unequal treatment: Confronting racial and ethnic disparities in healthcare.* Washington, DC: The National Academies Press.

Smith, D., & Spraggins, R. (2001). *Gender 2000 census 2000 brief.* Washington, DC: US Census Bureau.

Society for Women's Health Research. (nd). *Inclusion of women in medical research.* Retrieved from http://www.womenshealthresearch.org/site/PageServer?pagename=hs_learn

US Census Bureau. (2008). *An older and more diverse nation by midcentury.* Retrieved from http://www.census.gov/newsroom/releases/archives/population/cb08–123.html

US Census Bureau. (2010). *Language use in the United States.* Retrieved from www.census.gov/hhes/socdemo/language/

Williams, D. (1999). Race, socioeconomic status, and health. The added effects of racism and discrimination. *Annals of the New York Academy of Science, 896,* 173–188.

Wizemann, T. M., & Pardue, M. L. (Eds.). (2001). *Exploring the biological contributions to human health: Does sex matter?* Washington, DC: National Academy Press.

Zemke, R., Raines, C., & Filipczak, B. (2000). *Generations at work.* New York: AMACOM.

Chapter 2

SYSTEMATIC ATTENTION TO

HEALTH CARE DISPARITIES

LEARNING OBJECTIVES

- To appreciate the difference between health care disparities that are inequitable and those that are not

- To become familiar with the data and data sources for describing health care disparities

- To become aware of the different roles played by the public, private, and philanthropic sectors as they pertain to reducing health care disparities

- To understand how legislation, accreditation, and advocacy are mobilizing action to reduce disparities

- To understand how data, evidence-based health care, cultural competence, and comparative effectiveness research are all part of a systems approach to reducing disparities

- To become familiar with how a variety of health care organizations are systematically addressing disparities

Not all disparities are alike. Health care disparities differ in kind and in source. This chapter is focused on the different types of health care disparities that exist across groups in the United States and the varied sources of those disparities. These include gender differences, differences related to sexual orientation, and differences occasioned by the special needs of the elderly. However, major attention is given to disparities of health status and access across racial and ethnic groups because these constitute a critical issue facing health care in the United States. We will ultimately see that most disparities can be addressed systematically, though the specific approach may differ depending on the disparity and its source. Frequently, addressing disparities will involve a culturally competent approach. More often than not, a systematic approach will depend on the acquisition of appropriate data and measures. The information so acquired should provide an evidence base for planning and structuring culturally appropriate health services that meet the needs of specific populations. We will look at several cases of health care organizations that illustrate systematic approaches to eliminating disparities.

WHAT ARE HEALTH CARE DISPARITIES?

The National Institute of Health's (NIH, 2002) definition of disparities as "differences in the incidence, prevalence, mortality, and burden of diseases and other health conditions that exist among several populations in the United States" contains no judgments as to inequities with respect to the sources of disparities, only that they exist. This is appropriate because, on reflection, there are significant differences in the sources of disparities, that is, the etiological basis for differences in health status across groups. Researchers who have looked carefully at the sources of disparities note that they are the result of many interacting variables: biological, environmental, social, and idiosyncratic. Epidemiology is the study of the onset, course, outcomes, incidence, and prevalence of diseases and disorders in populations and epidemiological studies provide the data for determining disparities in health care. Differences in health status based in biology include gender differences, differences related to the natural process of aging, and genetic differences in risk for various diseases and disorders across ethnic and racial groups. Clearly, these biologically based disparities in health status are primarily unavoidable differences. However, just because they are unavoidable does not mean they should be ignored or can't be ameliorated by awareness and systematic attention. There are also differences in health status that arise out of lifestyle, dietary, or religious practices that are a matter of cultural practices or personal choice. Differences become disparities when their effect on the health care of a group is ignored or the sources of difference are not considered in the delivery of health care services to the group. Differences become disparities when they are the result of bias, discrimination, or a preexisting inequality.

The interaction between socioeconomic class, race, and ethnicity in producing disparities in health status is a striking instance in which one dimension of diversity crosscuts another with very critical results. The health disparities that arise out of this interaction are the largest and have received the most attention because they are the major type of health disparity and because they are largely seen as unfair or **inequitable health care disparities** (Carter-Pokras & Baquet, 2002). Equity in health care is seen as care of equal quality for all based solely on need and clinical factors. The National Institute of Medicine in its landmark book *Unequal Treatment: Confronting Racial and Ethnic Disparities in Health Care* (Smedley, Stith, & Nelson, 2003) called attention to disparities in treatment as "racial or ethnic differences in the quality of health care that are not due to access-related factors or clinical needs, preferences, and appropriateness of intervention" (p. 4). The focus of that book centered on structural and regulatory factors as well as discrimination at the individual provider level, all of which were shown to result in lower levels of care for some racial and ethnic groups. However, equitable health care has been defined as "care that does not vary in quality by personal characteristics such as ethnicity, gender, geographic location and socioeconomic status" (Disparity Solutions Center, 2010, p. 6). Notice that it is the quality of care that is addressed, not necessarily the same type of care. Many health care managers and providers aver that they give the same kind of care to everyone. However, appropriate care may mean assessing the different needs of patients and addressing those needs. Other literature makes clear that access to treatment, not just the quality of treatment alone, contributes significantly to disparities in health care status across groups (National Business Group on Health, 2011).

RACE AND ETHNIC DISPARITIES IN HEALTH STATUS

The categories that have been used to define race in governmental health care research and reporting are the same as those used in the Census: black or African American; American Indian/Alaska Native (AI/AN); Asian, Hawaiian, or Pacific

TABLE 2.1   US Race and Ethnicity Demographics, by Percent

Non-Hispanic white	64.0
Black or African American	12.6
Asian	4.8
Native Hawaiian and other Pacific Islander	0.2
American Indian/Alaska Native	0.9
Some other race	5.5
Two or more races	1.9
Hispanic	16.0

Source: US Census Bureau (2011).

Islander; and white. Hispanics/Latinos are defined as an ethnic group made up of persons from any Spanish-speaking country in the Americas and Spain and can be of any race, hence the subcategories *non-Hispanic whites* and *Hispanics* used in much reporting. The 2000 census was the first that allowed persons to indicate that they had multiracial background (Jones, 2001). It is helpful in interpreting disparity data to keep in mind the relative size of each of these groups with respect to their representation in the total US population. See Table 2.1 for the most recent racial and ethnic demographics from the 2010 US Census.

In most of the health literature and disparities statistics, racial and ethnic groups are identified only as non-Hispanic white, Hispanic, African American or black, Asian, Hawaiian, or other Pacific Islander, or American Indian or Alaska Native. These categories may be useful for broadly describing the demographic make-up of the US population but are not always very useful from an epidemiological perspective in health care because they are too broad, and each category encompasses subgroups that are significantly different from each other along many dimensions. For example, the Hispanic/Latino category includes Cubans, Puerto Ricans, and Mexican Americans. Data from the Hispanic Health and Nutrition Study (National Center for Health Statistics, 1985), which had a sample divided into these subgroups, demonstrated that, in terms of health issues, the three groups differed from each other substantially. Part of this variation can be attributed to the very different characteristics of the three groups with respect to age, education, social class, and migration history. Cubans migrated to the United States as a result of revolution and were primarily middle to upper-middle class and as a group were significantly older and better educated than Puerto Ricans and Mexican Americans. Their health status and needs were different as a result. Similarly, most data that capture the generally superior health status and access to health care enjoyed by much of the Asian population fails to discriminate among Chinese, Japanese, Koreans, South Asians (e.g., Indians, Sri Lankans, Pakistani), and Southeast Asians (e.g., Vietnamese, Hmong, and Mien). Many Southeast Asians, for example, have significant health problems and particular difficulty accessing the health system. Aggregating data into broader racial or ethnic "glosses" has the effect of obscuring important health disparities within the larger categories, as is the case with Southeast Asians.

Additionally, national-level figures are somewhat less useful at the local level, where care is actually delivered, because each locale will differ in its population make-up. If, say, a hospital or health care plan draws its patients from a large Vietnamese settlement, looking at statistics for the broader Asian population is not likely to yield helpful epidemiological data. As a result of analyses by critics (Ulmer, McFadden, & Nerentz, 2009) and directed by the Affordable Care Act, the Office of Management and Budget and the Department of Health and Human Services are revising the minimum standards for reporting race and ethnicity and language data (Office of Minority Health, 2011b). The new data standards, summarized in Table 2.2, enable greater granularity in categorizing population subgroups and should make more accurate and useful summaries of health care information across population subgroups available. The new standards enable health care organizations to document granular variation in the populations of their catchment area and still allow them to roll those data into the major categories for broader comparisons.

Sources of disparities statistics include the Nation Center for Health Statistics (NCHS), the Centers for Disease Control (CDC), the Agency for Healthcare Research and Quality (AHRQ), the various annual or semiannual disparities reports issued by the NIH and the DHHS, as well as a variety of other government documents. A major criticism of this veritable flood of information is that there has been little standardization in the way data are gathered and reported (Institute of Medicine, 2010a). Since about 2005, most US government agencies use the categories summarized in the 2011 data standards in the foregoing collections standards format. Nongovernmental agencies and some states may not use the exact same nomenclature. In data cited in this chapter, the nomenclature used in the sources is preserved.

Often health statistics are reported in tables that are highly complex and difficult for the average reader to decipher. The different agencies collect data in

TABLE 2.2 Data Collection Standards for Ethnicity and Race

Ethnicity Data Standard	Categories
Are you of Hispanic, Latino/a, or Spanish origin? (One or more categories may be selected) a. No, not of Hispanic, Latino/a, or Spanish origin b. Yes, Mexican, Mexican American, Chicano/a c. Yes, Puerto Rican d. Yes, Cuban e. Yes, another Hispanic, Latino, or Spanish origin	These categories roll-up to the Hispanic or Latino category of the OMB standard.

Race Data Standard	Categories
What is your race? (One or more categories may be selected) a. White b. Black or African American c. American Indian or Alaska Native	These categories are part of the current OMB standard.
d. Asian Indian e. Chinese f. Filipino g. Japanese h. Korean i. Vietnamese j. Other Asian	These categories roll-up to the Asian category of the OMB standard.
k. Native Hawaiian l. Guamanian or Chamorro m. Samoan n. Other Pacific Islander	These categories roll-up to the Native Hawaiian or Other Pacific Islander category of the OMB standard.

Source: Office of Minority Health (2011b).

discrepant categories and for different health conditions. The subgroup categories under which data are arranged often differ from year to year and across agencies. Comparisons are often made between African Americans and whites and sometimes Hispanics but information on Asians is harder to find, as is that for Pacific Islanders and American Indians/Alaska Natives. Straight across comparisons of all the groups are very difficult to locate because not all of the data summaries focus on all races and ethnicities. The more recent National Health Care

Disparities Reports published by AHRQ contain helpful charts and graphs (AHRQ, 2010a). Much more useful and helpful, however, are the chart books, graphs, and summaries produced by the Kaiser Family Foundation (www.kff.org) and The Commonwealth Fund (Mead et al., 2008) that summarize and interpret data from the national data bases. The following are common sources of health care disparities data:

- Agency for Health Care Quality and Research (AHRQ)

- Centers for Medicaid and Medicare Services (CMS)

- The Commonwealth Fund Chart Cart and other fund publications

- Centers for Disease Control (CDC)

- Institute of Medicine (IOM)

- Kaiser Family Foundation

- National Institutes of Health (NIH)

- National Center for Health Statistics (NCHS)

- Office of Minority Health (OMH)

- Society for Women's Health Research

- US Census Bureau

The following data reflect only a small portion of the extant statistical data on disparities but will be sufficient to demonstrate the sizeable differences in health status across racial and ethnic groups. As a rule, the health status data follow a consistent pattern across many health indicators going from the best health status to the worst: Asian Americans have the best health, whites next, Hispanics follow, and American Indians/Alaska Natives (AI/AN) and African Americans have the poorest health (Aries, 2010). This general pattern is shown across all age groups. The gaps between Asians and African Americans are striking on many indicators, as shown in the following examples:

- Infant mortality per 1,000 births in 2003 was 4.8 for Asians, 14 for African Americans, 8.7 for American Indian/Alaska Native, 5.6 and 5.7 for Hispanics and whites, respectively; thus, an African American baby is three times more likely to die in its first year of life than an Asian baby and more than two times more likely to die than a white or Hispanic baby (Mathews & Mac-Dorman, 2006).

- Life expectancy for a girl born in 2006 or 2007 was eighty-seven years for an Asian female, seventy-seven for an African American girl, eighty-one for a white female, and eighty-three for a Hispanic girl (US Census Bureau, 2011).

- Life expectancy for an Asian boy was eighty-two years, seventy for an African American male, seventy-eight for a Hispanic boy, and seventy-six for a white (US Census Bureau, 2011).

- In terms of age-adjusted death rates per 100,000 from 2005 to 2007, the rate for Asian/Pacific Islanders was 432; for African Americans, 987; for American Indian/Alaska Native, 643; for whites, 767; and for Hispanics, 567 (Centers for Disease Control and Prevention, 2010a).

- African Americans have the highest death rates from heart disease, stroke, cancer, influenza, diabetes, pneumonia, and HIV, whereas Asians have the lowest rates of all these diseases, with whites, Hispanics, and American Indian/Alaska Native falling between (CDC, 2010a).

Thus, in terms of the most basic life-and-death issues, the variation across population groups is quite astonishing. A somewhat similar pattern exists with respect to chronic and infectious diseases:

- Data from the 2004 National Health Interview Survey as reported in 2006 revealed that the percentages of different races and ethnicities among persons who ever had asthma were 16 percent for American Indian/Alaska Native, 11 percent for African Americans, 10 percent for whites, and 8 percent for both Asians and Hispanics (*The Commonwealth Fund Health Quality Survey*, 2006).

- Data from the national survey from 2007 to 2009 showed the following prevalence data for persons with diabetes: 12.6 percent of African Americans, 11.7 percent of Hispanics; 8.4 percent of Asians; and 7.1 percent of whites (National Diabetes Information Clearinghouse, 2011).

- In 2007, deaths per 100,000 for diabetes were 42.8 for African Americans, 37.2 for American Indian/Alaska Native, 28.9 for Hispanics, 20.5 for whites, and 16.2 for Asians (CDC, 2010a).

- A multiethnic study (African Americans, Hispanics, Chinese Americans, and whites) of congestive heart failure (CHF) found that African Americans had the highest incident rate of CHF, followed by Hispanic, white, and Chinese Americans. The authors concluded that the higher risk of incident CHF was related to differences in the prevalence of hypertension, diabetes mellitus, and socioeconomic stress (Bahrami et al., 2008).

- Data from the Third National Health and Nutrition Examination Survey showed that Hispanic men had the highest age-adjusted prevalence of metabolic syndrome among adults twenty years or older, 28 percent; followed by whites, 25 percent; and African Americans, 16 percent (Ford, Giles, & Dietz, 2002).

- Seven out of ten African Americans are either overweight or obese; they are also substantially more likely to be obese than any other group. Being overweight is a major risk factor for diabetes, cardiovascular disease, and other chronic conditions (*The Commonwealth Fund Health Quality Survey*, 2006).

Overall, then, there is substantial variation in the percentage of persons in each racial and ethnic group suffering from a chronic condition or disability. *The Commonwealth Fund Health Care Quality Survey* (2006) reports that, in a study of Americans eighteen to sixty-four years of age, 48 percent of African Americans, 40 percent of whites, 29 percent of Hispanics, and 25 percent of Asians had a chronic condition or disability. The burden of chronic disease is costly and these diseases adversely affect the persons and their families who have to cope with them.

Patterns of infectious disease are similar to those for chronic disease:

- In 2009, the Centers for Disease Control and Prevention reported that 52 percent of those infected by HIV in the United States were African American, 28 percent white, 18 percent Latino, 1.5 percent Asian or Pacific Islander, and less than 1 percent American Indian/Alaska Native (Centers for Disease Control and Prevention, 2010b).

- For tuberculosis, the rates per 100,000 were Asians, 23.3; Hispanics, 7; African Americans, 7.3. Of the total cases 59 percent were foreign born, primarily Asians and Hispanics (National Center for HIV/AIDS/Viral Hepatitis, STD, and TB Prevention, 2010).

- For hepatitis A in California in 2007, rates per 100,000 cases were Hispanics, 13.3; African Americans, 4.8; whites, 4.9; American Indian/Alaska Native, 3.4; and Asians, 2.7 (California Pan Ethnic Health Network, 2000).

- African Americans and Latinos had the highest rates of new HIV infections per 100,000 in 2009: 103.9 for African American men and 39.7 for African American women, and 39.9 for Latino males, accounting for 64 percent of new cases (Centers for Disease Control and Prevention, 2010b, 2011a).

Substantive health problems exist for many US subpopulations but a uniform pattern of very poor health starting in infancy to dementia and reduction of life expectancy is found most particularly for African Americans.

Most critically, these racial and ethnic differences are also very much apparent when the use of preventive services is examined. For example, many racial and ethnic minority women are less likely than the general population to receive timely prenatal care. Optimal prenatal care should reduce rates of low birth weight and of infant and maternal death. About 83 percent of women start prenatal care in first trimester and 89 percent of white women get this early prenatal care. There are significantly lower rates of early prenatal care among African Americans, 26 percent; Hispanics, 25 percent; Pacific Islanders, 23 percent; and American Indian/Alaska Native, 31 percent (AHRC, *National Health Care Disparities Report*, 2006). A national study of persons over the age of sixty-five during the 2002–2003 influenza season determined that 67 percent of the sample had received the influenza vaccine and 60 percent had received the pneumococcal polysaccharide (pneumonia) vaccine. Coverage among African Americans and Hispanics was 15 percentage points below that of whites (Singleton, Santibanez, & Wortley, 2005).

In recent years it has been possible to screen for many diseases early enough to prevent them from growing into more dangerous or deadly conditions. Early screenings make it possible to intervene in many disease processes or to make lifestyle changes that will prevent worsening of a condition. However, many persons in minority groups do not know about or do not avail themselves of screening tests. In 2003, 25 percent of Hispanic and 32 percent of Asian women were more likely to have gone without a Pap smear to screen for cervical cancer in the past three years than were whites (21 percent) and African American women (16 percent) (CDC, 2005). Despite high rates of diabetes mellitus, only 37 percent of Hispanic diabetics received the recommended annual tests necessary for the proper management of diabetes (AHRC, *National Health Care Disparities Report*, 2006). Colorectal cancer is the third most common cancer diagnosed in men and women in the United States, accounting for an estimated 143,000 new cases in 2010. Because of increased screening, death rates have dropped 31 percent since about 1990. However, Hispanics lagged far behind other racial and ethnic groups in obtaining colorectal screening tests (Mead, Cartwright-Smith, Jones, Ramos, & Woods, 2008). Lacking good preventive health care, diseases and disorders can progress to more severe late stages, causing disability, more intractable symptoms, and higher costs of care.

Use of mental health services by minorities show patterns similar to those for other health care services. Available evidence suggests that the prevalence of mental health conditions among racial and ethnic minorities is no greater than in the general population. However, minorities have less access to mental health services and subsequently are less likely to receive those services. They are also underrepresented in mental health research. Safety net providers furnish a disproportionate share of mental health services to minorities (Department of Health and Human Services, 2001). Language barriers are particularly problematic in mental health services because diagnosis and treatment relies heavily on verbal communication. Additionally, cultural differences in the perception and interpretation of mental disorders and a scarcity of mental health practitioners from ethnic and racial groups exacerbate this problem (Mezzich, Kleinman, Fabrega, & Parron, 1996).

Socioeconomic Sources of Racial and Ethnic Differences in Health Status

The causes of these racial and ethnic health care disparities are complex, stemming from socioeconomic, environmental, and biological factors and their interactions. The first two of these factors are linked: persons with low incomes and education are more likely to live in substandard, unhealthy housing, often in crowded urban areas or underserved rural locales (CDC, 2011a). These factors are called **social determinants of health** because the socioeconomic situations of persons and the places where they live and work strongly influence their health status (American College of Physicians, 2010). The risk for mortality, morbidity, limited access to care, and inferior care increases with decreasing socioeconomic level. This association is cumulative over the life course, thus affecting the elderly segments of each racial and ethnic group.

To begin with, many racial and ethnic minorities lack the funds to pay for private health insurance, which is growing more costly by the year (DeNavas, Proctor, & Smith, 2010). In their new *Action Plan to Reduce Racial and Ethnic Health Disparities*, the Department of Health and Human Services (2011a) states that lack of insurance, more than any other demographic or economic barrier, affects the quality of care received by minorities, and points out that though minorities are just one-third of the US population, they make up more than half of the uninsured. Minorities are less likely to have employer-sponsored coverage (Kaiser Family Foundation, 2010). Many low-income families make too much money to be eligible for Medicaid but not enough to afford private coverage. According to the Centers for Disease Control and Prevention (2011b), 29 percent of Hispanics and 32 percent of American Indian/Alaska Natives were without coverage in 2011 compared to 17 percent of African Americans, 15 percent of Asians, and 11 percent of whites. The OMH makes the point that though minorities are one-third of the nation's population, they are over half of the uninsured (OMH, 2011a).

Lack of coverage translates to lack of care: 21 percent of African Americans and 43 percent of Hispanics compared to 15 percent of whites and 16 percent of Asians had no regular provider or medical home in 2006 (*The Commonwealth Fund Health Care Quality Survey*, 2006). Having a medical home or regular source of care means that individuals have providers they can contact by phone or with whom they can easily set up an office visit. A medical home provides a significant degree of continuity of care inasmuch as records of health status, prior visits, referrals, treatments, tests, and medications are kept in one place (Agency for Healthcare Research and Quality, 2010b). Persons without medical insurance receive less preventive care and are thus diagnosed at more advanced disease stages. They are more likely to receive their care in a hospital outpatient clinic or emergency rooms. They are more likely to be readmitted after a hospital stay. They are more likely to seek care in different locales, further fragmenting their care.

Medicaid and Medicare are major sources of care for African Americans and Hispanics. In 2008 and 2009, 27 percent of African Americans and Hispanics were covered by Medicaid and 9 percent of African Americans and 5 percent of Hispanics were covered by Medicare (Kaiser Family Foundation Commission on Medicaid and the Uninsured, 2010). Medicaid or the State Children's Health Insurance Program (SCHIP) provided coverage for 50 percent of poor African American children and nearly that proportion of poor Hispanic children in 2009. **The Patient Protection and Affordable Care Act of 2010** will expand coverage to most individuals with incomes up to 133 percent of the family poverty line. This will mean a large influx of minority populations into health care venues over the coming years, presenting a unique opportunity to reduce disparities if appropriate and culturally competent care is undertaken.

Genetic Differences as a Source of Racial and Ethnic Variation in Disease Risk

Looking at the broad and consistent patterns of disease risk across racial and ethnic populations and knowing that human "races" tend to fall into semidistinctive subunits within the human genome based on historic geographical distribution (Risch, Burchard, Ziv, & Hua, 2002) raises the possibility of variation in diseases due to genetic factors. Expectations about finding genetic links to diseases have also been increased by successes in linking single genes to disorders in specific populations, such as sickle cell disease among African Americans and Mediterranean groups, Tay Sachs and Goucher's disease among Jews with a European background, and cystic fibrosis among white persons of European heritage. However, it is much easier to find a single gene with one big effect than to find the multiple genes that add up to risk for the complex chronic diseases that show variation across population groups. Thus, the molecular geneticists are turning their attention to the challenge of finding clusters of genes that combine to create disease risk. Genomewide scans are underway to discover evidence of linkages between health conditions and particular chromosomal regions. However, many genes need to interact with the environment in order to be expressed, and it is clear that the environments associated with racial and ethnic groups in the United States vary in quite consistent ways with socioeconomic variables, so environmental factors are likely to play a major role. Attributing the substantial differences in disease risk across populations solely to genetic disadvantage is untenable because genetics would not explain this general pattern across many disorders. For example, the African American disadvantage that is seen across many diseases is likely to be a combination of **genetic risk** factors and a common-source exposure to a disease-promoting environment (Anderson, Bulatao, & Cohen, 2004). In the near future, the issue of racial and ethnic distribution of genetic risk factors may become moot as personalized medicine begins to make use of more accurate individual genome analysis. At present, however, confronting disease disparities by addressing poverty, education, lifestyle factors, and access is likely to yield the most certain benefits.

Racial and Ethnic Disparities in Health Status as the Focus of National Attention

The disparities that are visible across racial and ethnic populations in the United States are the subject of national attention and goal setting because health care disparities are seen to be a nationwide economic and quality-of-care problem. Since the establishment of the Office of Research on Minority Health in 1990, the federal government has steadily increased funds to investigate and develop strategies to reduce racial and ethnic disparities. In 2000, in a bill introduced by the late Senator Edward Kennedy, Congress mandated the implementation of a strategic plan for health disparities research with the Minority Health and Health Disparities Research and Education Act (2000). attention In 2003, the first National Healthcare Disparities report, developed by the AHRQ, was the initial comprehensive effort to measure differences in access and use of services across all racial and ethnic groups and has been followed by yearly reports on disparities (see, for example, AHRQ, 2010a, 2011); attention to disparities also was prominent in the CDC's *Healthy People 2010* and other Department of Health and Human Services (DHHS) reports. These reports document that racial and ethnic health disparities exist in all regions of the country, among the insured and uninsured and across multiple medical conditions and at all levels of service. They are clear in the health data related to gender and to the elderly.

Recent actions by the federal government demonstrate that concern for health care disparities is receiving increased focus. The federal government made elimination of disparities an overarching goal of the *Healthy People 2010* initiative. The Medicare Improvement Plan for Patients and Providers Act of 2008, the Children's Health Insurance Program Reauthorization Act (2009), and the Health Information Technology Act of 2009 all contain many provisions addressing cultural and linguistic competence and health care disparities. As we have seen, the Patient Protection and Affordable Care Act of 2010 also directly mandates strategies to address disparities.

However, despite unmistakable evidence of disparities for at least two decades, little concrete progress has been made in eliminating them. When the Institute of Medicine examined the efforts made at the federal level in *Examining the Health Disparities Research Plan of the National Institutes of Health: Unfinished Business* (Thomson, Mitchell, & Williams, 2006), the evaluators made clear that many gaps still exist in the ability to provide a full, actionable evidence base on disparities and their sources, and the hoped-for coordination of research and data gathering across the various DHHS institutes and centers had been very imperfectly realized, in part because the funds that were to support the strategic plan had not actually been allocated! Even the Department of Health and Human Services, in its 2011 action plan to reduce disparities, notes that there has been little improvement in health care disparities during the previous decade. Overall, however, the extensive literature suggests that racial and ethnic disparities *can be* greatly reduced by altering the structure of the health care system, by changing the way health care services are delivered, by training health care personnel in culturally competent care, and by carefully measuring the results of these interventions. There is consensus that culturally competent care and reduction of disparities should be viewed as quality-of-care issues and be subject to measurement and evaluation similar to all other quality factors. Not only would reduction of health care disparities diminish the burden of poor health on many Americans, but, because it has been estimated that racial and ethnic disparities resulting in direct medical costs and low productivity in the United States also result in substantial costs to the nation (between 2003 and 2006 these costs were estimated at $1.24 trillion), reducing disparities would reduce the overall cost of health care to public and private sectors (LaVeist, Gaskin, & Richard, 2009).

Recently, as part of the Patient Protection and Affordable Care Act of 2010, the National Center on Minority Health and Health Disparities was upgraded to become the National Institute on Minority Health and Health Disparities (NIH, 2010) and has as its responsibility the planning, coordinating, and evaluation of all disparities research activities conducted or supported by the National Institutes of Health institutes and centers. Further, several major philanthropic organizations, including the Kaiser Family Foundation, The Commonwealth Fund, the Robert Wood Johnson Foundation, and The California Endowment, have made disparities reduction a major research and funding focus.

DISPARITIES ACROSS OTHER DIVERSITY DIMENSIONS: GENDER, SEXUAL ORIENTATION, THE ELDERLY

Although the health disparities across racial and ethnic groups dwarf all others by comparison, this doesn't mean that disparities or differences related to other dimensions of diversity are unimportant. Many of the disparities in health status related to gender, sexual orientation, and age are the product of inattention to or ignorance of the special needs of these groups.

Health Care Disparities Associated with Gender

Historically, discrepancies in the quality of care between men and women have resulted from lack of research and discounting the possibility that male-female differences in health and illness might be centered on issues other than reproductive health. However, recent research has demonstrated that gender-related physiological and health care needs go far beyond reproductive issues. "Over the past decade new discoveries in basic human biology have made it increasingly apparent that many normal physiological functions—and, in many cases, pathological functions—are influenced either directly or indirectly by sex-based differences in biology" (Wizemann & Pardue, 2011, p. 13). Then, too, in what was once male-dominated medical practice, women's legitimate and common health concerns (for example, menstrual problems and menopause) were trivialized and frequently attributed to emotion or somatization. Because women were often excluded from medical and pharmaceutical research, gender differences in the expression of common disorders and response to medication remained obscure. Now it is known that gender-based differences are found at the system, organ, tissue, cellular, and subcellular levels. These differences, in combination with possible differential environmental exposure, have their effect on health. Some of the important differences listed by the Society for Women's Health Research (2010) in their fact sheet summaries include the following:

- Heart disease strikes women on average ten years later than men and women are more likely than men to have another heart attack within a year of the first.

- Cardiac arrest is about three times greater in men than women but women have lower recovery and survival rates than men.

- Until recently, only men were considered at risk for myocardial infarction (MI) and the typical MI symptom for men is chest pain. Women are more likely to have subtle symptoms of MI such as nausea, vomiting, fatigue, mid-back pain, and indigestion.

- Women constitute 80 percent of the population suffering from osteoporosis.

- Women are two times more likely than men to contract a sexually transmitted infection. HIV is among the leading causes of death for US women aged twenty-five to fifty-four and is the number one cause of death for African American women aged twenty-five to thirty-four.

- Three out of four people suffering from autoimmune diseases, such as multiple sclerosis, rheumatoid arthritis, and lupus, are women.

- Each year approximately forty thousand more women than men suffer from a stroke. This is related to women's greater life expectancy and the higher rates of stroke in older age groups.

Clearly, the biochemical make-ups of men and women differ, for example, in terms of hormones and their various effects on organ systems, developmental processes, and behavior. Efforts are now being made to tease out the separate influences of hormones and genes on susceptibility to disease and disease processes among men and women. For example, as we have seen, although actual life expectancy differs among ethnic groups, women in all ethnic and racial groups tend to live longer than men. Though these differences cannot be considered inequitable because they are believed to be biological in basis, they are important to be aware of in diagnosing and treating male and female patients.

Unquestionably, women have many more issues than men around reproductive health. One researcher points out that women's reproductive health represents 16 percent of overall health plan costs, which is more than cardiovascular disease, diabetes, and asthma combined (Owens, 2008). Maternity concerns include prenatal and postnatal care, childbirth itself, and breastfeeding, all of which require health services. Throughout their lives, women are more likely to experience cancers of various reproductive organs, which require preventive screening such as mammograms and Pap screening for cervical cancer. Consequently, women require significantly more ongoing preventive health services than men. Men over fifty, particularly African American men, who are much more likely to have prostate cancer, undergo screening for this disease, but late in life and not as regularly as women are screened for cancer of their reproductive organs. Even outside the area of reproductive health, it has been noted that women tend to use significantly more health care services and spend more health care dollars than men; this is particularly true among women older than forty-five and in association with chronic illness (Owens, 2008).

The new Patient Protection and Affordable Care Act decrees that individuals covered through new small and large group plans by 2011 will have coverage—without cost sharing—for preventive services that are deemed "highly effective" by the US Preventive Services Task Force. In the case of mammography, all qualified health plans will need to cover annual mammography for women starting at age forty. For immunizations, those recommended by the Advisory Committee on Immunization Practices (ACIP) of the Centers for Disease Control and Prevention will be required by law to be covered without cost sharing. For women and girls under twenty-six, this will mean that the HPV vaccine for prevention of cervical cancer must be covered free of cost sharing (no co-pays, deductibles, or co-insurance can be applied). Reproductive health issues most relevant to women, such as birth control, the HPV vaccine, and abortion, are still highly controversial; men's issues around birth control and erectile dysfunction seem far less subject to debate.

In terms of access to health care, women have experienced some particular problems (Rustgi, Doty, & Collins, 2009). A Commonwealth Fund Biennial Health Insurance Survey (2007) disclosed that women have higher rates of public coverage than men, and more men than women have employer-based coverage. Even women who have employer-based insurance are very likely to be covered as dependents. Thus they can be more vulnerable to losing their insurance than men if they are widowed or divorced or if their husbands lose their jobs. The same study showed that 45 percent of women and 39 percent of men were underinsured or uninsured for a time in the past year. More than three in five of the women reported a problem paying medical bills compared with about half of the men. Currently, about 6 percent of women purchase coverage through the individual insurance market. Historically, these plans have been able to deny coverage to individuals with a "preexisting condition" such as pregnancy, mental illness, or a chronic condition. In this market, women typically have had to purchase a separate rider to cover maternity care, which can be extremely costly and often requires a waiting period before the benefits are covered. Furthermore, in many states, insurers have been able to charge women who purchase individual insurance more than men for the same coverage, a practice called *gender rating*. The Patient Protection and Affordable Care Act of 2010 makes many changes to this market that will benefit women. It subjects new individual insurance market plans to the same regulations as plans sold in state-based exchanges. Therefore, it will ban the practices of gender rating. Furthermore, all plans sold on the individual market will have to cover a minimum level of services, which includes maternity care.

The 2010 legislation also establishes offices on women's health in major federal agencies, including the Department of Health and Human Services, Centers for Disease Control and Prevention, the Food and Drug Administration, Health Resources and Services Administration, and an Office of Women's Health and Gender-Based Research at the Agency for Health Care Research and Quality. These agencies are designed to establish goals, provide information on women's health activities, and identify women's health priorities within their respective agencies. The law also authorizes the establishment of a Department of Health and Human Services Coordinating Committee on Women's Health to oversee the activities of these offices as well as a National Women's Health Information Center to facilitate exchange of information regarding health promotion, prevention, major advances in research, and other relevant developments in women's health.

Health Disparities Among Lesbian, Gay, Bisexual, and Transgender (LGBT) People

LGBT people share with the larger society the full range of health risks, though they tend to have unique issues related to sexual identity. First, because of the social stigma that has historically been attached to their sexual identity, LGBTs may not wish to disclose their orientation to researchers or health care personnel. At present, most health data on LGBTs are submerged in the research on the general population. For researchers there are also problems of definition, for example, identifying the concept of "transgender" in a way that is recognized by a study population. There are methodological difficulties in working with small study samples (2 to 3 percent of the overall population) and nonprobability samples. Thus there are few good studies of overall health conditions in these varied subpopulations. Additionally, though often lumped together because of small sample sizes or the concept that this entire group is defined in contrast with the majority population in terms of sexual orientation, the health issues of each of these subpopulations are likely to be unique. The Patient Protection and Affordable Care Act of 2010 contains provisions to strengthen federal data collection efforts on LGBTs by convening experts to address definitional issues surrounding sexual identification and orientation with the goal of requiring that all national data collection should cover these populations by 2013 (Office of

Minority Health, 2011a). DHHS has announced plans to include sexual orientation identifiers and gender identity in the next National Health Interview Survey (HealthCare.gov, 2011). Additionally, the Institute of Medicine has carefully studied the issue of research in these populations (Committee on Lesbian, Gay, Bisexual and Transgender Health Issues and Research Gaps and Opportunities, 2011) and has produced many excellent suggestions about how to proceed.

One recent statewide study conducted by the Massachusetts Department of Public Health (Conron, Mimiaga, & Landers, 2010), which used the state's behavioral risk factor surveillance system, has produced important data:

- Gay men and women were more likely to be current smokers than their heterosexual counterparts.

- Lesbian women and bisexuals were more likely to have multiple risk factors for heart disease.

- Sexual minorities as a whole were more likely to report having had some form of sexual assault during their lifetime.

- Gay men were about 33 percent less likely than heterosexual men to be obese and lesbians were about 50 percent more likely than heterosexual women to be obese.

- Bisexuals in particular were found to be burdened by poor health.

Similar findings for lesbians were revealed in an examination of sexual orientation, health risk factors, and physical functioning in the Nurses' Health Study (Case et al., 2004). Based on a sample of 90,823 women, lesbian women (694) were found to have a higher prevalence of risk factors for breast cancer, cardiovascular disease, higher body mass index, smoking, and depression. Results for bisexual women were similar.

A recent statewide study conducted in California by the UCLA Center for Health Policy Research showed that aging (fifty to seventy year olds) lesbian, gay, and bisexual adults had higher rates of chronic disease, mental distress, and isolation than heterosexuals of similar age though their access and use of health care services was little different (Lin, 2011). Clearly, there are significant differences in the health status of LGBTs and the larger population; however, there is a paucity of research that explores the source of these differences.

The exception to the general lacunae of research on the etiology of disease and disorder in the LGBT is the extensive research on sexual behavior and IV drug use on the transmission of HIV/AIDS. Gay and bisexual men remain the population most heavily affected by sexually transmitted diseases in the United States. Whereas CDC (2010b) estimates that men who have sex with men make up 2 to 3 percent of the total US population, this group accounts for more than 50 percent of all new HIV infections annually from 2006 to 2009. As noted earlier, HIV/AIDS is heavily skewed toward the African American population, partially because there is more transmission of HIV/AIDS through drug use than in other populations. Unfortunately, the incidence among young African American males is on the increase. With the exception of the costs of HIV/AIDS, the costs or other sequelae of health care disparities among the LGBT population have not been studied.

Health Issues Unique to the Aging Population

Age as a dimension of diversity is playing an increasingly critical role in health care in terms of economics and medical attention. The good news is that people in the United States are living much longer. The US population of age sixty-five plus is expected to double by 2033. More people were sixty-five years and over in 2010 than in any previous census. Between 2000 and 2010, the population sixty-five and over increased at a faster rate than the total US population as a whole. Among the older population, the eighty-four- to ninety-year-old age group showed the fastest growth of any group between the 2000 and 2010 census, growing by 30 percent (He & Muenchrath, 2011; He, Sengupta, Velkoff, & DeBarros, 2005). The bad news is that this means that an ever-growing percentage of the population will suffer from the diseases of aging. Currently, about 80 percent of seniors have one chronic health condition and 50 percent have two. Chronic health conditions include, in the order of their prevalence, diseases of the heart, malignant neoplasms, cerebrovascular disease, chronic obstructive pulmonary disease (COPD), diabetes, and Alzheimer's disease. As noted earlier, significant differences exist across race and ethnic groups in the prevalence of chronic lifestyle diseases. These differences only exacerbate with age, leading to multiple chronic conditions and different life expectancy. Age-related disorders such as crippling osteoarthritis and blinding macular degeneration also require medical care. The National Institute on Aging Alzheimer's Disease Progress Report (2011) notes that at present 2.4 to 5.1

million people have Alzheimer's disease (AD) and that the number of people with AD doubles for every five years past sixty-five. Studies indicate that prevalence rates for persons over sixty-five are highest for African Americans and Hispanics, about the same for Asians and whites, and somewhat lower for American Indians but the reason for these differences is yet to be determined (Manly & Mayeux, 2004).

As the population of the nation ages, more and more health care dollars, research, and expertise will be devoted to prevention of chronic diseases and maintaining the health of persons already suffering from one or more chronic diseases. These efforts will require a greater focus on continuity of care and greater knowledge of the patient's sociocultural environment, hence an approach that will include cultural competence and attention to diversity. The increasing costs of Medicare will be an ongoing issue in assessing how the nation views differences in the health care needs of the old and the young.

STAKEHOLDER ATTENTION TO HEALTH CARE DISPARITIES

Aside from the social and moral implications of wide disparities in health status and access, disparities in health status among minorities are very costly to the nation. Waidmann (2009), for example, estimated that $23.9 billion would have been saved in 2009 alone if minority health equaled that of whites. A study commissioned by Washington-based think tank The Joint Center for Political and Economic Studies (LaViest, Gaskin, & Richard, 2009) found that the United States lost $1.24 trillion between 2003 and 2006 through disparities in minority care. These researchers also estimated that during these three years, the direct medical costs associated with health disparities amounted to $229.4 billion, and when indirect costs such as lost productivity were added in, the three year total increased to $1.24 trillion. Given that minority populations are increasing in size much faster than whites, the costs will accelerate if disparities are not quickly addressed. Because minorities constitute a large portion of the US population, the poor health care they receive adds substantively to the nation's low standing among developed nations across many indices of health status. Recent international comparisons, for example, show that life expectancy in the United States ranks forty-ninth among all nations and infant mortality rates are higher than in many poorer nations (Institute of Medicine, 2010b).

Awareness of and need to address disparities in health care has taken an unconscionably long time to come. As noted earlier, the federal government began to collect data on health statuses of different population groups in the mid-1980s and began then to require that federally funded research address minority populations and women. Actionable regulations and guidelines did not begin to surface until around the beginning of the twenty-first century. The national Cultural and Linguistically Appropriate Services (CLAS) standards were published in 2000 by the Office of Minority Health, and the Office of Civil Rights (OCR) guidelines on the provision of language services were published a few years before that. Some state governments, seeking to address the needs of minorities on their Medicaid rolls, began to look at language and cultural issues in the care of their minority patients in the late 1990s. However, with the exception of several of the larger nonprofit health plans, such as Kaiser Permanente, Harvard Pilgrim, and Group Health of Puget Sound, health management organizations and health plans largely ignored disparities in the health of different groups within their patient bases until well into the twenty-first century. Additionally, because minorities were generally less affluent than whites, most for-profit health plans did not consider them a viable market for health insurance and some still do not. The administrators of many health plans and hospitals rarely took notice of disparities in the care of their diverse patients; most were reluctant to believe that such differences in care existed or, if they did, that they could not be addressed without too costly changes in delivery structures. In 2008, for example, one of the authors of this book was told by an upper level manager of a health plan in a state with a highly diverse population that the addition of extra keystrokes to capture racial and ethnic data on their **demographic data set** was "too costly" for the value of the information gained.

Instigation of change in attitudes toward disparities came from advocacy groups and philanthropic organizations that prompted government regulations and from frontline care providers. A prime example was a task force that was created by the California Department of Health in 1996 that was formed at the request of an advocacy group when California decided to set up state-supported health plans through which all Medicaid persons would receive their care (Brach, Paez, & Frazer, 2006). The state would identify minorities through enrollment procedures and the plans then would address their cultural and linguistic needs according to contract stipulations. Other states followed suit in terms of requiring that government-funded health care services recognize the special cultural and linguistic needs of minority patients. Health care providers that didn't serve Medicaid, State Children's Health Insurance Program (SCHIP), or that served very few minorities largely ignored the regulations. Growing advocacy came through local and state organizations such as the California Pan Ethnic Health Network (CPEHN) and Diversity Rx, a national advocacy organization that publicized the needs of minorities through conferences and Internet education. Several large foundations, including the Robert Wood Johnson Foundation, The California Endowment, The Commonwealth Fund, and the Kaiser Family Foundation, underwrote research and development efforts as well as major convenings on the issue. Accreditation organizations such as the National Committee on Quality Assurance (NCQA) and the Joint Commission began to view disparities as a quality and care delivery issue and gradually instigated requirements and guidelines that forced health care organizations to pay attention to disparities. NCQA has sought to increase specific strategies to address disparities by offering annual awards to health care organizations that have adopted innovative strategies to address the needs of diverse groups (NCQA, 2006, 2007, 2008, 2009).

Clinicians, that is, doctors and nurses and other frontline care providers, found it increasingly difficult to meet the needs of cultural and linguistic minorities as well as the newly recognized needs of patients of diverse sexual orientation. The practice associations, such as the American Academy of Family Physicians, the American College of Emergency Physicians, the American Academy of Pediatrics, and the American Nurses Association, began including guidelines for the provision of care to persons from diverse groups and including information on treatment of specific populations in their discipline focused journals (for example, *Academic Medicine*, 2003; *Annals of Internal Medicine*, 1996; *Journal of Nursing Education*, 2003). From the point of view of clinicians, adoption of strategies to care for diverse patients was a practical matter, and they needed the administrative backup of health plans, clinics, and hospitals to mobilize structural and service delivery changes, such as interpretation and translation services, for providing quality care to diverse constituencies.

Finally, employer associations such as the National Business Group on Health (National Business Group on Health, 2011; Trahan & Williamson, 2009) have begun to make clear to employers that it is in their interest as health insurance purchasers to make sure that health care organizations attend to the needs of their diverse employees. Their surveys show that employers' concern about health care disparities is low but growing (National Business Group on

Health, 2009a, 2009b, NCQA, 2011). Employers are beginning to see that it is in their interest that health plans address health care disparities (Higgins, Au, & Taylor, 2009). In 2012, the National Business Group on Health provided employers with the *Health Disparities Cost Impact Tool* so that they could actually assess the cost of health care disparities among their employees to their businesses. Gradually, as accreditation agencies such as NCQA and the Joint Commission (2009) began to view reduction of disparities as a quality and accreditation issue and health plan purchasers began to see it as important, the management side of health care organizations began to slowly come on board.

Health care organizations thus are being moved to address disparities by advocates, their frontline providers, governmental regulations, purchasers, and accreditation agencies. However, up to 2011, action taking to address disparities has been fragmented and lacking in institutionalization through systems of accountability or assessments of health outcomes. Many toolkits and conceptual frameworks for addressing disparities have been developed and published but it is unknown to what extent the health care organizations for which they are designed actually have knowledge of them or how widely they are used.

A recent scan of disparities reduction activities (NCQA, 2011) cites three key themes:

- Growing awareness but limited commitment of resources

- Disjointed leadership with diffuse plans and fragmented efforts to reduce disparities

- Absence of key stakeholders, such as consumers and communities, from the conversation

Admittedly, the disparities issue has grown even more serious as minority populations have increased in proportion of the US population and as the income gap between the nation's well-off and its poor has also increased. It is expected that some of the new strategies either required by law or accrediting agencies or recommended by powerful research and advocacy organizations may help change this still rather discouraging picture (Beach, 2004; Committee on Public Health Strategies to Improve Health, 2011). As will be seen, there is no dearth of strategies to address health care disparities—there is only the will to implement them.

SYSTEMATIC STRATEGIES FOR REDUCING HEALTH CARE DISPARITIES

The first step in reducing disparities in a culturally competent, systematic way is to develop a sound evidence base (National Quality Forum, 2008a; Regenstein & Stickler, 2006) Accountability in reducing disparities will not be possible without acquiring data as a basis for measuring progress. Health care organizations have generally collected and entered gender and age as patient variables in their data systems, but the systematic entry of racial and ethnic data, now required by the Patient Protection and Affordable Care Act of 2010 (DHHS, 2011b), has only occurred in the last few years. Though more and more health plans (NCQA, 2007), hospitals (Siegel, Regenstein, & Jones, 2007), and clinics have begun to include race, ethnicity, and language data in their demographic data sets, this activity has primarily been voluntary, nonstandardized, and fragmented. At first, many health care organizations were reluctant to collect these data from patients for fear that they would offend them (Burke, Stewart, & Harty, 2008). Others believed that it was against the law to ask patients about these matters (Rosenbaum, Burke, Nath, Santos, & Thomas, 2006). Still others were unsure of valid and reliable categories in which to record race and ethnicity (Lurie & Fremont, 2006) or didn't know what to do with these data once collected. These impediments have been cleared up by research, regulation, and model programs (Institute of Medicine, 2009; National Quality Forum, 2009a). Far from being illegal or an abridgement of patients' civil rights, collecting data on ethnicity, race, and language has been deemed to advance the purposes of the Civil Rights Act of 1964 and would operate as evidence of compliance with the law rather than be a violation of it (Burke, Stewart, & Hardy, 2008; Rosenbaum, Burke, & Nath, 2006). Many state governments agree with that concept and have included legislation that requires collection of these data (Au, Taylor, & Gold, 2009). The routine collection of information on the sexual orientation of patients is still rarely undertaken.

Health care organizations have tried a variety of ways of approximating the race and ethnicity of their client populations, such as staff assessment (staff guesses of patients' identities), analysis of census tract data, and geocoding, but the most useful and accurate method by far has been to ask the patients to self-identify (Kelmer, 2011). Data gathered by the latter method are at the individual level and can become part of the patient's medical record, allowing medical practitioners to consider language access and cultural factors in addressing patient needs. Capturing the race and ethnicity of patients can also be used in varying aggregates for analyzing geographic concentrations, health status, and intervention outcomes. Researchers have determined that, although a small segment of minority patients would be concerned that their health care provider collects such data, most, when told that the data were going to be used to improve quality of care, are not reluctant to agree (Baker et al., 2006).

The federal government clearly considers the evaluation of a patient's quality of care by race and ethnicity as a necessary step toward quality improvement or it wouldn't have mandated that all federally funded health programs and population surveys collect these data (Andrulis, Siddiqui, Purtle, & Duchon, 2010). Going further, the Patient Protection and Affordable Care Act requires that organizations receiving federal funding monitor and report disparities to the Department of Health and Human Services and to the public (DHHS, 2011b). Because most health care organizations receive at least some federal funding through Medicaid, SCHIP, or Medicare, this means that there are few health care providers or systems that aren't covered by this regulation (Bonito & Eidheldinger, 2005).

Fortunately, a number of efforts have been made to help health care organizations collect and use racial and ethnic and language data. A particularly good aid, a toolkit, was developed by the Health Research and Educational Trust supported by the Robert Wood Johnson Foundation and The Commonwealth Fund (Hasnain-Wynia, Hague, Hedges-Greuing, Prince, & Reiter, 2007). The toolkit contains step-by-step instructions about where and how to collect racial and ethnic data from patients and staff training in the importance and use of the data, with specific sections for management, legal affairs, quality improvement, clinicians, and information technology. Another toolkit that is useful is the National Health Plan Collaborative's *Toolkit to Reduce Racial and Ethnic Disparities* (2008; Lurie et al., 2008). The Disparities Solutions Center at Massachusetts General Hospital (2006) published *Improving Quality and Achieving Equity: A Guide for Hospital Leaders* (2006) and *Creating Equity Reports* (Weinick, Flaherty, & Bristol, 2008). The latter document also includes strategies for collecting socioeconomic data from patients. Recently, the National Commission on Quality Assurance (NCQA), in support of their new multicultural health care standards, issued a publication providing ideas and examples of how to implement those standards, including a detailed set of how-tos in collecting racial and ethnic data (National Committee on Quality Assurance, 2010). Here is a summary of available models and methods for racial and ethnic data collection and use:

- *HRET Disparities Toolkit for Collecting Race, Ethnicity and Primary Language Information from Patients* (Hasnain-Wynia, Hague, Hedges-Greuing, Prince, & Reiter, 2007)

- *Implementing Multicultural Health Standards: Ideas and Examples* (NCQA, 2011)

- *Tools to Address Disparities in Health Care: Data as Building Blocks for Change* (America's Health Insurance Plans, 2005)

- *Improving Quality and Achieving Equity: A Guide for Hospital Leaders* (Massachusetts General Hospital, 2006)

- *Advancing Effective Communication, Cultural Competence, and Patient- and Family-Centered Care: A Road Map for Hospitals* (The Joint Commission, 2010)

- *Creating Equity Reports: A Guide for Hospitals* (Weinick, Flaherty, & Bristol, 2008)

- *Implementing Multicultural Health Care Standards: Ideas and Examples* (National Commission on Quality Assurance, 2010)

- *National Voluntary Consensus Standards for Ambulatory Care; Measuring Disparities* (National Quality Forum, 2008b)

Ultimately it is hoped that the collection of race, ethnicity, language, and LGBT data will be standardized as part of health information technology so that measurement of needs, interventions, and quality of care can be assessed across organizations and data sets. Health information technology will make it possible to assess disparities across national data sets, health plans, hospitals, clinics, and even practice-based primary care (Cusack, Knudson, Kronstadt, Singer, & Brown, 2010; Institute of Medicine, 2009). The growing focus on **comparative effectiveness research** (CER), which is designed to compare different prevention and treatment interventions as well as medications in terms of their impact on health outcomes (Begley, 2011), can yield insights into the most effective strategies across population groups if health care organizations take the important step of stratifying their quality and **outcome measures** by race, ethnicity, and, where useful, gender, age, and sexual orientation (Gibbs, Nsiah-Jefferson, McHugh,

Trivedi, & Praothrow-Stith, 2006) The final step of such as systematic approach will be the feedback loop: using the data to improve and target interventions. The measurement and evaluation of outcomes will be an important step in verifying the efficacy of culturally informed interventions, which, to date, have not often been systematically evaluated (Committee on Public Health Strategies to Improve Health, 2011; DHHS, 2011c).

The ultimate and most important use of race, ethnicity, language, and LGBT data, therefore, is to enable organizations to identify and address the health care needs of individuals in these underserved groups and to track their performance with these subpopulations, that is, to use these data as a primary strategic driver of systematic cultural competence (America's Health Insurance Plans, 2005). The work of Aetna and its HMO affiliates is a case in point. In 2002 Aetna became the first national for-profit commercial health plan to begin collecting voluntary racial and ethnicity and language preference data from its members, doing so on enrollment forms, health-risk assessment systems, and its Aetna navigator website, using strict policies against inappropriate disclosure to protect the privacy of its members. Members in forty-seven states and the District of Columbia have signed up. Over 80 percent of members who had the opportunity to produce their racial and ethnic identifier data did so. Then by integrating these data with claims data, the organization was able to identify, for example, African American and Hispanic women who had not had a necessary mammogram and conducted a successful outreach program. Aetna has used their racial and ethnic data to better understand the make-up of their membership and to develop preventive health, early detection, targeted interventions, and disease management programs based on member characteristics (NCQA, 2007). The organization has created a racial and ethnic equality dashboard, which takes self-reported race and ethnicity information and combines it with medical claims, pharmacy information, quality measures, and member satisfaction to provide a detailed view of disparities in Aetna's membership. By using this dashboard, the organization has been able to identify where disparities exist and intervene with culturally and linguistically appropriate strategies (Kelmar, 2011).

The L.A. Care Plan (Los Angeles) is the largest public plan in the nation, a local initiative established over a decade ago when California determined that its Medicaid population would be served by specially organized HMOs. In 2008, the organization analyzed its NCQA Health Care Effectiveness Data and Information Set (HEDIS) rates by race and ethnicity and learned that African

American members were significantly less likely to have postpartum visits compared to whites and Latinas and were also less likely to receive breast cancer screening. They conducted focus groups to determine the reasons for such differences and learned that African American women lacked knowledge about the importance of these health care interventions and some tended to distrust the health care system. This experience led the plan to create its Health Disparities Improvement Project. This broad-based plan included ongoing collection and analysis of data, community education classes, engagement and mobilization of community health workers, and empowerment of regional community advisory committee members, as well as opening a family resource center to collaborate with local community organizations to offer education and screenings to primarily African American and Latino members (NCQA, 2009).

The National Health Plan Collaborative (NHPC), a public-private partnership among nine health plans covering nearly ninety-five million lives, leading research organizations, the DHHS Agency for Health Care Research and Quality, and the Robert Wood Johnson Foundation, was formed in 2003 with the goal of reducing disparities (Lurie et al., 2008). By linking their data on the racial and ethnic identity of their members to their clinical measures on diabetes, the plans were able to locate disparities and address specific issues by designing, piloting, and evaluating culturally and linguistically appropriate interventions ranging from disease management to targeted preventive screening and community collaboration to meeting patients' linguistic needs.

The Disparities Solutions Center, operating in association with Massachusetts General Hospital, reports on a variety of disparities reduction efforts at the community, state, and national levels (www.disparitiysolutions.org). Taken together, all of these model programs show that addressing health care disparities is far from impossible if systemized knowledge of the needs of different patient populations is used.

Moreover, the structure of health care delivery in the United States is undergoing significant and exciting change. The growing emphasis on personalized health care and patient-centered medical homes that coordinate care—concepts that involve long-term partnership relations between patients, their families, and their providers—requires attention to and understanding patients' cultures and unique needs (Beach, Saha, & Cooper, 2006). Actively engaging patients in their own care will require cultural understanding and good communication. In order for communication to take place, accommodation to diverse patients' languages and cultures will be critical. Strategies that are culturally competent and evidence based will be indispensable.

SUMMARY

The importance of cultural competence to disparities reduction and the emerging new delivery processes is clear. Cultural competence in health care has been described as "the ongoing capacity of health care systems, organizations, and professionals to provide for diverse patient populations high-quality care that is safe, patient-centered, **evidence based**, and equitable" (National Quality Forum, 2009b, p. 3). Over time, as the nation enters into an era of comparative effectiveness research, and learning from these early data gathering and analysis models, it easily will be possible to determine if interventions, treatments, and medicines are effective for all or if there is variation at the group as well as individual levels. Data and measurement should become the strongest and most systematic tools of cultural competence and disparities reduction. Although the cultural competence movement of the turn of the twenty-first century began more as a recognition that the health care system needed to address the cultural and linguistic needs of an increasingly diverse patient population, cultural competence is now being refined as a set of tools to address costly and burdensome disparities in health status and access. We have moved from an awareness of cultural differences to recognition and acknowledgment of inequity. Because of this change in emphasis, the concepts and interventions labeled *culturally competent care* and *diversity management* will be increasingly important, but more and more, they will be subject to the requirements of being systematic, evidence based, measurable, and cost effective.

KEY TERMS

comparative effectiveness research

demographic data sets

epidemiology

evidence-based medicine

genetic risk

HEDIS

inequitable health care disparities

outcome measures

Patient Protection and Affordable Care Act of 2010

social determinants of health

REVIEW QUESTIONS AND ACTIVITIES

1. Clearly, disparities in health status have existed among groups in the United States for a long time. Why do you think the nation has been so slow in addressing them?

2. There were many federal agencies mentioned in this chapter. What role does the federal government play in disparities reduction? Could the individual states do the work to address disparities without the federal government? Why or why not?

3. Much of US health care is in the hands of the private sector. Could the private sector address disparities issues better than state or federal governments? Why or why not?

4. Discuss the proposed categories for identifying persons by race and ethnicity. Are these categories appropriate and efficient? Why or why not? How would you change them if you could?

5. Two accreditation organizations, the National Committee on Quality Assurance and the Joint Commission, are playing a significant role in disparities reduction activities. What is it that these organizations do? Why is their joining in the effort important?

6. What is evidence-based medicine and health care? What do data have to do with it? How does comparative effectiveness research figure into evidence-based care?

7. Have members of the class examine the how-to guides developed by the various organizations. How are they different? Similar? Which one is the best?

REFERENCES

Academic Medicine, 78(6). (2003). Cultural competence theme issue.

Agency for Health Care Research and Quality. (2005). *National health care disparities report, 2005.* Retrieved from http://archive.ahrq.gov/qual/nhdr05/nhdr05.htm

Agency for Health Care Research and Quality. (2006). *National health care disparities report.* Retrieved from http://archive.ahrq.gov/qual/nhdr06/nhdr06.htm

Agency for Healthcare Research and Quality. (2010a). *National healthcare quality report.* Retrieved from http://fodh.phhp.ufl.edu/files/2011/05/AHRQ-disparities-2010.pdf

Agency for Healthcare Research and Quality. (2010b). *What is the PCMH? AHRQ's definition of the medical home.* Retrieved from http://pcmh.ahrq.gov/portal/server.pt/community/pcmh__home/1483/what_is_pcmh

Agency for Healthcare Research and Quality. (2011). *Healthcare quality and disparities in women: Selected findings from the 2010 national quality and disparities reports.* Retrieved from http://www.ahrq.gov/qual/nhqrwomen/nhqrwomen.htm

American College of Physicians. (2010). *Racial and ethnic disparities in health care: Updated 2010.* Philadelphia: American College of Physicians.

America's Health Insurance Plans. (2005). *Tools to address disparities in healthcare: Data as building blocks for change. A data collection toolkit for health insurance plans/healthcare organizations.* Washington, DC: Author.

Anderson, N. B., Bulatao, R. A., & Cohen, B. (Eds.). (2004). *Critical perspectives on racial and ethnic differences in late life.* Washington, DC: The National Academies Press. Retrieved from http://www.nap.edu/openbook.php?record_id=11086&page=R1.

Andrulis, D. P., Siddiqui, N. J., Purtle, J. P., & Duchon, L. (2010). *Patient Protection and Affordable Care Act of 2010: Advancing health equity for racially and ethnically diverse populations.* Washington, DC: Joint Center for Political and Economic Studies.

Annals of Internal Medicine, 124(6). (1998). Cultural competence theme issue.

Aries, E. (2010). United States life tables by Hispanic Origin. *Vital Health Statistics, 2*(152). Retrieved from http://www.cdc.gov/nchs/data/series/sr_02/sr02_152.pdf

Au, M., Taylor, E. F., & Gold, M. (2009). *Improving access to language services in health care: A look at national and state efforts.* Washington DC: Mathematica Policy Research. Retrieved from http://www.ahrq.gov/populations/languageservicesbr.pdf

Bahrami, H., Kronmal, R., Bluemke, D., Olson, J., Shea, S., Liu, K., Burke, G., & Lima, J. (2008). Differences in the incidence of congestive heart failure by ethnicity. *Archives of Internal Medicine, 168*(19), 2138–2146.

Baker, D. W., Cameron, K. A., Feinglass, J., Georgas, P., Foster, S., Pierce, D., Thompson, J., & Hasnain-Wynia, R. (2005). Patients' attitudes toward health care providers collecting information about their race and ethnicity. *Journal of General Internal Medicine, 20*(10), 895–900.

Baker, D. W., Cameron, K. A., Feinglass, J., Georgas, P., Foster, S., Pierce, D., Thompson, J., & Hasnain-Wynia, R. (2006). A system for rapidly and accurately collecting patients' race and ethnicity. *American Journal of Public Health, 96*(3), 532–537.

Beach, M. C., Saha, S., & Cooper, L. A. (2006). *The role and relationship of cultural competence and patient centeredness.* The Commonwealth Fund. Retrieved from http://www.commonwealthfund.org/usr_doc/Beach_rolerelationshipcultcomppatient-cent_960.pdf

Begley, S. (2011). The best medicine: Cutting healthcare costs with comparative effectiveness research. *Scientific American, 305*(7), 50–55.

Bonito, A. J., & Eicheldinger, S. (2005). *Health disparities: Measuring health care use and access for racial/ethnic populations.* Washington, DC: Center for Medicare and Medicaid Services.

Brach, C., Paez, K., & Frazer, I. (2006). *Cultural competence California style.* Working Paper 06. Rockville, MD: Agency for Healthcare Research and Quality.

Burke, T., Stewart, A., & Harty, M. E. (2008). The legal context for employer health care quality improvement initiatives that collect and report information by member race and ethnicity. *Bureau of National Affairs and Health Quality Report, 16*(25).

California Pan Ethnic Health Network. (2000). *Health charts, California 2000.* Retrieved from http://www.cpehn.org/healthcharts.php.

Cameron, K. A., Feinglass, J., Georgas, P., Foster, S., Pierce, D., Thompson, J. A., & Hasnain-Wynia, R. (2005). Who, when, and how: The current state of race, ethnicity, and primary language data collection in hospitals. *Journal of General Internal Medicine, 20*(10), 895–900.

Carter-Pokras, O., & Baquet, C. (2002). What is a health disparity? *Public Health Reports, 117*(5), 426–434.

Case, P., Austin, S. B., Hunter, D. J., Manson, J. E., Malspeis, S., Willet, W. C., & Spiegelmen, D. (2004). Sexual orientation, health risk factors, and physical functioning in the Nurses' Health Study II. *Journal of Women's Health, 23*(9), 1033–1047.

Centers for Disease Control and Prevention. (2005). *Summary health statistics for US adults. National health interview survey, 2003.* Retrieved from http://www.cdc.gov/nchs/data/series/sr_10/sr10_225.pdf

Centers for Disease Control and Prevention. (2010a). *Healthy People 2010.* Retrieved from http://www.cdc.gov/nchs/data/hpdata2010/hp2010_final_review.pdf

Centers for Disease Control and Prevention. (2010b). *HIV incidence, statistics and surveillance.* Retrieved from http://www.cdc.gov/hiv/topics/surveillance/incidence.htm

Centers for Disease Control and Prevention. (2011). *The early release program.* Retrieved from www.cdc.gov/nchs/nhis.htm

Committee on Lesbian, Gay, Bisexual and Transgender Health Issues and Research Gaps and Opportunities. (2011). *The health of lesbian, gay, bisexual, and transgender people: Building a foundation for better understanding.* Institute of Medicine. Retrieved from http://www.iom.edu/Reports/2011/The-Health-of-Lesbian-Gay-Bisexual-and-Transgender-People.aspx

Committee on Public Health Strategies to Improve Health. (2011). *For the public's health: The role of measurement in action and accountability.* Washington, DC: National Academies Press.

The Commonwealth Fund. (2006). *The Commonwealth Fund health quality survey.* Retrieved from http://www.commonwealthfund.org/Surveys/2006/The-Commonwealth-Fund-2006—Health-Care-Quality-Survey.aspx

The Commonwealth Fund. (2007). *The Commonwealth biennial insurance survey, 2007.* Retrieved from http://www.commonwealthfund.org/Grants/2006/Dec/The-Commonwealth-Fund-2007-Biennial-Health-Insurance-Survey.aspx

The Commonwealth Fund. (2010). *States in action archive. State and federal efforts to enhance access to basic health care.* Retrieved from http://www.commonwealthfund.org/Newsletters/States-in-Action/2010/Mar/March-April-2010/Feature/Feature.aspx

Conron, K., Mimiaga, M. J., & Landers, S. J. (2010). A population-based study of sexual orientation, identity, and gender differences in adult health. *American Journal of Public Health, 100*(10), 1953–1960.

Cusack, C. M., Knudson, A. D., Kronstadt, J. L., Singer, R. F., & Brown, A. L. (2010). *Practice-based population health information technology to support transaction to proactive primary care.* AHRQ Publication No. 10–0092-EF. Rockville, MD: Agency for Healthcare Research and Quality.

DeNavas-Walt, C., Proctor, B. D., & Smith, I. (2010). *Income, poverty and health insurance coverage in the United States: 2009.* US Census Bureau Current Population reports, PG60–238. Washington, DC: US Government Printing Office.

Department of Health and Human Services. (2001). *Mental health: Culture, race and ethnicity. A supplement to mental health: Report of the surgeon general.* Retrieved from http://www.olc .edu/ ~ jolson/socialwork/OnlineLibrary/Surgeon%20General%20Report%20on%20Mental %20Health%20%20(2001)%20%20Page%2077.pdf

Department of Health and Human Services. (2011a). *Action plan to reduce racial and ethnic disparities: A nation free of disparities.* Office of Minority Health Disparity Reduction Efforts. Retrieved from http://minorityhealth.hhs.gov/npa/files/Plans/HHS/HHS_Plan_ complete.pdf

Department of Health and Human Services. (2011b). *Affordable Care Act to improve data collection, reduce health disparities.* Retrieved from www.hhs.gov/news/press/2011pres/06/ 20110629a.html

Department of Health and Human Services. (2011c). *National stakeholder strategy for achieving health equity.* National Partnership for Action. Retrieved from http://minorityhealth.hhs. gov/npa/templates/content.aspx?lvl=1&lvlid=33&ID=286

Disparities Solutions. (2010). *Improving quality and achieving equity: A guide for hospital leaders.* Massachusetts General Hospital. Institute for Health Policy. Retrieved from http://www2 .massgeneral.org/disparitiessolutions/guide.html

Ford, E. S., Giles, W. H., & Dietz, W. H. (2002). Prevalence of the metabolic syndrome among U.S. adults: Findings from the third national health and nutrition examination survey. *Journal of the American Medical Association, 287*(3), 356–359.

Gibbs, B. K., Nsiah-Jefferson, L., McHugh, M. D., Trivedi, A. N., & Praothrow-Stith, D. (2006). Reducing racial and ethnic health disparities: Exploring and outcome-oriented agenda for research and policy. *Journal of Health Politics, Policy and Law, 31*(1), 185–218.

Hasnain-Wynia, R., Hague, H., Hedges-Greuing, C., Prince, V., & Reiter, J. (2007). *Collecting race, ethnicity, and language data: A how-to guide.* Health Research and Educational Trust. Retrieved from http://www.hretdisparities.org/.

He, W., & Muenchrath, M. N. (2011). *American community survey reports, ACS-17, 90+ in the United States: 2006–2008.* US Census Bureau. Washington, DC: US Government Printing Office.

He, W., Sengupta, M., Velkoff, V. A., & DeBarros, K. A. (2005). *Current population reports, P23–209,65+ in the United States: 2005.* US Census Bureau. Washington, DC: US Government Printing Office.

HealthCare.gov. (2011). *Improving data collection for the LGBT community.* Retrieved from http://www.healthcare.gov/news/factsheets/2011/06/lgbt06292011a.html

Health insurance plans address disparities in care: Highlights of a 2004 AHIP/RWJF quantitative survey collection and use of race and ethnicity. America's Health Insurance Plans. Washington, DC. Retrieved from http://www.ahip.org/content/default.aspx?docid=5859

Higgins, P. C., Au, M., & Taylor, E. F. (2009). *Reducing ethnic disparities in partnerships between employers and health plans.* Princeton, NJ: Mathmatica Policy Research.

Institute of Medicine. (2009). *Race, ethnicity, and language data: Standardization for health care.* Retrieved from http://www.iom.edu/Reports/2009/RaceEthnicityData.aspx

Institute of Medicine. (2010a). *Future directions for the national health care quality report.* Retrieved from http://www.nap.edu/catalog.php?record_id=12846

Institute of Medicine. (2010b). *The healthcare imperative: Lowering costs and improving outcomes.* Retrieved from http://iom.edu/Reports/2011/The-Healthcare-Imperative-Lowering-Costs-and-Improving-Outcomes.aspx

The Joint Commission. (2009). *The Joint Commission 2009 requirements that support effective communication, cultural competence, and patient-centered care.* Retrieved from http://www.jointcommission.org/assets/1/6/2009_CLASRelatedStandardsHAP.pdf

The Joint Commission. (2010). *Advancing effective communication, cultural competence, and patient-and family-centered care: A road map for hospitals.* Retrieved from http://www.jointcommission.org/assets/1/6/aroadmapforhospitalsfinalversion727.pdf

Jones, N. A., & Symens-Smith, A. (2001). *The two or more races population: 2001.* Retrieved from http://www.census.gov/prod/2001pubs/c2kbr01–6.pdf

Journal of Nursing Education, 42(6). (2003). Cultural competence theme issue.

Kaiser Family Foundation Commission on Medicaid and the Uninsured. (2010). *The uninsured: Primer: Supplemental charts.* Retrieved from http://www.kff.org/uninsured/7451.cfm

Kelmer, S. B. (2011). *Letter to Secretary Kathleen Sebelius re: Notice of availability of proposed data collection standards for race, ethnicity, primary language, sex, and disability required by section 4302 of the Affordable Care Act.* Letter submitted during comments period prior to enactment of the proposed legislation.

LaViest, T. A., Gaskin, D. J., & Richard, P. (2009). *The economic burden of health inequalities in the United States.* Washington, DC: The Joint Center for Political and Economic Studies. Retrieved from http://www.jointcenter.org/hpi/sites/all/files/Burden_of_Health_FINAL_0.pdf

Lin, J. (2011, March 4). Isolation, chronic disease more common among older gays, lesbians. *California Watch.* Retrieved from http://californiawatch.org/dailyreport/isolation-chronic-disease-more-common-among-older-gays-lesbians-9524

Lurie, N., & Fremont, A. (2006). Looking forward: Crosscutting issues in race/ethnicity data collection. *Health Services Research, 41*(4 pt. 1), 1519–1533.

Lurie, N., Fremont, K. A., Somers, S. A., Coltin, K., Gelzer, A., Johnson, R., Rawlins, W., Ting, G., Wong, W., & Zimmerman, D. (2008). The national health plan collaborative to reduce disparities and improve quality. *The Joint Commission Journal on Quality and Patient Safety, 34*(5), 256–265.

Manley, J. J., & Mayeux, R. (2004). Ethnic differences in dementia and Alzheimer's disease. In N. B. Anderson, R. A. Bulatao, & B. Cohen (Eds.), *Critical perspectives on racial and ethnic differences in health in late life*. Washington, DC: The National Academies Press.

Massachusetts General Hospital Institute for Health Policy. (2006). *Improving quality and achieving equity: A guide for hospital leaders*. Retrieved from http://www.rwjf.org/files/research/3695.pdf

Mathews, T. J., & MacDorman, M. F. (2006). Infant mortality statistics from the 2003 period linked birth/infant death data set. *National Vital Statistics Reports, 54*(16) 1–29. Retrieved from http://www.cdc.gov/nchs/data/nvsr/nvsr54/nvsr54_16.pdf

Mead, H., Cartwright-Smith, L., Jones, K., Ramos, C., Woods, K., & Siegel, B. 2008. *Racial and ethnic disparities in U.S. health care: A chartbook*. Retrieved from http://www.common wealthfund.org/Publications/Chartbooks/2008/Mar/Racial-and-Ethnic-Disparities-in-U-S—Health-Care—A-Chartbook.aspx

Mezzich, J. E., Kleinman, A., Fabrega, H., & Parron, D. L. (1996). *Culture and psychiatric diagnosis. A SSM=IV perspective*. Washington, DC: The American Psychiatric Press.

Minority Health and Health Disparities Research and Education Act of 2000. (2000). Retrieved from http://www.govtrack.us/congress/bills/106/s1880

National Business Group on Health. (2009). *Eliminating racial and ethnic health disparities: A business case update for employers*. Retrieved from http://minorityhealth.hhs.gov/Assets/pdf/checked/1/Eliminating_Racial_Ethnic_Health_Disparities_A_Business_Case_Update_for_Employers.pdf

National Business Group on Health. (2011). *National business group on health honors six employers with inaugural awards for reducing health care disparities*. Retrieved from http://www.busi nessgrouphealth.org/pressrelease.cfm?ID=174

National Center for Health Statistics. (1985). Plan and orientation of the Hispanic health and nutrition survey, 1984–1985. *Vital Health Statistics, Series 1*(19). DHHS Publication No. (PHS) 85–1321. Washington, DC: US Government Printing Office.

National Committee on Quality Assurance. (2006). *Innovative practices in multicultural health care*. Retrieved from http://www.ncqa.org/Portals/0/HEDISQM/CLAS/CLAS_Innovative Prac06.pdf

National Committee on Quality Assurance. (2007). *Innovative practices in multicultural health care*. Retrieved from http://www.ncqa.org/Portals/0/HEDISQM/CLAS/CLAS_Innovative Prac07.pdf

National Committee on Quality Assurance. (2008). *Innovative practices in multicultural health care.* Retrieved from http://www.ncqa.org/Portals/0/HEDISQM/CLAS/CLASInnovative Prac_08.pdf

National Committee on Quality Assurance. (2009). *Innovative practices in multicultural health care.* Retrieved from http://www.ncqa.org/Portals/0/HEDISQM/CLAS/CLAS_InnovPrac_09.pdf

National Committee on Quality Assurance. (2010). *Implementing multicultural health standards: Ideas and examples.* Retrieved from http://www.ncqa.org/Portals/0/Publications/ Implementing%20MHC%20Standards%20Ideas%20and%20Examples%2004%2029% 2010.pdf

National Committee on Quality Assurance. (2011). *National scan of CLAS and disparities reduction activities.* Retrieved from www.ncqa.org/tabid/451/Default.aspx

National Diabetes Information Clearinghouse. (2011). Statistics on race. Retrieved from http:// diabetes.niddk.nih.gov/dm/pubs/statistics/#Racial

National Institute on Aging. (2011). *Alzheimer's disease progress report: A deeper understanding.* NIH Publication No. 11–7829. Washington, DC: US Department of Health and Human Services.

National Institutes of Health. (2000). *National Institutes of Health strategic research plan & budget to reduce and ultimately eliminate health disparities, Vol. I, fiscal years 2000–2006.* Retrieved from www.nimhd.nih.gov/our_programs/strategic/pubs/volumei_03103edra.pdf

National Institutes of Health. (2010). NIH announces Institute on Minority Health and Health Disparities. *NIH News.* Retrieved from www.nih.gov/news/health/sep2010/nimhd-27.htm

National Quality Forum. (2008a). Closing the disparities gap in healthcare quality with performance measurement and public reporting. *Issue Brief, 10,* 1–6.

National Quality Forum. (2008b). *National voluntary consensus standards for ambulatory care— Measuring disparities.* Retrieved from http://www.qualityforum.org/Publications/2008/03/ National_Voluntary_Consensus_Standards_for_Ambulatory_Care%E2%80%94Measuring_ Healthcare_Disparities.aspx

National Quality Forum. (2009a). *A comprehensive framework and preferred practices for measuring and reporting cultural competency: A consensus report.* Retrieved from http://www.quality forum.org/Publications/2009/04/A_Comprehensive_Framework_and_Preferred_Practices_ for_Measuring_and_Reporting_Cultural_Competency.aspx

National Quality Forum. (2009b). Cultural competency: An organizational strategy for high-performing delivery systems. *Issue Brief, 13,* 1–6.

Office of Minority Health. (2000). *National standards on cultural and linguistically appropriate services.* Retrieved from http://minorityhealth.hhs.gov/assets/pdf/checked/finalreport.pdf

Office of Minority Health. (2011a). *Assessment of state laws, regulation and practices affecting the collection and reporting of racial and ethnic data by health insurers and managed care plans. Improving data collection for the LGBT.* Retrieved from http://www.healthlaw.org/images/ stories/issues/nhelp.lep.state.law.chart.final.0319.pdf

Office of Minority Health. (2011b). *Data collection standards for race, ethnicity, primary language, sex, and disability status.* Retrieved from http://minorityhealth.hhs.gov/templates/content. aspx?ID=9227&lvl=2&lvlID=208

Owens, G. M. (2008). Gender differences in health care expenditures, resource utilization, and quality of care. *Journal of Managed Care Pharmacy, 14*(3, sup. S), S2–S6. Retrieved from http://www.amcp.org/data/jmcp/JMCPSupp_April08_S2-S6.pdf

Regenstein, M., & Sickler, D. (2006). *Race, ethnicity, and language of patients: Hospital practices regarding collection of information to address disparities in health care.* Washington, DC: The National Public Health and Hospital Institute.

Risch, N., Burchard, E., Ziv, E., & Hua, T. (2003). Categorization of humans in biomedical research: Genes, race and disease. *Genome Biology, 3*(7). Retrieved from http://genome-biology.com/2002/3/7/comment/2007/

Robert Wood Johnson Foundation. (nd). *Finding answers: Disparities research for change.* Retrieved from www.solvingdisparities.org

Rosenbaum, S., Burke, T., Nath, S., Santos, J., & Thomas, D. (2006) *Policy brief: The legality of collecting and disclosing patient race and ethnicity data.* The George Washington University School of Public Health Services Department of Health Policy. Retrieved from www.rwjf .org/files/publications/other/RaceEthnicDisparitiesData06222006.pdf

Rustgi, K S., Doty, M. M., & Collins, S. R. (2009). *Women at risk: Why many women are foregoing needed health care.* The Commonwealth Fund. Retrieved from http://the commonwealthfund.com/ ~ /media/Files/Publications/Issue%20Brief/2009/May/Women% 20at%20Risk/PDF_1262_Rustgi_women_at_risk_issue_brief_Final.pdf

Siegal, B., Regenstein, M., & Jones, K. (2007). *Enhancing public hospitals reporting of data on racial disparities in care.* Washington, DC: Robert Wood Johnson Foundation.

Singleton, J. A., Santibanez, T. A., & Wortley, P. M. (2005). Influenza and pneumococcal vaccination of adults aged $\geq$ 65: Racial/ethnic differences. *American Journal of Preventive Medicine, 29*(5), 412–420.

Smedley, B. D., Stith, A. Y., & Nelson, A. R. (Eds.). (2003). *Unequal treatment: Confronting racial and ethnic disparities in healthcare.* Washington, DC: National Academies Press.

Society for Women's Health Research. (2010). *Women and men: 10 differences that make a difference.* Retrieved from http://www.womenshealthresearch.org/site/PageServer?pagename= hs_sbb_10diff&printer_friendly=1

Thomson, G. E., Mitchell, R., & Williams, M. B. (2006). *Examining the health disparities research plan of the National Institutes of Health: Unfinished business.* Washington, DC: National Academies Press.

Trahan, L. C., & Williamson, P. (2009). *Elimination racial and ethnic disparities: A business case update for employers.* National Business Group on Health. Retrieved from http://minority health.hhs.gov/Assets/pdf/checked/1/Eliminating_Racial_Ethnic_Health_Disparities_A_ Business_Case_Update_for_Employers.pdf

Ulmer, C., McFadden, B., & Nereng, D. P. (2009). *Race, ethnicity and language data: Standardization for health care quality improvement.* Washington, DC: National Academies Press. Retrieved from www.nap.edu/catalog/12696.html

US Census Bureau. (2011). *Statistical abstracts of the United States, 2011.* Retrieved from http://www.census.gov/prod/2011pubs/11statab/pop.pdf

Waidmann, T. (2009). *Estimating the cost of racial and ethnic health disparities.* Washington, DC: The Urban Institute. Retrieved from www.urban.org/uploadedpdf/411962_health_disparities.pdf

Weinick, R. M., Flaherty, K., & Bristol, S. J. (2008). *Creating equity reports: A guide for hospitals.* Boston: The Disparities Solutions Center, Massachusetts General Hospital. Retrieved from http://www.rwjf.org/files/research/050608hospitalequityreport.pdf

Wizemann, T. M., & Pardue, M. L. (2001). *Exploring the biological contribution to human health: Does sex matter?* Washington, DC: National Academy Press. Retrieved from http://www.nap.edu/catalog.php?record_id=10028

Chapter 3

WORKFORCE
DEMOGRAPHICS

LEARNING OBJECTIVES

- To identify the three major labor force trends that are driving change in US workforce demographics

- To characterize the gender, racial, and ethnic demographics of the health care workforce

- To discuss the impact of social, human capital, and organizational factors on health care workforce demographics

- To identify recommended organizational-level actions that are consistent with the systems approach and suggested by the American College of Healthcare Executives (ACHE), American Hospital Association (AHA), Institute for Diversity in Health Management (IFD), and National Center for Healthcare Leadership (NCHL)

- To appreciate the challenges of managing a diverse workforce n Chapter One, we provided an overview of diversity in the United States, paid special attention to the impact of diversity on health and health care, and introduced an organizing framework (Figure 1.2) for the systems approach to diversity and cultural competence. In Chapter Two, we focused on the etiology of disparities in health and health care, emphasizing how a systems approach can help ameliorate disparities that are too often associated with key dimensions of diversity, including race, ethnicity, gender, sexual orientation, and socioeconomic status.

Chapter Three builds on this foundation by zeroing in on the health care workforce. Even a cursory look at Figure 1.2 reveals the key role that the workforce plays in improved health outcomes for diverse patients. After all, it is the health care workforce that is charged with the responsibility of delivering care to diverse patients. And a culturally competent health care workforce that mirrors the diversity of patients served is best positioned to successfully ameliorate the disparities in health and health care discussed in Chapter Two.

This chapter begins with a description of three general trends in US labor force demographics and an overview of the challenges these trends present to health care organizations in workforce recruitment and retention. Then, the racial, ethnic, and gender demographics of the health professions are outlined and the social, human capital, and organizational factors that contribute to these demographics are discussed. Finally, actions that health care organizations can take to recruit and retain a diverse and culturally competent workforce are overviewed and the special challenges that a diverse workforce presents are discussed.

TRENDS IN THE US LABOR FORCE

Toossi (2009) identified three trends in the US labor force that will dominate through 2018:

- Slower growth
- Increasing numbers of older workers
- Continuing growth in racial and ethnic diversity

Due to slower growth of the labor force, health care organizations will face stiffer competition from other industries and will, therefore, need to pay more attention to improving working conditions and the quality of work life or risk losing scarce labor to other industries that workers may view as more accommodating to their needs and less stressful. The mismatch between the increasingly higher level of educational preparedness and skills required for available jobs and workforce preparedness exacerbates this challenge.

Additionally, labor force representation of older workers will continue to grow even as the participation rate of the overall labor force is projected to decline (Toossi, 2009). To recruit and retain older workers, health care organizations will need to ensure that their culture, climate, and human resource policies and procedures result in an environment in which older workers can thrive and work productively with their younger colleagues. A registered nurse, for example, with a national average age of forty-seven, is estimated to lift a total of 1.8 tons during a single shift! Increasingly, hospitals are opting to provide assistive devices for lifting such as double-layered sheets to lessen friction when patients are repositioned in bed or moved to a stretcher and to invest in equipment to assist in lifting and transferring patients (Burling, 2007). Changes such as these will help enable older nurses to provide bedside care longer as well as reduce the rate of preventable injuries among younger nurses, making staying in the field more appealing.

Furthermore, to build a satisfied, loyal, and engaged workforce, health care organizations must understand and respond effectively to generational differences in work style, preference, and values. Four generations are now working together in today's health care organizations:

- Veterans (1922 to 1943)

- Baby boomers (1944 to 1960)

- Gen X (1961 to 1980)

- Gen Y or the millennials (1981 to 2000)

Members of the veterans generation, fifty-two million strong, are now age sixty-eight and higher and are remaining in the workforce longer due in part to the Great Recession. Similarly, baby boomers, the largest of the four generational cohorts, boast 73.2 million individuals who are now in their fifties and sixties. Gen X members, fewer in number at 70.1 million, are in their thirties and forties, and the newest generation entering the workforce, Gen Y, is 69.7 million members and in their twenties and younger (Zemke, Raines, & Filipczak, 2000).

Tamara Erickson, author of three recently published books on generational differences and the workplace (2008a, 2008b, 2010), explains that each generational cohort approaches work differently, as follows (2008a):

1. Veterans: "I want to join the world and benefit accordingly."

2. Boomers: "I want to help change the world but I also must compete to win."

3. Gen X: "I can't depend on institutions—I must keep my options open."

4. Gen Y: "I must live life now—and work toward long-term shared goals." (p. 37)

Health care organizations that are responsive to these generational differences will be more effective at recruitment, retention, leadership succession planning, and, ultimately, patient care. Strategies for responding to generational diversity are discussed later in this chapter.

The third and final major workforce demographic trend noted by Toossi (2009) is the growing racial and ethnic diversity of the workforce, which was first broadly publicized in the landmark 1987 Hudson Institute report entitled *Workforce 2000: Work and Workers for the 21st Century* (Johnston & Packer, 1987) and propelled the managing diversity movement in corporate America. This trend will continue not only because population diversity is increasing but also because of the different balance in each racial and ethnic group between those who are entering and those who are leaving the workforce.

As Table 3.1 reveals, between 1998 and 2008 almost five times as many Hispanics entered the workforce as left, and this trend is projected to continue through 2018. For the black workforce, the balance between entrants and leavers is projected to be roughly equivalent. Non-Hispanic whites will have only 72 percent as many entrants as leavers and the projected proportion of Asian entrants is over two and one-half times that of leavers.

These trends, together with differences in birthrates and immigration rates by racial and ethnic group, underlie the workforce composition developments outlined in Table 3.2. Asian immigrants, for example, account for 23 percent and Hispanics for 52 percent of recent net migration to the United States (Franklin, 2007). By 2018 non-Hispanic whites are expected to constitute less than 65 percent of the workforce, compared to about 80 percent in 1986. The relative representation of men and women in the workforce is projected to change very little (Toossi, 2009).

TABLE 3.1   Comparisons of Labor Force Entrants and Leavers by Race and Ethnicity, 1998–2008 and 2008–2018, Projected

Group	1998–2008 (actual percent)		2008–2018 (projected percent)	
	Entrants	Leavers	Entrants	Leavers
White non-Hispanic	54.4	83.2	55.4	76.9
Hispanic	24.3	5.3	24.5	7.8
Black	12.1	13.3	14.4	11.6
Asian	5.3	5.1	7.5	2.8

Note: Numbers may add up to more or less than 100 percent because individuals may report membership in more than one group and data on American Indian and Alaska Native and Native Hawaiian and other Pacific Islanders are not displayed in this exhibit.

Source: Toossi, M. (2009). Labor force projections to 2018: Older workers staying more active. *Monthly Labor Review, 132*(11), 30–51.

TABLE 3.2   Composition of US Labor Force by Gender, Race, and Ethnicity, 1998, 2008, 2018, Projected, by Percent

	1998	2008	2018
Men	53.7	53.5	53.1
Women	46.3	46.5	46.9
White non-Hispanic	73.9	68.2	64.0
Hispanic	10.4	14.3	17.6
Black	11.6	11.5	12.1
Asian	4.6	4.7	5.6

Note: Numbers may add up to more or less than 100 percent because individuals may report membership in more than one group and data on American Indian and Alaska Native and Native Hawaiian and other Pacific Islanders are not displayed in this exhibit.

Source: Toossi, M. (2009). Labor force projections to 2018: Older workers staying more active. *Monthly Labor Review, 132*(11), 30–51.

Responding to these three trends is a business imperative for health care organizations that strive to improve health outcomes for diverse communities. As Figure 1.2 indicates, strategic diversity management results in the inclusion of a diverse workforce, which in turn leads to enhanced patient satisfaction and culturally and linguistically appropriate care delivery, thus improving patient outcomes.

For those seeking career opportunities in health care fields, the outlook is positive. Employers in health services will see continuing need to hire across a broad range of clinical specialties and clinical support roles in particular. Health care organizations that operate with a commitment to the systems approach to diversity and cultural competence will be well positioned to compete with other sectors of the US economy to recruit and retain a well-qualified, culturally competent, and diverse workforce.

The Bureau of Labor Statistics' (BLS) *Career Guide to Industries, 2010–2011 Edition* reports that ten of the twenty fastest-growing occupations are in health care, estimating that health care will add 3.2 million new wage and salary jobs between 2008 and 2018, which is more than any other industry. The health care sector is composed of more than 595,000 organizations that vary in size, staffing, and structure. More than three of every four are offices of physicians, dentists, or other health practitioners. And, even though hospitals represent only about 1 percent of health care organizations, they employ 35 percent of the health care workforce. The health care sector's 22 percent projected employment growth rate is twice the BLS' estimate across all industries. Growth in hospital employment is projected to be the lowest in the health care sector at 10 percent, with home health care services employment the highest at 46 percent.

Registered nursing, the largest of the health professions at nearly three million, is projected to grow in number by over 23 percent by 2018. Projected growth in employment for physicians and surgeons is similar at 26 percent, with a projected growth rate of 14 percent for pharmacists. For more information about health care industry careers and employment projections visit www.bls.gov/ooh and click on *healthcare.*

Not all occupations within health services are in clinical or clinical support roles. This growing industry also employs medical and health services managers, and business operations and financial specialists, among others. Management, business, and financial operations occupations account for about 4 percent of employment in the health care sector with an additional 18 percent in office and administrative support personnel. Thus, a considerable amount of the projected 2008 to 2018 growth in management, business, and financial occupations is attributable to the health care industry as well, as the BLS's *Occupational Outlook Handbook, 2010–2011 Edition* confirms (www.bls.gov/ooh). Additionally, the BLS projects a 20 percent increase in health information technology (IT) positions between 2008 and 2018, due in large part to broader-based implementation of the electronic medical record and related initiatives to improve quality and efficiency through replacing paper-based systems with integrated IT solutions.

DIVERSITY AND THE HEALTH PROFESSIONS

Workforce diversity is important because it plays a role in the delivery of culturally and linguistically appropriate care, is a key indicator of an organization's commitment to the systems approach to diversity management, and allows for **concordance**, that is, a match between the group identities of a patient and his or her caregiver, which research associates with patient preference and satisfaction (see, for example, Laveist & Nuru-Jeter, 2002; Saha, Taggart, Komaronmy, & Bindman, 2000).

Table 3.3 presents the gender and racial ethnic demographics for a number of key health professional and support roles and displays each occupation's gender and racial and ethnic demographics and that of the employed workforce overall. The source of these data is the Current Population Study (CPS), a joint project of the US Census Bureau and the Bureau of Labor Statistics, and the primary source of labor force statistics for the population of the United States. The Census Bureau, using a statistical sample of occupied households, administers the CPS on

TABLE 3.3 Health Professions Gender, Racial, and Ethnic Demographics and Representation Relative to Workforce Representation, 2011

Profession	Women	Black	Asian	Hispanic
Overall US workforce representation	46.9	10.8	4.9	14.5
Medical and health services managers*	71.4+	11.2=	5.0=	8.4−
Physicians and surgeons	33.8−	5.3−	16.1+	6.6−
Physician assistants	69.8+	9.6−	2.7−	10.1−
Registered nurses	91.1+	10.4−	7.3+	5.1−
Licensed practical and licensed vocational nurses	90.5+	23.7+	3.9−	8.3−
Nursing, psychiatric, and home health aides	87.7+	33.1+	4.3−	13.3−
Occupational therapists	92.0+	2.7−	7.6+	4.6−
Physical therapists	67.8+	5.2−	8.9+	5.0−
Physical therapist assistants and aides	60.8+	10.4−	3.5−	9.7−
Speech-language pathologists	95.6+	1.5−	1.5−	6.4−
Pharmacists	55.7+	7.1−	15.3+	4.4−
Dentists	22.2−	1.0−	11.0+	5.8−
Dental hygienists	97.5+	0.5−	5.5=	7.2−
Emergency medical technicians and paramedics	36.0−	4.5−	0.9−	6.4−

Note: Persons whose ethnicity is identified as Hispanic may be of any race. The source document does not report data for races other than black and Asian.

Percent representation relative to overall representation: + overrepresented, = proportionally represented, − underrepresented.

Source: Bureau of Labor Statistics (June 2012).

a monthly basis and combines the results to create an annual report. The basic CPS questionnaire records the race and ethnicity of each respondent. With respect to race, a respondent can be white, black, Asian, American Indian and Alaskan Native (AI/AN), native Hawaiian and other Pacific Islander (NHOPI), or combinations of two or more of the preceding. The CPS uses BLS-defined categories to collect information on the occupation of employed persons and reports these by gender, race, and Hispanic ethnicity. Because a respondent's ethnicity can be Hispanic or non-Hispanic, regardless of race, there is likely to be overlap between the racial and ethnic categories reported in Table 3.3. For example, a survey respondent might self-identify as black and Hispanic.

Table 3.3 reveals that women are overrepresented relative to workforce representation for all but three occupations listed: physicians and surgeons, dentists, and emergency medical technicians and paramedics. Hispanic representation is low in every listed occupation. Blacks are underrepresented in professional roles such as physicians and surgeons, pharmacists, and the allied health professions, including occupational and physical therapists and speech-language pathologists, and overrepresented in support staff roles such as "licensed practical and licensed vocational nurses" and "nursing, psychiatric, and home health aides." Asians, however, are overrepresented among physicians and surgeons and pharmacists but underrepresented among speech-language pathologists and "nursing, psychiatric, and home health aides," for example.

A deeper look at the physician workforce can highlight some of the challenges presented by the workforce demographics in Table 3.3. Although women are entering medical school in record numbers, pipeline problems will continue to challenge health care organizations striving for racial and ethnic concordance among physicians in particular. For example, data released by the American Association of Medical Colleges (AAMC) (2011) show that women represented 47 percent of first-year medical students in 2011, which is roughly equivalent to women's representation in the overall workforce. However, AAMC statistics (2011) document continuing underrepresentation of blacks and Hispanics and overrepresentation of Asians among 2011 first-year medical students, with Asians, Hispanics, and blacks represented at 22.6 percent, 8.5 percent, and 7.2 percent, respectively.

International medical school graduates (IMGs) in the physician workforce also help explain the racial and ethnic demographics presented in Table 3.3. In a 2010 report, the American Medical Association (AMA) estimates the percentage of IMGs in the United States to be 25 percent, with IMGs representing more than 127 nationalities. Just over 14 percent of IMGs are US citizens who attended medical school in another country. Almost half of the physicians of Asian ethnicity practicing in the United States in 2008 were IMGs. As the AMA notes, language and acculturation challenges are presented by these physician workforce demographics (AMA, 2010).

Increasingly, these acculturation challenges are being addressed through education and training that is focused on understanding the culture and norms of the United States and US health care. For example, Creighton University School of Medicine's internal medicine program in Omaha, Nebraska, developed a one-week orientation program for foreign-born IMGs. Topics covered ranged from how to work with nurses in a way that nurses perceive as respectful to speaking up during grand rounds, which are a routine part of a US medical residents' training during which physicians discuss patients' diagnosis and treatment, often at bedside. US cultural norms are openly shared and discussed, which helps IMGs understand and meet expectations. Myriad other cultural issues are addressed during orientation, including the physician-patient relationship, which differs significantly from the unquestioned authority many foreign-born IMGs experience in their country of origin (Croasdale, 2006).

As Table 3.4 attests, health care workers vary widely in earnings. In hospitals, for example, 28 percent of employees are registered nurses with median weekly earnings of $1,251 and 21 percent are in a support role, such as "nursing, psychiatric, and home health aides" with median weekly earnings of $434. Consider the challenges this represents in the context of multidisciplinary health care teams. When role diversity is strongly associated with gender and racial and ethnic diversity as well as income and other indicators of socioeconomic status such as education and household wealth, conflict can be exacerbated and teamwork made more challenging, thus impeding the delivery of culturally and linguistically appropriate care.

DRIVERS OF DISPARITIES IN THE HEALTH PROFESSIONS

Health care organizations that are committed to the systems approach to diversity and cultural competence focus on goals such as building representation of racial and ethnic minorities in the highly paid health professions and increasing representation of men in nursing. But challenges abound because a plethora of social, human

TABLE 3.4 Median Weekly Earnings by Gender for Selected Health Professions, 2010

	2010 Overall Median Weekly Earnings in Dollars	2010 Median Weekly Earnings, Men	2010 Median Weekly Earnings, Women
Medical and health services managers	1,251	1,510	1,163
Physicians and surgeons	1,975	2,278	1,618
Physician assistants	1,312	Not calculated	1,129
Registered nurses	1,055	1,201	1,039
Licensed practical and licensed vocational nurses	718	Not calculated	716
Nursing, psychiatric, and home health aides	434	488	427
Occupational therapists	1,059	Not calculated	1,094
Physical therapists	1,304	Not calculated	1,208
Physical therapist assistants and aides	622	Not calculated	Not calculated
Speech and language pathologists	1,207	Not calculated	1,184
Pharmacists	1,880	1,930	1,605
Emergency medical technicians and paramedics	732	825	597

Source: Bureau of Labor Statistics (January 2012).

capital, and organizational factors drive the patterns of representation by gender, race, and ethnicity in the health professions, discussed in the previous section of this chapter. Some of these factors can be directly controlled or indirectly influenced by health care organizations, and others must necessarily be addressed by the broader society. Figure 3.1 is a graphic representation of the role that **social factors, human capital factors,** and **organizational factors** play in career disparities:

- Social factors include social attitudes, socioeconomic disparities, and the sociopolitical context.

- Human capital factors include education, experience, and technical and interpersonal competencies.

- Organizational factors include policies, procedures, plant and technology, and people.

FIGURE 3.1 Model of Factors Affecting Career Advancement of Women and People of Color

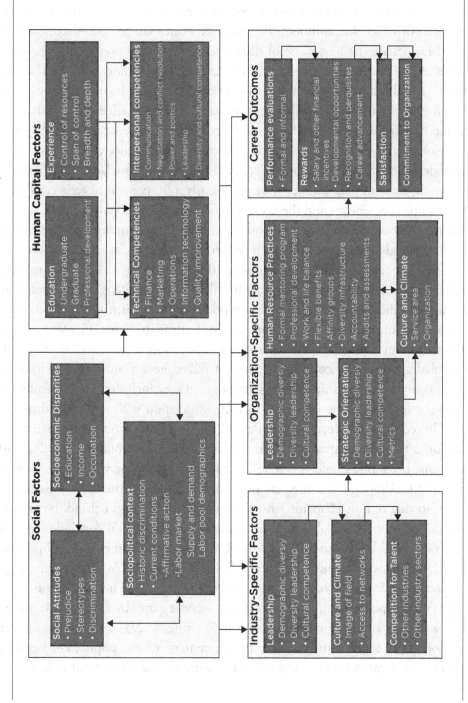

Source: Dreachslin and Foster Curtis (2004). Reprinted and adapted with permission.

Figure 3.1 is the organizing framework from a comprehensive study of factors that affect career advancement for women and people of color in health care management in which the authors (Dreachslin & Foster Curtis, 2004) conclude that social factors are the root cause of disparities in representation and career accomplishment in the health professions. Furthermore, the authors contend that detrimental social factors are systemic or institutionalized in the broader society and also found evidence that organizational factors can counter the adverse effect that social factors have on human capital factors and can ultimately ameliorate career disparities.

Consider, for example, how social factors might influence career choice. Social attitudes, including bias or prejudice, can lead to the association of a particular career choice with race, ethnicity, or gender. Over 90 percent of registered nurses, for example, are women and the association of nursing with gender in our society is among the factors that might discourage a man from entering the nursing profession. Social attitudes will be discussed in greater depth later in this book.

Another social factor, socioeconomic disparities, can make access to higher education and high-quality public education more challenging for individuals from lower-income families and affect workers of color disproportionately due to the association between wealth and race and ethnicity. This, in turn, adversely affects human capital by limiting access to education, thus reducing the pool of qualified applicants of color for the highly skilled health professions. Household wealth, or the net worth of the household's assets including home equity and savings after subtracting debt, has a strong association with race and ethnicity in the United States. According to a Pew Hispanic Center study (Kochhar, Fry, & Taylor, 2011), the median net worth of a Hispanic household was $6,325, a non-Hispanic black household was $5,677, and a non-Hispanic white household was $113,149. Although the median net worth of Asian American households is closer to that of non-Hispanic white households, it still lags behind. Based on an analysis of publicly available data, Ong and Patraporn (2006) conclude that Asian American wealth is more unevenly distributed among Asian ethnic groups than is non-Hispanic white wealth, with households of Southeast Asian ethnicity lagging behind Asian Indian, Chinese, and Japanese households. The US Census Bureau (2011) also reports that household median income varies by racial ethnic group as follows: Asian and Pacific Islander, $65,637; white, $52,312; Hispanic, $37,913; and black, $34,912. Furthermore, the percentage of the population below the poverty level varies by race and ethnicity, with almost 25 percent of blacks and

Hispanics living below 125 percent of the poverty line compared to less than 12 percent of whites and Asian and Pacific Islanders.

The third social factor identified in Figure 3.1, sociopolitical context, also affects the demographics of the health professions. For example, the impact of historic discrimination and the continuing tendency toward racial, ethnic, and socioeconomic homogeneity in housing patterns, when combined with the association among race, ethnicity, wealth, and household income discussed previously, affects aspiration levels, awareness of career options, and access to high-quality affordable educational opportunities. The result: a **skills gap** that operates to the relative disadvantage of workers of color by reducing the store of human capital that these workers bring to the labor market.

The Pew Hispanic Center (Fry, 2007, pp. 6–7) reports that "a high proportion of Hispanic and black students attended a school that had not only relatively few white students but relatively few students of any racial or ethnic identity other than their own . . . Asian students were less likely than Hispanic or black students to be heavily concentrated in schools largely comprised [sic] of students of their own race and ethnicity." Furthermore, as the Education Trust (2006) reports, school districts serving high-poverty communities or communities with high concentrations of people of color are underfunded relative to communities with high concentrations of wealthier non-Hispanic white households. The Education Trust (2006) concludes, "Our low-income and minority students, in particular, get less of what matters most; these students get the fewest experienced and well-educated teachers, the least rigorous curriculum, and the lowest quality facilities" (p. 1). Funding gaps, The Education Trust explains (2006), "are compounding the disadvantages that low-income students face outside of school and undercutting public education's ability to act as an engine of social mobility" (p. 6).

Together, these social factors help explain the demographics of the health professions, as presented in Table 3.3. And a key connection is education, which is perhaps the most important human capital variable. Table 3.5 illustrates the significant differences in educational levels by race and ethnicity. Almost one-third of whites and over half of Asians have a bachelor's degree or higher, with Hispanics and blacks at about 14 percent and 20 percent, respectively. Hispanic educational attainment differs by ethnicity. For example, whereas 26.2 percent of those reporting Cuban ethnicity have a bachelor's degree or higher, the comparable

TABLE 3.5   Educational Attainment for People over Twenty-Five by Gender, Race, and Ethnicity, 2010, by Percent

	Not High School Graduate	High School Graduate	Some College	Associate's Degree	Bachelor's Degree	Advanced Degree	Bachelor's Degree or Higher
Men	13.4	31.9	16.5	8.0	19.4	10.9	30.3
Women	12.4	30.7	17.1	10.2	19.4	10.2	29.6
White	12.4	31.3	16.7	9.2	19.6	10.7	30.3
Hispanic	37.1	29.6	12.9	6.5	10.1	3.8	13.9
Black	15.8	35.2	19.8	9.4	13.3	6.5	19.8
Asian	NC[1]	NC[1]	NC[1]	NC[1]	NC[1]	NC[1]	52.4

Source: US Census Bureau Statistical Abstract of the United States (2012).
[1]Not calculated for Asian ethnicity.

statistic for those reporting Mexican ethnicity is 10.6 percent and for Puerto Rican ethnicity 17.5 percent (US Census Bureau, 2012).

Not surprisingly, higher education is associated with higher earnings in the health professions. The association between low educational attainment and Hispanic ethnicity or black race is, thus, a key social factor that must be addressed to improve low representation of these groups in the higher earning health professions.

The flow of students into a professional occupation is often called a **career pipeline**. The federal government and the associations representing the health care professions are aware of the narrowness of the pipeline for African American, Hispanic, and Native American students. Title VII and Title VIII of the Public Health Service Act have for several years provided grants, stipends, and scholarships to minority students seeking training or career advancement in the health professions. Title II funding supports the education and training of more than ten thousand minority graduates, residents, and faculty members each year. Additionally, a program designed to ready minority students who wish to enter training in a health care profession, the Health Careers Opportunity Program, provides students with an opportunity to develop the skills needed to successfully compete, enter, and graduate from health professions schools prior to entry into the regular course of instruction. The program collaborates with school districts and community-based organizations and offers counseling, work experience, and information on the sources of financial assistance. The Affordable Care Act of 2010 has reauthorized and expanded programs for health workforce diversity under Titles VII and VIII. In 2011 the Health Resources and Services Administration (HRSA) spent close to ten million dollars on diversity-related programs to increase the number of minority nurses, physicians, dentists, and pharmacists. Information about these programs can be found on HRSA's website at http://bhpr.hrsa.gov/grants/diversity/index.html. HRSA also maintains the National Center for Health Workforce Analysis, where updated information on diversity in the health care workforce can be obtained.

However, health care organizations do not have to wait for the larger society to address the social factors discussed in this section in order to recruit and retain a highly skilled and diverse workforce that more closely mirrors community demographics. As is the case with health disparities, organizational-level action that is strategically driven by leadership through the systems approach can move the organization toward a more representative workforce despite the challenges that social factors represent.

CHECKLIST OF RECOMMENDED ORGANIZATIONAL-LEVEL ACTIONS

What organizational-level actions are recommended to improve diversity in the health care workforce and counter the deleterious effects of the systemic social factors discussed previously? A checklist of actions, based on a review of research and best practices (Dreachslin & Foster Curtis, 2004), was developed collaboratively by the American College of Healthcare Executives (ACHE), American Hospital Association (AHA), Institute for Diversity in Health Management (IFD), and National Center for Healthcare Leadership (NCHL). The checklist can be used to assess a hospital or other health care organization's performance against best practices in four areas: community responsiveness, culturally proficient care, workforce diversity, and leadership team diversity.

Each question asks whether a specific best practice in strategic diversity management and cultural competence is followed in the organization. The results are used to identify strengths, target areas for action, and determine whether the organization employs the systems approach to diversity management and cultural competence. Organizations with a majority of "yes" answers concentrated in only one or two of the four major areas assessed have not yet linked their diversity and cultural competence initiatives through a systems approach, which is a hallmark of high-performing organizations.

DIVERSITY PRACTICES CHECKLIST

As Diverse as the Community You Serve

☐ Do you monitor at least every three years the demographics of your community to track changes in gender, racial, and ethnic diversity?

☐ Do you compare the results among diverse groups in your community and act on the information?

□ Do you actively use these data for strategic and outreach planning?

□ Has your community relations team identified community organizations, schools, churches, businesses, and publications that serve racial and ethnic minorities for outreach and educational purposes?

□ Do you have a strategy to partner with them to work on health issues important to them?

□ Has a team from your hospital met with community leaders to gauge their perceptions of the hospital and seek their advice on how you can better serve them in patient care and community outreach?

□ Are the individuals who represent your hospital in the community reflective of the diversity of the community and your organization?

□ When your hospital partners with other organizations for community health initiatives or sponsors community events, do you have a strategy in place to be certain you work with organizations that relate to the diversity of your community?

□ As a purchaser of goods and services in the community, does your hospital have a strategy to ensure that businesses in the minority community have an opportunity to serve you?

□ Are your public communications, community reports, advertisements, health education materials, websites, and so on accessible to and reflective of the diverse community you serve?

☐ Have you done focus groups and surveys within the past three years in your community to measure the public's perception of your hospital as sensitive to diversity and cultural issues?

Culturally Proficient Patient Care

☐ Do you regularly monitor the racial and ethnic diversity of the patients you serve?

☐ Do your organization's internal and external communications stress your commitment to culturally proficient care and give concrete examples of what you're doing?

☐ Do your patient satisfaction surveys take into account the diversity of your patients?

☐ Has your hospital developed a language resource, identifying qualified people inside and outside your organization who could help your staff communicate with patients and families from a wide variety of nationalities and ethnic backgrounds?

☐ Are your written communications with patients and families available in a variety of languages that reflect the ethnic and cultural fabric of your community?

☐ Based on the racial and ethnic diversity of the patients you serve, do you educate your staff at orientation and on a continuing basis on cultural issues important to your patients?

☐ Do you compare patient satisfaction ratings among diverse groups and act on the information?

☐ Are core services in your hospital such as signage, food service, chaplaincy services, patient information, and communications attuned to the diversity of the patients you care for?

☐ Have your patient representatives, social workers, discharge planners, financial counselors, and other key patient and family resources received special training in diversity issues?

☐ Does your hospital account for complementary and alternative treatments in planning care for your patients?

☐ Does your review of quality-assurance data take into account the diversity of your patients in order to detect and eliminate disparities?

Strengthening Your Workforce Diversity

☐ Do your recruitment efforts include strategies to reach out to the racial and ethnic minorities in your community?

☐ Have you made diversity awareness and sensitivity training available to your employees?

☐ Does the team that leads your workforce recruitment initiatives reflect the diversity you need in your organization?

☐ Is the diversity of your workforce taken into account in your performance evaluation system?

☐ Do your policies about time off for holidays and religious observances take into account the diversity of your workforce?

☐ Do you acknowledge and honor diversity in your employee communications, awards programs, and other internal celebrations?

☐ Have you done employee surveys or focus groups to measure their perceptions of your hospital's policies and practices on diversity and to surface potential problems?

☐ Do you compare the results among diverse groups in your workforce? Do you communicate and act on the information?

☐ Does your human resources department have a system in place to measure diversity progress and report it to you and your board?

☐ Do you have a mechanism in place to look at employee turnover rates for variances according to diverse groups?

☐ Do you ensure that changes in job design, workforce size, hours, and other changes do not affect diverse groups disproportionately?

Expanding the Diversity of Your Leadership Team

☐ Has your board of trustees discussed the issue of the diversity of the hospital's board? Its workforce? Its management team?

☐ Have sufficient funds been allocated to achieve your diversity goals?

☐ Is there a board-approved policy encouraging diversity across the organization?

☐ Is your policy reflected in your mission and values statement? Is it visible on documents seen by your employees and the public?

☐ Have you told your management team that you are personally committed to achieving and maintaining diversity across your organization?

☐ Does your strategic plan emphasize the importance of diversity at all levels of your workforce?

☐ Has your board set goals on organizational diversity, culturally proficient care, and eliminating disparities in care to diverse groups as part of your strategic plan?

☐ Is diversity awareness and cultural proficiency training mandatory for all senior leadership, management, and staff?

☐ Have you made diversity awareness part of your management and board retreat agendas?

☐ Is your management team's compensation linked to achieving your diversity goals?

☐ Does your organization have a mentoring program in place to help develop your best talent, regardless of gender, race, or ethnicity?

☐ Do you provide tuition reimbursement to encourage employees to further their education?

☐ Does your organization have a process in place to ensure diversity reflecting your community on your board and subsidiary and advisory boards?

☐ Do you have a succession or advancement plan for your management team linked to your overall diversity goals?

☐ Have you designated a high-ranking member of your staff to be responsible for coordinating and implementing your diversity strategy?

☐ Are search firms required to present a mix of candidates reflecting your community's diversity?

Source: American College of Healthcare Executives, American Hospital Association, Institute for Diversity in Health Management, and National Center for Healthcare Leadership. (2004). Reprinted with permission.

As the checklist communicates, isolated efforts to strengthen workforce diversity are not sufficient to recruit and retain a diverse and culturally competent workforce in a health care organization. Attention must also be paid to community responsiveness, culturally proficient care, and leadership team diversity because only the systems approach will ensure the commitment of the whole organization to a shared purpose: improved community health and well-being through the delivery of culturally and linguistically appropriate care to every patient.

WORKFORCE DIVERSITY CHALLENGES

Workforce diversity, although essential to culturally and linguistically appropriate care, is not a panacea and presents its own unique challenges to health care organizations—even to those who take the recommended strategic approach to managing diversity and cultural competence. Research discussed in detail in Chapter Ten reveals that a diverse workforce is more complex to manage than a homogeneous workforce. Chapter Eleven describes how high-performing health care and other organizations are successfully managing diversity to improve outcomes such as patient care and profitability. In this section, we will explore three common diversity dilemmas in the health care workforce: generational differences, languages other than English in the workplace, and responding to patient preferences. How health care organizations and their leaders address dilemmas like these will affect employee satisfaction, performance, and ultimately patient care.

Consider first the challenges of managing a generationally diverse workforce. Tamara Erickson (2008a, 2008b, 2010), a nationally renowned expert in generational diversity management, recommends a high degree of customization, essentially the workforce management equivalent of patient-centered care for the generationally diverse workforce. Others may counter that taking her approach will fuel perceptions of special treatment and exacerbate intergenerational conflict. Erickson's recommendations for customization are highlighted as follows. What do you think? Will Erickson's recommendations enhance the performance of a generationally diverse health care workforce and improve patient care or will they fuel conflict and resentment?

TAMARA ERICKSON'S PRESCRIPTION FOR RECRUITMENT AND RETENTION OF A GENERATIONALLY DIVERSE WORKFORCE (2008A, 2008B, 2010)

- *Retire retirement:* Eliminate mandatory retirement age policies and create opportunities for older employees to stay in the workforce through phased retirement, job sharing, moving from full-time to part-time employment, and implementing a bell-shaped career curve that allows individuals to decelerate their careers in their fifties and sixties rather than abruptly end them.

- *Design cyclic work:* Allow workers to blend work, education, leisure, and other interests throughout their careers as an alternative to the traditional approach: first education, then career, and finally retirement to pursue leisure or other interests.

- *Recruit at multiple entry points:* Actively recruit not only younger workers but also mid-career and older workers and ensure that your organization's policies and practices will enable workers from all four generations to achieve their potential.

- *Invest in development:* Ongoing attention to education and professional development is essential to high-performing organizations, especially as knowledge increases exponentially. Organizations that invest in development through tuition reimbursement, training, and educational-leave policies engage employees and improve performance.

- *Offer lateral career opportunities:* As baby boomers near retirement and a declining proportion of younger workers express an interest in assuming more responsibility at work, the opportunity to learn and contribute through taking on a new but parallel assignment rather than moving up in the organizational hierarchy can motivate across the generations. For example, a forty-something bedside nurse might move into a role in the organization's quality improvement initiative or a seasoned community relations manager might move into a parallel role managing the organization's diversity initiative.

- *Engage hearts and minds:* Move from a focus on employee satisfaction to employee engagement. Erickson (2008a) puts it this way: "Satisfaction is about sufficiency—enough pay, adequate benefits, and no major problems or unfair treatment to sour one's attitude toward the employer . . . Engagement is about passion and commitment—the willingness to expend one's discretionary effort to achieve success" (p. 88). Of course, what engages one employee won't necessarily engage another. So, organizations must have policies that are flexible enough to accommodate diversity and an organizational culture that capitalizes on each employee's preferences in service to a common purpose that is shared throughout the organization.

Next, consider this: a growing number of health care professionals speak languages other than English as their first language. Sometimes employees who share a language other than English want to speak to one another in that language in the workplace. And some organizations have responded with English-only rules. How would you have handled the dilemma that confronted Bon Secours Baltimore where three Filipino American nurses and a health unit coordinator were fired for speaking their first language, Tagalog, in the workplace, a violation of the health system's English-only policy? The fired health care workers filed suit with the EEOC (Equal Employment Opportunity Commission), the US agency that enforces workplace antidiscrimination laws. The EEOC ruled in favor of the workers, who said in their affidavits that they only spoke Tagalog to each other during breaks and not within earshot of patients. The August 16, 2011, ruling found that the workers were victims of "unequal terms and conditions of employment, a hostile work environment, disciplinary action and discharge because of their national origin in violation of Title VII (of the Civil Rights Act of 1964)" (Rueda, 2011, p. 1). Attorney Martin J. Burns (2011) offers the following advice to organizations: "When an English-only rule applies only at certain times, for example, when employees are engaged in certain activities or in the presence of customers, the EEOC interprets this employer action as permissible under Title VII, provided that the employer can show that the rule is justified by business necessity" (pp. 1–2).

Finally, consider the question, Is the customer always right? How would you have handled Abington Hospital's dilemma described in the following?

IS THE CUSTOMER ALWAYS RIGHT?

A Philadelphia-area hospital received some national attention it didn't want, including charges that it violated the Civil Rights Act of 1964 when it complied with the request of a patient's husband that only white hospital staff members care for his pregnant wife. Officials of Abington Memorial Hospital in Abington, Pa., have issued a public apology, apologized individually to the employees involved, formed a diversity task force to develop plans to avoid future incidents and are holding employee forums on revising the hospital's nondiscrimination policy.

Source: Robeznieks (2003).

What if the husband were Muslim and requested only female caregivers for his wife due to religious restrictions? Would you have accommodated that request?

How should leaders address diversity dilemmas such as the case examples discussed here? There are no easy answers. But, as Dreachslin (2007) explains,

> The most notable advice that research offers to healthcare executives is this: Manage diversity. If left unmanaged, demographic diversity will interfere with team functioning. Identify a common ground among diverse groups, because similarity can pull different team members together. Invest in professional development so that team members have the tools they need to navigate their differences. Other elements that can improve team and organizational decision making include group-process and conflict-management skills, self-awareness and understanding of cultural style differences, ability to validate alternative points of view, and efforts to surface and manage implicit bias. (p. 84)

And, most important, adopt the systems approach to ensure that diversity management is sustainable and inclusion is built into the health care organization's culture.

SUMMARY

The three trends in the labor force that are dominant between now and 2018 (Toossi, 2009) include slower growth overall coupled with a skills gap, increasing numbers of older workers, and continuing growth in racial and ethnic diversity.

Health care organizations that take a systems approach to strategic diversity management will be better positioned to compete with other industries to address these trends and recruit and retain an increasingly diverse workforce. Social and human capital factors, including socioeconomic disparities, which are associated with race and ethnicity as well as education, will continue to present challenges to health care executives as they strive to ameliorate underrepresentation of people of color in the highly paid health professions such as medical and health services managers, physicians and surgeons, and speech and language pathologists, recruit more men into nursing, and address myriad diversity dilemmas.

Health care organizations can assess and improve their responsiveness to workforce diversity using publicly available tools such as the diversity management checklist presented in this chapter. Health care managers, staff, and providers can improve their personal performance and develop their own self-awareness by understanding how their own group identities and biases can influence their behavior in the workplace, by learning more about communication style differences that are associated with race and ethnicity or gender, and by learning how to communicate and resolve conflict more effectively in the multicultural healthcare organization. These are explored in depth in Part Two, "The Development of Cultural Competence."

KEY TERMS

career pipeline

concordance

human capital factors

organizational factors

skills gap

social factors

workforce diversity

REVIEW QUESTIONS AND ACTIVITIES

1. What challenges does the workforce skills gap pose to health care organizations?

2. Identify three policies and practices that would help in the recruitment and retention of older workers by a health care organization. Describe how and why these policies and practices would be beneficial. Then, describe how the same policies might benefit employees from other groups, for example, gender, race, ethnicity, religion, and so on.

3. Imagine that you are the director of human resources for a health system that has a strategic goal of recruiting and retaining more Hispanic nurses and your annual merit increase is dependent on your success. Given the workforce demographic and educational accomplishment data presented in Tables 3.3 and 3.5 what challenges will you experience? How will you address these challenges? What actions will you take to increase representation of Hispanics in your nursing staff? Now imagine that your goal is to increase representation of male nurses and answer the same questions.

4. Referring to Figure 3.1, can the social factors that contribute to disparities in workforce representation and career accomplishment for people of color be

overcome? What policy actions by government do you recommend and why? What private sector initiatives do you recommend and why? What actions by other stakeholders such as individuals, families, communities, school systems, and health care providers can mitigate the effects of the social factors discussed in this chapter? How would these actions, in turn, affect human capital factors?

5. Go to www.diversityinc.com and search for three organizational-level best practices in recruiting and retaining a diverse workforce. Explain why you selected each of these best practices and how you would justify their implementation to the CEO of a health care organization in your community.

6. If you work in a health care organization, use the assessment checklist in this chapter to evaluate the organization's responsiveness to diversity. What are the organization's areas of strength? Which areas need the most improvement?

REFERENCES

AAMC. (2011). *Number of first-time medical school applicants reaches new high.* Washington, DC: Author.

AMA. (2010). *International medical graduates in American medicine: Contemporary challenges and opportunities: A position paper by the AMA-IMG Section Governing Council AMA.* Chicago: Author.

American College of Healthcare Executives, American Hospital Association, Institute for Diversity in Health Management, National Center for Healthcare Leadership. (2004). *Strategies for leadership: Does your hospital reflect the community it serves?* Chicago: American Hospital Association, 2004.

Bureau of Labor Statistics. (January 2012). Table 39: Median weekly earnings of full-time wage and salary workers by detailed occupation and sex. Retrieved from http://www.bls.gov/cps/tables.htm#empstat

Bureau of Labor Statistics. (June 2012). *Table 11: Employed persons by detailed occupation, sex, race, and Hispanic or Latino ethnicity.* Retrieved from http://www.bls.gov/cps/tables.htm#empstat

Burling, S. (2007, December 8). Giving patients, and nurses, a lift. *Philadelphia Inquirer*, pp. A1, A7.

Burns, M. J. (2011). Be wary of English-only policies in workplace. *Connecticut Law Tribune*, *37*(30), 1–2.

Croasdale, M. (2006, December 11). Classes teach new IMGs American-style medicine. *American Medical News.* Retrieved from http://www.ama-assn.org/amednews/2006/12/11/prl21211.htm

Dreachslin, J. L. (2007). Diversity management and cultural competence: Research, practice, and the business case. *Journal of Healthcare Management, 52*(2), 79–96.

Dreachslin, J. L., & Foster Curtis, E. (2004). Factors affecting the career advancement of women and racially/ethnically diverse individuals in healthcare management. *Journal of Health Administration Education, 21*(4), 441–484.

The Education Trust. (2006). *Funding gaps 2006.* Retrieved from http://www.edtrust.org/dc/publication/the-funding-gap-0

Erickson, T. (2008a). *Retire retirement: Career strategies for the boomer generation.* Boston: Harvard Business Press.

Erickson, T. (2008b). *What's next gen X? Keeping up, moving ahead, and getting the career you want.* Boston: Harvard Business Press.

Erickson, T. (2010). *Plugged in: The generation Y guide to thriving at work.* Boston: Harvard Business Press.

Franklin, J. (2007, November). *An overview of BLS projections to 2016.* Monthly Labor Review. Retrieved from http://www.bls.gov/opub/mlr/2007/11/art1abs.htm

Fry, R. (2007). *The changing racial and ethnic composition of U.S. public schools.* Pew Hispanic Center. Retrieved from http://pewhispanic.org/files/reports/79.pdf

Johnston, W. R., & Packer, A. H. (1987). *Workforce 2000: Work and workers for the 21st century.* Indianapolis: Hudson Institute.

Kochhar, R., Fry, R., & Taylor, P. (2011). *Wealth gaps rise to record highs between whites, blacks, and Hispanics.* Washington, DC: Pew Research Center.

Laveist, T. A., & Nuru-Jeter, A. (2002). Is doctor-patient race concordance associated with greater satisfaction with care? *Journal of Health and Social Behavior, 42*, 296–306.

Ong, P., & Patraporn, R. V. (2006). *Asian Americans and wealth: The role of housing and non-housing assets.* Paper prepared for the Closing the Wealth Gap Research Forum, Assets Learning Conference, Phoenix, September.

Robeznieks, A. (2003, October 27). Hospital apologizes for complying with racial request. *American Medical News.* Retrieved from http://www.ama-assn.org/amednews/2003/10/27/prsb1027.htm

Rueda, N. U. (2011, August 21). Fil-Ams win US racial suit. *Philippine Daily Inquirer.* Retrieved from http://globalnation.inquirer.net/9763/fil-ams-win-us-racial-suit

Saha, S., Taggart, S. H., Komaronmy, M., & Bindman, A. B. (2000). Do patients choose physicians of their own race? *Health Affairs, 19*, 76–83.

Toossi, M. (2009). Labor force projections to 2018: Older workers staying more active. *Monthly Labor Review, 132*(11), 30–51.

US Census Bureau. (2012). *Statistical abstract of the United States.* Retrieved from http://www.census.gov/compendia/statab/

Zemke, R., Raines, C., & Filipczak, B. (2000). *Generations at work: Managing the clash of veterans, boomers, Xers, and Nexters in your workplace.* New York: AMACOM.

THE DEVELOPMENT OF

CULTURAL COMPETENCE

The chapters in Part Two develop the concept of cultural competence in theory and application to health care. In Chapter Four, "Foundations for Cultural Competence in Health Care," we clarify the concept of culture, looking carefully at its complexities and its impact on health and health care seeking. Noting that to have culture is a universal attribute of human beings, but that no one culture *is* human nature, we see that culture is expressed at personal and organizational levels. Culture is pervasive and affects every aspect of life. Health care organizations in the United States are charged with providing services to a diverse people with deeply held but various culturally derived expectations about illness and appropriate treatment. The health care workforce is made up of persons whose workplace values and norms may also be varied. We discuss how the strategies of cultural competence as an important way to validate differences and at the same time reconcile them in the service of good health care have gained acceptance in the discourse about health care institutions. Fortunately, helped by advocacy of institutional change in the public and private sectors, some very good models of what culturally competent health care looks like have been created, are being applied, and are being evaluated in the systems approach.

Chapter Five, "Hallmarks of Cultural Competence in Health Care Professionals," centers on the development of a reflective cultural competence at the personal and professional levels. Along with learning about the beliefs of other cultures and acquiring skills for working with diverse patients, becoming culturally competent requires health care professionals to reflect on themselves as being the product of their own cultures so as to better understand and appreciate the cultures and needs of others. Self-reflection is often difficult in the face of multiple professional responsibilities and the competing challenges of day-to-day work life. In terms of personal philosophy, becoming culturally competent can be a transformative experience and a process of self-discovery. It may involve dealing with personal biases, implicit and explicit. We address these challenges and ask the reader to participate in this journey to cultural competence.

In the final chapter of Part Two, Chapter Six, "Training for Knowledge and Skills in Culturally Competent Care for Diverse Populations," we turn to the kinds of training that are necessary for acquiring the knowledge and skills needed to provide culturally competent care. Here we emphasize what people working in health care need to know and do in order to provide culturally competent health care. Again we stress that acquiring the practical knowledge base and strategies of hands-on cultural competence in everyday practice is developmental and requires time. A one-size-fits-all set of knowledge and skills is inappropriate in the health care setting because the training needs to be relevant to the functions of people performing the vastly different functions of a health care organization. A number of process-related concepts and tools useful in organizing and providing care to patients from different cultures are presented for the reader to consider, evaluate, and perhaps try out. The results of cultural competence training at the various functional levels of an organization need to be evaluated by different indicators, a complicated matter indeed. We describe some models and concepts for different types of assessment for the reader to consider.

Chapter 4

FOUNDATIONS FOR
CULTURAL COMPETENCE
IN HEALTH CARE

LEARNING OBJECTIVES

- To understand what is meant by the term *cultural competence*

- To become familiar with the complexity of the culture concept and its meaning in the context of health care

- To recognize the impact of cultural differences on the delivery of health care services

- To understand how cultural competence is basic to the new directions being taken in health care delivery

- To become aware of the interaction of organizational and personal cultural competence in the provision of health care

- To become aware of US health care as a workforce culture with cultural competence dimensions

When, as is happening in the United States today, many cultures and subcultures from across the globe come in contact with each other, individuals from these cultures bring different ideas and expectations into their interactions: ideas and expectations about work, family, education, governance, the marketplace, and health care, to name just a few areas. The need to work through these differences in a positive and constructive way to achieve mutual understanding and effective action taking underlies the concept of cultural competence in the delivery of services in health care. When, as was discussed in Chapter Two, there are significant disparities in health care access and status across population groups, cultural competence becomes even more critical.

This chapter first presents comprehensive definitions of cultural competence that emphasize the concept as integrating culture, epidemiology, and treatment, linking it to heath care quality and positive health outcomes. Very frequently, people use the terms *culture* and *cultural competence* without comprehending the full meaning of the culture concept as it applies to health care. The core of the chapter is devoted to clarifying the broader culture concept, an understanding of which is central to grasping the meaning of *cultural* competence in health care. The tendency to categorize groups along dimensions of race, ethnicity, and national origin raises issues in determining just where culture is located, and these questions are explored. The chapter includes a brief history of how concepts central to cultural competence in health care evolved over time, culminating in the present understanding of the construct.

Cultural competence can be expressed at the individual and organizational levels and, as will be described, both levels are important and each should be supportive of the other. Since about 2000, theoretical and action frameworks for cultural competence in health care delivery have been developed, and several of the most useful of these will be described.

The US health care system itself can be considered a culture, with learned values, norms, and structural arrangements that center on patient care and the interactions of the vast array of occupations that support care. Reflecting these norms and values, a health care organization can also be considered a culture with culturally competent work relations which are also a foundational aspect of cultural competence in health care. Finally, an important aspect of applied culturally competent care is evaluation. Attention will be called to some excellent and easily accessible assessment tools that are also heuristic in nature.

WHAT *IS* CULTURAL COMPETENCE IN HEALTH CARE?

A particularly comprehensive definition of the term explicitly focused on health care is the one given by Lavizzo-Moury and MacKenzie (1996): "Cultural competence is the demonstrated awareness and integration of three population-specific issues: health-related beliefs and cultural values, disease incidence and prevalence, and treatment efficacy. But perhaps the most significant aspect of this concept is the inclusion and integration of the three areas that are usually considered separately" (p. 919). Davis (1997) gave another operational definition of the term by saying that cultural competence is the "integration and transformation of knowledge about individuals and groups of people into specific standards, policies, practices and attitudes used in appropriate cultural settings to increase quality of services, thereby producing better health outcomes" (p. 3). The Centers for Disease Control (CDC) in 2011 pointed out that the term *competence* implies not just a mind-set or attitudes but also a set of knowledge and practical skills. Note that all of these definitions emphasize integration and confluence, a systemic coming together of several elements:

- Knowledge of a group's culture

- Information about the epidemiology of disease and disorder characteristic of the group

- Use of this information to design services and implement practices that provide measureable benefits to the group

The Meaning of *Culture* in Cultural Competence

In order to get a comprehensive understanding of *cultural* competence, we must first consider what we mean by culture. A widely accepted definition of culture used in anthropology, the discipline that specifically focuses on the study of cultures, is that culture is the learned and shared knowledge and symbols that specific groups use to interpret their experience of reality and to guide their thinking and behavior. A distinct way of looking at the world, people, relationships, and events that make up a culture may be unique to a small tribal or **ethnic group** or it may be a worldview that is shared by a nation, that is, a national culture. Cultural understandings are conveyed through language and transmitted by the processes of **socialization** within a cultural group. They are reflected in the religions, morals, norms, values, rules, social roles, customs, technologies, and survival strategies of the group. Culture largely determines how people adapt to their social and material environments, work, parent, love, worship, marry, and understand health, illness, and death. Usually, the multiple aspects of a culture interrelate and support each other and make up a unique worldview. It is important to remember that culture is learned, not inherited biologically. Typically, an individual draws a significant part of his or her sense of self from the cultural group in which he or she grew up and was socialized into. This aspect of identity is often called a person's **cultural identity**.

Much of a group's culture resides in the heads of its constituents; thus, it is invisible and often hard to detect. One way to understand culture is to think of it as the "software" of the mind. Essentially, individuals are "programmed" by their cultural group to interpret and evaluate behavior, events, relationships, ideas, and other people in ways that are specific to their group. Another way to understand culture is to call it the "lens" through which people in a specific group view the world. You will have noticed that these analogies imply that culture exercises a kind of invisible control over members of the group. This is correct; psychologists call this process *internalizing* the cultural norms and concepts. The invisibility of culture makes cultural differences hard to recognize unless they are made visible by outward signs such as dress, language, and behavior.

Further, because a great deal of an individual's lifelong cultural learning occurs out of consciousness as that person interacts with others and is influenced by what they say and do, they learn much of their culture without realizing they are doing so. Humans all do this very naturally while acquiring their cultures; however, this ongoing process often has the effect of rendering their own culture invisible to them, though they can readily identify cultures that differ from their own. Frequently when a new idea, phenomenon, or practice is experienced by members of a cultural group, they tend to interpret it in the context of their familiar worldview. If it can't be fitted into that view, it is likely to be rejected. Additionally, and not too surprising, when a culture is **internalized**, it tends to be seen by its members as *the* natural and right way of viewing the world. People tend to see their own culture as "human nature" and often see the cultures of other groups as less legitimate and sometimes as unnatural. This bias is called **ethnocentrism**. It takes considerable introspection and self-analysis for individuals to discover how deep and strong an influence culture exercises over their thoughts and actions and how ethnocentrism biases their thinking processes.

Doing this work is an essential part of cultural competence training, and it becomes a lifelong process for someone who encounters people from various cultures in the work they do. For now, it's a good thing to remember that to *have* culture is human nature, but no one culture *is* human nature.

Cultures are not at all static. They are dynamic and changing, maybe even disappearing, as the individuals within them innovate, have different experiences, and have contact with people from other cultures. It can be said that a culture is constantly under construction by its members as well as by powerful environmental, economic, technological, political, and religious forces that affect it. Rates of culture change can be gradual, incremental, and peaceful or rapid through coercion, war, or revolution. For this reason, understanding a culture can't be simply knowledge of a list of cultural traits but an understanding of how a group and individuals interact with each other and their social, material, and spiritual environments. Because a patient's cultural worldview greatly influences his or her concepts of health, disease, and treatment, cultural competence on the part of health care professionals and organizations requires an understanding of these dimensions of the culture concept. Recognizing the profound effects of culture on oneself and others is a challenge but it is also foundational to competently caring for a diverse patient population.

Culture and Concepts of Health and Illness

The provision of health care services touches on issues that, throughout history and for all cultures, have been deeply meaningful and important: illness, pain, congenital abnormalities, crippling physical accidents, mental illness, birth, and death. Most all societies devote significant amounts of time and treasure to preventing and treating ill health and maintaining good health among their members, whether this is done by ritual practices, purification rites, social healing, scientific research, or sometimes a combination of all of these methods. Every group has its theories of bodily function and disease etiology, treatment, and death as well as its specialists or healers that are charged with dealing with these important issues. Because health and illness are critical to all cultures, they are often imbued with religious and moral overtones. And, because different cultures have, historically and currently, faced different challenges to the health of their members, their understandings of what constitutes good health, its preservation, and maintenance, often vary widely from one locale to another and from one culture to another. Adding to the complexity, epidemiological differences, that is, differences in the onset, prevalence, and course of adverse health conditions, have varied in the historic experience of different cultural groups, and these differences have created significant divergence in the understanding of causal factors, treatments, and health beliefs.

It is important to understand that although cultural understandings about health, the body, and causes of illness are important in the health care context, they are certainly not the only aspects of a culture that critically affect health care. For example, cultural ideas about same-sex sexuality may affect prevention of and compliance with treatment of sexually transmitted diseases. Traditional family roles may dictate caregiver relationships and treatment decision making. Marital roles may affect notions of what constitutes spousal abuse or even affect a woman's ability to alter family dietary practices that are unhealthful. Health and disease are often given meaning and viewed through a culture's religious prism. These nuances of a cultural worldview may be even more important and difficult to discover than health beliefs or traditional ideas about treatment but they are equally important.

Culture, Categories, Complexity, and Confusion

If the concept of culture weren't complex enough, additional complication occurs when groups of people are categorized. Cultural groups are often correctly referred to as ethnic groups because, by definition, an ethnic group is identified as a group that is bound together by a unique worldview with sets of behaviors and ideas that correspond to that worldview. In discussing groups of people, much confusion has arisen because there has been a tendency to confound ethnicity, race, national origin, and linguistic groups. For example, the Chinese, a **national origin group**, are categorized in the US Census and DHHS statistics as Asian, a *race*. So are the Japanese. *Race* is a word commonly used to differentiate groups of people by their biological, physiological, or genetic background. However, as was pointed out earlier, culture is *learned*, not inherited genetically, so a race, such as Asian, is not a culture.

It is certainly the case that the Chinese share a worldview and language different from the Japanese: they are culturally different, though of the same race. These differences at the national level are often referred to as "national cultures." However, within China, there are fifty-six recognized ethnic groups, each one incorporating several million people, with the Han Chinese being the largest. Each of these ethnic groups is *culturally* unique, though each shares to a greater or lesser degree the national Chinese culture and all are categorized as part of the Asian race. The same can be said of the all of the national origin groups subsumed under "Asian" in the US Census and DHHS statistics. And, among African American populations in the United States, black persons born in this country are culturally and linguistically quite different from immigrant Haitians, Nigerians, and Somalis, who all differ dramatically from each other in terms of culture. But these groups are all lumped together as "African American." The term *Middle Eastern*, basically a geographically derived category, includes cultures from Iran, Turkey, Tunisia, Iraq, Morocco, and others. All of these cultures share a major religion, Islam, but these national groups differ culturally and linguistically from each other in important ways and have within them distinct ethnic groups; even the way they practice Islam differs significantly. The US Census and DHHS treat Hispanics (sometimes called *Latinos*) as a monolithic ethnic group, subsuming persons from Mexico, Cuba, Puerto Rico, and other Spanish-speaking peoples into different sub-groups. Even though Hispanics are treated as an ethnic group, these national groups differ greatly from each other though they speak different versions of the same language. Clearly, the Census categories used across government agencies don't tell us very much about culture: *Asian* is not a learned culture nor is *Hispanic*.

Subcultures: An Important Part of Most Cultures

Adding to the complexity brought about by lumping dissimilar groups together as described previously is that within any cultural group there is significant within-group variability as to how extensively individual members internalize the many aspects of the culture into which they have been socialized. For starters, major cultures almost always contain subcultures. These subcultures are formed by such things as social class, gender, age, race, religion, occupation, region, generation, and sexual orientation. A **subculture** shares much of the overarching culture of the larger group within which it occurs, but also has characteristics that are unique and identifiable. These subcultures are a very important source of diversity *within* a cultural group. Subcultures often have names such as *youth culture, middle class culture,* and *gay culture*. The subcultures will share some like characteristics of similar subcultures in other major cultures but also will be unique. Thus, the gay Vietnamese subculture will be different from the gay Mexican subculture, though their members share the same sexual orientation, and each will relate to their own larger cultures in different ways. Health care providers in an HIV clinic in Orange County, California, for example, found it important to understand the distinct characteristics of the Vietnamese gay subculture in order to mount effective outreach efforts to that group. Outreach efforts designed to communicate with non-Vietnamese gays, both Mexican and Anglo, had not been effective.

Acculturation as an Aspect of Cultures in Contact

Because humans are constantly learning and having new experiences, a single individual can alter his or her cultural identity over time through a variety of processes. One of these is **acculturation**, which occurs when a person socialized in one culture comes in contact with people or organizations of another culture and begins to internalize aspects of the new culture. Obviously, this happens in varying degrees, and it's very hard to tell how much acculturation has taken place in each individual. Usually the outward aspects of culture such as clothing and foods change more rapidly than norms for behavior, gender roles, family orientations, religions, and health beliefs.

Acculturation is often reflected in general distance from immigrant status, when a person from one nation immigrates to another. The first generation is the immigrant generation, the second generation is American-born of immigrant parents, and the third generation is American-born children of American parents. (Interestingly, Japanese Americans have names for each of these generations: Issei, Nisei, and Sansei, respectively.) In health care it is common for traditional health beliefs acquired in the country of origin to be shared and strongly held by the immigrant generation, less pervasive in their adult children, and nearly absent in the third. With so many people immigrating to the United States from so many different nations, there are millions of people in varying stages of acculturation. The use of hyphenated designations, such as *Mexican-American, Chinese-American,* and *Polish-American,* acknowledges the enduringness of a nation-of-origin culture and the acquisition of a shared American culture.

When an individual can operate very well in two cultures, that person is called **bicultural**. When circumstances create a situation in which a person has difficulty operating well in either culture, it is called *marginalization* and many poor immigrants face this problem because their poverty severely limits their access to the institutions of the larger society. This situation is further exacerbated when immigrants settle or are pushed into areas heavily populated by persons of their same background. Whereas immigrants in these circumstances benefit by being able to speak their native language, and their norms and values are understood by those around them, such social isolation tends to limit their knowledge of institutions and instrumentalities of the larger society.

All of these dynamic social forces give rise to significant differences among people within each cultural group and make it important not to generalize features of a culture to individuals within the group. This process is called *stereotyping*. Everyone does this faulty generalizing from time to time; however, the culturally aware person is far less likely to fall into this fallacious way of thinking. An awareness of subcultural and individual variation within cultures is a good antidote to stereotypical thinking.

Cultural Competence and Immigrant Populations

The history behind the cultural competence thrust in US health care is somewhat complex. In the 1960s, 1970s, and 1980s, with the civil rights movement, changes in the immigration laws, and large-scale Southeast Asian, Armenian, Iranian, African, and Afghani refugee resettlement occurring on the heels of an era marked by assumed cultural homogeneity, the United States began to recognize a culturally diversifying population and growing schisms in health status across different population groups in the country. According to the US Census (Acosta & de la Cruz, 2011), immigrants make up 13 percent of the US population and come predominantly from Latin America (53 percent), Asia (28 percent), and other non-European populations (7 percent). In sum, 88 percent of immigrants come from cultures that are different from US national culture in many ways.

Because many of the new immigrants and refugee groups were made up of people different in culture from the managers and caregivers of primarily western background that dominated the health care (and other) institutions of the United States, culture clashes were bound to occur. During the 1980s and 1990s, there was a growing awareness of the difficulties involved when patients of varying backgrounds attempted to engage US health care systems. Medical anthropologists, physicians and nurses began to analyze issues arising out of cultural clashes and misunderstandings in medical settings (Chrisman & Maretzki, 1982; Kleinman,

1980; Kleinman, Eisenberg, & Goode, 1978; Leininger, 1978; *The Western Journal of Medicine*, 1983, 1992).

When patients and providers from different cultural and religious traditions interact in health care settings, there is a significant likelihood that their variant understandings about health, illness, and treatment may cause misunderstandings and miscommunication. There is the very real possibility that these difficulties can get in the way of trust between patients and providers and prevent effective health promotion and treatment. There have been many documented instances in which this has happened. One of the most famous instances was recounted in the book *The Spirit Catches You and You Fall Down: A Hmong Child, Her American Doctors, and the Collision of Two Cultures* (1997) by Ann Fadiman. This story of the cultural clash between the refugee parents of Lia Lee, a Hmong child with severe epilepsy, and her American doctors shows how radically variant cultural interpretations of illness and multiple failures of communication led to a tragic outcome for the little girl. The doctors attributed the cause of the toddler's disorder to strictly biological factors and the parents believed that spirits were to blame. The parents had a very different **explanatory model** of the problems afflicting their daughter than that held by her American physicians. These critical differences in the understanding of causes and symptoms, the parents' complete lack of familiarity with the health care system, together with the unwillingness and inability of the health care institutions to provide interpretation, led to the child's permanent vegetative state.

A major reason for some of the extreme differences in health beliefs among immigrant populations is that many areas of the world have not yet made what has been called the *epidemiological transition*. The concept refers to the enormous positive changes in life expectancy, incidence of infectious disease, and parasitic disease that followed the industrialization of Western society with its modern theories of disease, immunization, and sanitation. In the developed nations, morbidity and mortality are primarily caused by chronic diseases, such as diabetes, chronic pulmonary disease, and heart diseases, many of which can be prevented or moderated by lifestyle changes and modern medicines. Many countries still have not made this transition (Farmer, 2001; Omran, 1982).

When persons from these countries immigrate to the United States for economic reasons, asylum, or fleeing from wars in their own countries, their perceptions of disease are conditioned by experiences of disease and health that are very different from those prevalent in this country: diseases of sudden onset and quick death such as measles and smallpox; lingering diseases for which there seemed to be no explanation or cure, such as tuberculosis, hepatitis, and malaria; and diseases that followed natural disasters, such as cholera. Childbirth is still dangerous in many areas and instances of childbirth fever not uncommon. Infant mortality rates are high and many children do not live to adulthood. The causes of these problems are often not understood from a contemporary scientific perspective and modern preventive measures not undertaken. Folk healers and shamans are the health care experts and their treatments often intermingle religious and mundane concepts. The concept of disease prevention as understood in modern medicine is often not a strategy that has wide acceptance in the cultures of less-developed countries.

Additionally, there are traditional medical cultures, such as Chinese medicine and Ayurvedic medicine in India, that have complex theories of bodily function and systems of treatment that have been considered efficacious for many centuries by educated and uneducated persons alike. Acupuncture and herbal remedies derived from these traditions are common in the United States and are used by practitioners far from the cultures in which they originated.

A Buddhist mother and father from Jakarta gaze down at their twenty-one-year-old daughter as she breathes with the help of a respirator, tubes emerging from her body, and a monitor tracing her bodily functions. The young doctor is gently explaining that her injuries from the car crash have been so serious that her brain can no longer support cognitive functions and that she has suffered brain death. He begins to explain that the parents have some difficult decisions to make when the father, holding his daughter's warm hand, exclaims, "Thank you, thank you, doctor, for saving our daughter's life!"

What is understood as death and what criteria are used to signal it vary from culture to culture. What are some possible ways of handling this crosscultural dilemma?

Major differences may also occur in the manner in which the roles and interactional "rules" of the doctor-healer and the patient-family relationships are understood. Moreover, the organization and structuring of health care services, puzzling even to many Americans, can be incomprehensible to persons from a different background. For example, people from many cultures are accustomed to working with healers and medical doctors who care for the whole body and they may be unfamiliar with the specialties that, in the words of one Vietnamese patient, "cut the body in pieces," that is to say, ear, nose, and throat physicians who are different from cardiologists who differ from obstetricians and neurologists and so on. The ways in which one culture can differ from another in perspectives on health, disease, and treatment are many and complex.

Culture Is Best Discovered in Local Populations

So where does all this leave a hospital in Santa Maria, California, whose patients include a large number of immigrated Mixtecos, an indigenous group from Central Mexico who speak their own language, very little Spanish, and no English? Or the Minnesota and Fresno clinics and hospitals who serve Hmong from Vietnam and Laos, a group made famous in health care literature by Anne Fadiman (1997) and Culhane-Pera, Vawter, Xiong, Babbitt, and Solberg (2003)? Where does culture reside in these cases? The truth for the culturally competent providers and organizations in these locations and everywhere is that culture resides in the heads of individuals and in the mores or accepted traditions of their local communities. This is why those lists that say "The Japanese believe this" or that "the Armenians do that" are only marginally useful and can be viewed with caution only as a starting point. True cultural competence in health care requires that, although attending to the health care statistics describing disparities that the governmental agencies are using, providers and the organizations in which they work need to familiarize themselves with the cultures of local level populations—populations specific to their service areas.

An excellent example of how this is done can be found in the work of those affiliated with the Cross Cultural Health Care Program in Seattle, Washington, who went out into the local ethnic communities, talked with the elders, the shaman, and individuals within their city, and produced *Voices of the Communities* (The Cross Cultural Health Care Program, 1996). Although such a comprehensive project is more than many hospitals, health plans, clinics, and practitioners can undertake, there is no excuse for health care organizations and providers not knowing essential aspects of the various cultures residing in the catchment areas of practice: their languages, their specific health issues, and their internal systems for coping with maintaining health, treating disease, and facing death. This is an essential and baseline aspect of culturally competent health care.

The health issues that afflict local-level cultural groups show up in the national statistics. The problems suffered by the Mixtecos in California or the Haitians in Connecticut or the Hmong in Fresno roll up and disappear into the DHHS disparities statistics on Hispanics, African Americans, and Asians. These ethnic groups and their unique characteristics do not, however, disappear for the health providers who serve them. Whatever the national statistics, local level cultural competence is a major tool in the effort to end disparities.

LONG JOURNEY TOWARD CULTURAL COMPETENCE

Understanding the need for and developing culturally competent approaches in health care has been a long journey. The first early steps toward cultural competence involved **cultural awareness**. This involved recognizing that perhaps a melting pot ideology was not the best descriptor for what was occurring as the US population became more diverse. Many persons from other countries did not want or couldn't relinquish all their behaviors and ways of seeing the world. At the personal level, cultural awareness requires individuals to be able to actually "see" culture, that is, to become conscious of their own culture's effect on them and be aware that persons from other cultures have been socialized differently. Usually the first response to these discoveries takes one of two forms: denial of the legitimacy or rationality of the culture other than one's own or downplaying the differences between cultures by asserting that in most important ways, all cultures are alike. However, even cursory research, an opportunity to live in another country, or an introductory anthropology course will reveal large and important differences across cultures in many critical aspects of life. For example, people in every culture must eat and reproduce. However, *what* they eat and *how* they form unions to reproduce varies dramatically and can have major effects on health issues.

Cultural sensitivity was the next step in health care's journey toward cultural competence. This term came into vogue in the 1980s as various population groups—Latinos, African Americans, Asians, and Native Americans—began to organize to gain access to better health care, and the government initially recognized the legitimacy of their needs with documents such as the US Department of Health and Human Service's *Report of the Secretary's Task Force on Black and Minority Health* (1986). At the personal level, a culturally sensitive individual recognizes specific cultural needs and is sympathetic, not resistant, to them.

The next step forward involved the concept of **cultural relevancy**. This term was also prevalent during the 1980s and early 1990s. It engendered a more active stance: the notion of making health care services more meaningful and understandable to persons from nonmainstream cultures. Note that up to this point, most of the terms dealing with culture and health care focused on the *attitudes* and *state of mind* of health care providers and the stance of institutions vis-à-vis their patients.

Dr. Anderson, a well-regarded cardiologist, was frustrated at the beginning of a training session on clinical cultural competence: "I treat all of my patients the same," he stated. He was resistant to the idea of treating people differently, as it seemed to engender the idea of discrimination. The trainer asked if he treated a female heart attack victim differently from a man. "Of course I do," was his reply. An eighty-year-old differently from a fifty-year-old? "Yes," came his reply again. Was he aware that some medications worked differently for different racial groups? He was. He began to see that he in fact did treat his patients differently, and it was a sign of his expertise that he did. When clinicians state that they "treat all patients the same," most of the time what they really mean is that they give *all* of their patients the best care that they can. It becomes a short step then from recognizing that the individualized care that they feel is important could include cultural considerations as well as age and gender factors.

The term *cultural competency* was first used in 1989 by Cross, Bazon, and Isaacs at the Georgetown University Center Child Development Center following the use of the term *multicultural competency* by psychologist Paul Pedersen (1988). Adoption of the term occurred when people in the health care field began to understand that attitudes and states of mind were necessary but not sufficient to change practices, that specific kinds of knowledge and skills would also be required. The ability to work effectively across cultures would require the development of competencies at the organizational level and the level of individual care providers.

The notion of competencies implied concrete, informed behavior and sets of skills that could be taught, learned, and applied just like any other practice-related competency. By no means did the developers of the concept wish to exclude the very important attitudes of cultural awareness and sensitivity that were key to the willingness of care providers to acquire new information and skills; hence, most definitions of cultural competence emphasized the triad: attitudes, knowledge, and skills. However, the major difference is that cultural competence emphasized the idea of effectively operating in a multicultural context and required *action* (a new way of behaving) and *structural change* (a new way of organizing health care delivery).

A later, critical dimension to the set of ideas surrounding cultural competence was the addition of the concept of **cultural humility**. Coined by physicians Melanie Tervalon and Jann Murray-Garcia (1998), the term refers to a "lifelong process of self-reflection, self-critique, and respectful partnering with patients" (p. 118), reflecting a posture of continued openness toward the views of others as well as ongoing examination of one's own assumptions and biases. Cultural humility provides a framework for the health provider's active engagement with patients. Although challenging, this new dimension precludes the concept of cultural competence from being a static set of skills and information that is not constantly being refreshed by a humanizing perspective.

The term *cultural competence* has become widely accepted and used within the health care industry and the health care professions, though not without some resistance on the part of some. The very aspect of the concept that has made it most tangible, that of concrete, informed skills or competencies, has annoyed some professionals who feel that the term engenders the idea of cultural *in*competence, a notion inconsistent with their view of themselves as skilled professionals. The terms *cultural responsiveness* and *cultural proficiency* are therefore sometimes used instead of cultural competence.

Cultural Competence and Disparities Reduction

Cultural competence has been seen lately as one important factor in reducing the health care disparities in access, treatment, and health status across population groups in the United States. Thus, since about 2000, cultural competence has acquired a very strong social justice rationale. The National Institute of Medicine's study, *Unequal Treatment: Confronting Racial and Ethnic Disparities in Health Care* (Smedley, Stith, & Nelson, 2002), states that "any degree of uncertainty a physician has about the condition of a patient may, by itself, result in disparities in treatment" (p. 167). The study goes on to discuss how a physician's unfamiliarity with the life circumstances of a patient may affect his or her interaction with the patient and affect treatment decisions, causing the possibility of inadequate care.

Adding a social justice rationale since about 2000 gave a new and important dimension to cultural competence: in addition to being sensitive to the culture of patients, it was also important to consider the social determinants that surrounded their actions and ability to make healthy choices for themselves.

In conditions of social inequality such as chronic poverty, crowded and dilapidated housing, lack of transportation, intermittent or no employment, limited education, and low literacy, people have difficulty planning, and their lifestyle choices are dictated by a very narrow range of what they perceive is possible. Oscar Lewis, an anthropologist who studied the poor in Mexico (1959), coined the phrase *culture of poverty* to describe a set of actions and norms that emerge everywhere that people subject to the conditions of constant poverty and inequality try to cope with their life circumstances. Although the culture-of-poverty concept has been criticized with respect to its universality and the notion of its persistence even in the face of changed circumstances (Small, Harding, & Lamont, 2010), some of its aspects need to be considered as health care providers work with individuals whose behaviors and attitudes are formed by unhealthy life conditions and being forever poor: fatalism, apparent passivity, difficulty planning, impulse gratification, and feelings of powerlessness.

Long-term discrimination, marginality, and exclusion often foster distrust of society's institutions, even the health care system. Poverty unquestionably limits the choices that people can make and their access to society's resources. These social class–related attitudes and behaviors *are* amenable to change but not without acknowledgment and recognition on the part of providers of health care. If health care providers recognize the constraints forced on their patients by very limited resources, they can explore options and direct them to community resources. The large social class gulf that exists between many health care providers and members of minority and underserved patients is a class and cultural gap that has to be bridged by knowledge and compassion. Further, it is many times easier to conflate behaviors and attitudes formed in the crucible of poverty with those developed in a culture outside this country. Being able to differentiate the two different sources or even to see where the two sources interact is also foundational to cultural competence.

Cultural Competence and Changing Delivery Models

Changing health care delivery practices also contribute to the rationale for the adoption of cultural competence in health care. Among the more significant are patient-centered care, a growing focus on prevention, and the movement from in-patient to out-patient care.

Patient-Centered Care

Although the cultural and linguistic diversification of the nation's population and the existence of alarming disparities would be rationale enough for the adoption of cultural competence in health care, alterations in the philosophy of patient care across wide segments of the health care professions and systems also underscores the need for a change in the way services are structured and delivered along more personal lines. Since 2000, there has been a strong emphasis on patient-centered care as a key aspect of quality health care. The National Institute of Medicine (2001) defines patient-centered care as care that is respectful of and responsive to individual patient preferences, needs, and values. The Institute for Health Care Improvement (2011) notes on its website that "care that is truly patient-centered considers patients' cultural traditions, their personal preferences and values, their family situations, and their lifestyles. It makes the patient and their loved ones an integral part of the health care team who collaborate with health care professionals in making clinical decisions."

Health care has been moving away from a strictly disease-centered model and toward this patient-centered model. In the disease-centered model, health care providers make almost all treatment decisions based largely on medical and clinical experience and data from various medical tests. In the new, patient-centered model, patients become active participants in their own care and receive services designed to focus on their individual needs and preferences in addition to advice, treatment, and monitoring from teams of professionals. In order for such shared-control models to work, health care providers need to know their patients and their lifestyles much more comprehensively than has previously been the case. Good communication between providers and patients is critically important; thus ways to effectively surmount language barriers and bridge different **explanatory models** are crucial.

Prevention

Other recent changes that have occurred in the way health care services are delivered include a strong emphasis on prevention. This is because many of the health problems suffered by people in the United States are caused by chronic lifestyle diseases, such as type 2 diabetes, coronary artery disease, and congestive heart failure, to name just a few. These diseases are expensive to treat over their usually long duration and can negatively affect the lives of individuals and their families. Such diseases often require specialized home care, close medical monitoring, frequent hospital visits, and coordination of prescription medicines. However, many chronic diseases can be prevented or well managed by alterations in people's lifestyles. Even some forms of cancer, such as colon or cervical cancers, can be prevented or easily treated if discovered early enough with regularly scheduled preventive tests and exams. Operating within today's health care system requires that patients take on significant responsibility for preventing health problems by using information given to them by their doctors and health care organizations. Conversations with diverse patients about types of preventive care require culturally knowledgeable communication skills on the part of doctors.

Outpatient Procedures

Another change is that many conditions are now treated with procedures that are done on an outpatient basis whereas they used to be treated only in hospitals. This reduces the cost of treatment, but often requires that family members perform complicated caregiving duties. This means that patients and their families will be taking more responsibility for their own care. Providers will need to know much more about their patients' lifestyles in order to help them manage their own care within the context of their daily lives. All of these changes require health care providers and patients to communicate well and interact collaboratively.

National Institutional Support for Cultural Competence

The need for culturally competent health care providers and organizations is currently well recognized among accreditation and regulatory agencies. The Joint Commission, the major nongovernmental agency that assesses and accredits hospitals and health care organizations, takes the position that the issue of culturally and linguistically appropriate health care services is an important quality and safety issue and a key element in individual care (Wilson-Stronks, Lee, Cordero, Kopp, & Galvez, 2008,). The Joint Commission includes several standards involving cultural and linguistic competence as part of their assessment of health care organizations. As noted in preceding chapters, the National Commission on Quality Assurance (NCQA), another national agency that focuses on quality of care and health outcomes, strongly emphasizes cultural competence through its national awards program entitled *Innovative Practices in Multicultural Health*, now in its sixth year. The National Quality Forum (2010) has developed forty-five measurable and reportable competencies it deems necessary for providing safe and culturally responsive care to diverse patients.

At the federal government level, the Department of Health and Human Services, operating through the OMH, has instituted fourteen standards for health care organizations entitled *Culturally and Linguistically Appropriate Services in Health Care*. Known nationally as the **CLAS standards**, these fourteen benchmarks are used widely to evaluate services in all types of health care organizations and will be reviewed more extensively later in this chapter.

As an aid to health organizations and providers, the OMH established the Center for Linguistic and Cultural Competence in Health Care (CLCCHC), which continues to provide programs and guidance to individual providers and provider organizations. HRSA has also developed extensive resources to help health care organizations enhance their competencies in service delivery to diverse communities.

The complex of behaviors, skills, and knowledge subsumed under the term *cultural competence* has been endorsed widely across the spectrum of national health care organizations and professional and practice associations. This includes the American Medical Association, the American Nurses Association, the American

Psychological Association, the American Academy of Family Practice, the American College of Obstetrics and Gynecology, American College of Emergency Physicians, the American College of Health Care Executives, and the American Hospital Association with its affiliate organization, The Institute for Diversity in Health Care Management, among many others who have created policies and standards around cultural competence in health care directed toward their specific practice capabilities. There has been an extensive growth of literature within all health care disciplines that is directed to how cultural competence can inform care practices, how levels of individual and organizational cultural competence affect health care, how to implement specific practices, how cultural competence can be evaluated, and even whether or not culturally based practices are effective in producing better health care outcomes (Goode, Dunne, & Bronheim, 2006).

During the 1990s, as the movement toward health management organizations (HMOs) became important in the struggle to hold down health care costs, state and federal governmental agencies, realizing that many of the patients receiving government-subsidized care such as Medicaid and Medicare were increasingly diverse, began to require that health care organizations educate their providers in the care of patients from different cultures and structure their services in such a way as to consider the needs of these diverse patients. They also required that health care organizations provide language services to persons whose English was limited. California was the first state to enact these requirements and other states followed (Brach, Paez, & Fraser, 2006).

CULTURAL COMPETENCE AND THE HEALTH CARE PROVIDER ORGANIZATION

Cultural competence is expressed at the individual and the organizational levels. To be effective, the two levels have to support each other. For example, it is difficult for the individual clinician to communicate in a competent way with non-English speaking patients if the organization in which he or she works hasn't put in place an interpretation and translation program complete with policies and staff training on how they can be used. Conversely, if the clinician hasn't taken the opportunity to learn about these policies, remains uninformed, and resists using available language services, he or she is undercutting the cultural competence efforts of the organization that has made them available. Though cultural competence at the individual level is related to and enabled by the level of cultural competence in the organization for which an individual works, models of cultural competence tend to be structured differently depending on whether they are framed for individuals or organizations.

With respect to individuals, the emphasis is on the development of very specific communication and interaction skills and kinds of knowledge, buttressed by attitudes of openness. However, with respect to organizations, the emphasis is on developing policies and procedures that (1) enhance access to health care for diverse populations groups, (2) increase the quality and effectiveness of the care experience for diverse patients, (3) support the cultural competence of providers of services, and (4) enable culturally diverse health care workers to work effectively together. Because the cultural competence of individuals working within health care organizations is very closely linked to training models, individual cultural competence will be covered more extensively in Chapters Five and Six.

The most widely recognized framework for cultural competence in health care provider organizations is embodied in the *National Standards for Culturally and Linguistically Appropriate Services in Health Care* (Office of Minority Health, 2002). The fourteen CLAS standards are used by health care organizations to guide creation of policies and procedures related to cultural competence and by accreditation agencies, such as state departments of health and the Joint Commission, to assess the level of care provided by state and federally funded health care services. The CLAS standards are listed in the following. Standards Four, Five, Six, and Seven are mandates because they reflect current federal requirements for all recipients of federal funds, including Medicare reimbursement.

Standard One

Health care organizations should ensure that patients and consumers receive from all staff members effective, understandable, and respectful care that is provided in a manner compatible with their cultural health beliefs and practices and preferred language.

Standard Two

Health care organizations should implement strategies to recruit, retain, and promote at all levels of the organization a diverse staff and leadership that are representative of the demographic characteristics of the service area.

Standard Three

Health care organizations should ensure that staff at all levels and across all disciplines receive ongoing education and training in culturally and linguistically appropriate service delivery.

Standard Four

Health care organizations must offer and provide language assistance services, including bilingual staff and interpreter services, at no cost to each patient and consumer with limited English proficiency at all points of contact, in a timely manner, during all hours of operation.

Standard Five

Health care organizations must provide to patients and consumers in their preferred language verbal offers and written notices informing them of their right to receive language assistance services.

Standard Six

Health care organizations must ensure the competence of language assistance provided to limited English proficient patients and consumers by interpreters and bilingual staff. Family and friends should not be used to provide interpretation services (except on request by the patient or consumer).

Standard Seven

Health care organizations must make available easily understood patient-related materials and post signage in the languages of the commonly encountered groups and groups represented in the service area.

Standard Eight

Health care organizations should develop, implement, and promote a written strategic plan that outlines clear goals, policies, operational plans, and management accountability and oversight mechanisms to provide culturally and linguistically appropriate services.

Standard Nine

Health care organizations should conduct initial and ongoing organizational self-assessments of CLAS-related activities and are encouraged to integrate cultural and linguistic competence-related measures into their internal audits, performance improvement programs, patient satisfaction assessments, and outcomes-based evaluations.

Standard Ten

Health care organizations should ensure that data on the individual patient's and consumer's race, ethnicity, and spoken and written language are collected in health records, integrated into the organization's management information systems, and periodically updated.

Standard Eleven

Health care organizations should maintain a current demographic, cultural, and epidemiological profile of the community as well as a needs assessment to accurately plan for and implement services that respond to the cultural and linguistic characteristics of the service area.

Standard Twelve

Health care organizations should develop participatory, collaborative partnerships with communities and use a variety of formal and informal mechanisms to facilitate community and patient and consumer involvement in designing and implementing CLAS-related activities.

Standard Thirteen

Health care organizations should ensure that conflict and grievance resolution processes are culturally and linguistically sensitive and capable of identifying, preventing, and resolving crosscultural conflicts or complaints by patients and consumers.

Standard Fourteen

Health care organizations are encouraged to regularly make available to the public information about their progress and successful innovations in implementing the CLAS standards and to provide public notice in their communities about the availability of this information.

As can be seen, these standards, though general, are quite comprehensive and to implement them requires considerable effort and expense on the part of health care organizations. Nevertheless, many health care organizations have worked toward complying with them since their publication in the *Federal Register* in 2000. The OMH (2002) provides extensive guidance on the specific implementation of each standard, which can be accessed on the OMH website.

The impact of the CLAS standards cannot be underestimated and most of the organizational models for cultural competence in health care are based on these standards in one way or another. Some models emphasize specific sections of the CLAS standards. The model used by the National Center for Cultural Competence (NCCC) (nd) at Georgetown University states that cultural competence requires that organizations have a defined set of values and principles and demonstrate behaviors, attitudes, and structures that enable them to work effectively crossculturally and have the capacity to (1) value diversity, (2) conduct self-assessment, (3) manage the dynamics of difference, (4) acquire and institutionalize cultural knowledge, and (5) adapt to diversity and the cultural contexts of the communities they serve. They should incorporate these factors in all aspects of policy making, administration, practice, and service delivery, and systematically involve consumers, key stakeholders, and communities.

NCCC, recognizing that policy making and self-assessment are critically important to the development of organizational cultural competence, offers extensive guidance on these two aspects of their cultural competence model. They further offer help in devising cultural competence training curricula that focus on cultural awareness, cultural self-assessment, and communicating in a multicultural environment.

Other organizational models attempt to simplify and detail how-tos for implementing organizational cultural competence (Lewin Group, 2002). They are short on theory and long on specific action taking. The checklist included in Chapter Three is one such model. Another model, presented in the following outline, was used extensively in training and planning at a national health care organization and in organizational consulting (Gilbert, 1998).

Health care organizations, whether they are large or small, are consistently engaged in ongoing planning: for new services or modifications of existing services, for staffing, for new buildings or changes to the physical plant, and for information technology. Culturally competent planning involves high-level

ESSENTIAL STRUCTURAL COMPONENTS FOR BUILDING CULTURAL COMPETENCE IN HEALTH CARE ORGANIZATIONS

- Knowing who your patients are

  Comprehensive demographic data collection entering ethnicity, racial, and language data on IT systems

  Finding and mobilizing community contacts

- Tracking specific data by patient population subgroups

  Patient and member satisfaction data

  Health status data such as disease epidemiology within the distinct populations served

  Program and intervention data, for example, diabetic control per group

  Access of preventive tests, immunizations by group

  Geographic and service area distribution of racial and ethnic groups

  Use of data for HEDIS goal setting, structuring service delivery

- Assessing and addressing needs

  Understanding regulatory and accreditation requirements

  Integrating ethnic and racial epidemiological information into clinical goal setting and service delivery planning and practice

  Considering geographic distribution of specific groups for clinic placements, staffing needs

  Assessing language needs, setting up translation and interpretation services

- Providing ongoing, integrated cultural competence training

  For clinical staff: continuing medical education, focused seminars, grand rounds, practice specific, for example, pediatrics, OB/GYN, chemical dependency

  For management: culturally aware policy making, up-to-date knowledge of relevant legislation and accreditation requirements

  For frontline staff and support services: signage, communication, cultural food preferences, and so on

- Recruitment and staffing

  Staffing care teams and clinics for effective care of specific racial and ethnic groups

  Providing staff backup for bilingual providers

  Staffing for language concordance and provision of language access

  Staffing interpreters as required to provide language access

- Ongoing assessment

  Analyzing patient satisfaction data by gender, race, ethnicity, and other relevant patient descriptors

  Cutting health outcome data by patient descriptors

  Getting employee feedback on what is working and what isn't

  Getting community feedback

leadership consistently asking cultural competence questions, for example, How do the characteristics of our patient population or the population we wish to serve affect what we are planning? If, for example, a large portion of the population is made up of limited-English speakers, do we need to place connections for **telephonic or video interpretation** in our new exam rooms? Do the waiting rooms of the new clinic need to be enlarged to serve large families? Does our information technology capture the necessary demographic and informational data. For example, are there fields on the new electronic medical record for noting the provision of interpreter services at a patient encounter? Are our health education materials and classes reflective of the language needs of our patients? Does case management reflect cultural knowledge of the populations we serve? How can we include members from our ethnic communities in cultural competence trainings for our clinical and nonclinical staff? Are the signage and way-finding strategies we are employing really helpful to all of our patients? Are the consultants we are hiring to train our front office and reception personnel in communication skills knowledgeable about the multicultural character of our patient populations or do they just have an out-of-the-box training program? Are our food services or nutrition classes reflective of the foods familiar to the cultural groups we serve? Are our chaplains or spiritual leaders representative of the religious character of the communities we serve? True cultural competence resides in the service delivery details and supportive budgets as well as the grand vision and mission statements.

In fact, a leadership-driven strategic approach to cultural competence at the organizational level is so important that Chapters Ten and Eleven of this book focus on it. It is also important to remember that Figure 1.2, "Systems Approach to Diversity and Cultural Competence," is a visual representation of the inter-related processes that together will help ensure a culturally competent health care provider organization. Organizational assessment, including baseline assessment of cultural competence, is an essential component of the systems approach that will also be discussed in Chapters Six, Ten, and Eleven.

CULTURAL COMPETENCE AND THE MULTICULTURAL HEALTH CARE WORKFORCE

Health care in the United States is itself a discrete culture with politics, patient-centered values, workplace norms, multiple related systems, an economy, an occupational structure, and even a complex national discourse involving persons inside and outside the health care culture. Organizations within the health care culture share many common and distinguishing features, one of which is an occupational structure. The occupational structure is hierarchical: within each organization such as a hospital, clinic, health plan, or nursing facility, there are occupational positions at the top of the social class structure, such as surgeons, doctors, dentists, and pharmacists with higher levels of education, and there are entry-level positions such as medical assistants, cooks, janitors, and other service personnel who may have only a high school education and sometimes even less. In the middle of this hierarchy there are multitudes of occupations at varying levels of expertise: middle managers, department heads, nurses, health educators, social workers, audiologists, radiology technicians, and lab assistants, to name only a few of the allied health care providers. The larger the organization, the more multilayered is the occupational stratification.

Adding to the complexity of this class-based structural situation is significant stratification of positions by ethnicity: whites, predominantly, but also many persons of Asian background occupy the highest level clinical and management positions; middle-level positions are filled by a vast mix of ethnicities, but all are predominantly white; and lower-level positions are occupied primarily by Latinos and African Americans (Dione, Moore, Armstrong, & Martinano, 2006). To be sure, this is only the general occupational stratification of the health care work-force and is not representative of any one organization. However, as a result of this class, ethnic, and racial occupational structure, the dominant values and norms of the health care culture and workplace are those of the white middle to upper-middle class. Although upper and mid-level professionals and those who have to meet credentialing or accreditation standards are socialized into or become at least somewhat familiar with the overall cultural values of US health care, the vast array of service and entry-level employees, many of whom are for-eign born, are not and often receive a bare minimum of job-related training, remaining marginal to the patient-oriented culture of health care and its guiding values and norms (Thrall, 2006).

As discussed in Chapter Three, to some extent the stratification in US health care mirrors the class and ethnic structure in the US workforce overall, but there are some aspects of this occupational stratification that are peculiar to health care. Some health care occupations attract specific groups: Asians, for example, are represented in medicine and pharmacy in far greater numbers than their percentage in the overall workforce (Health Sciences Committee, 2004). Because of nursing shortages, large numbers of foreign-born, primarily Filipino, nurses have immigrated to the United States and are represented in significant numbers in that occupation (HRSA, 2010). Because of shortages in computer technologists, some health care organizations have recruited sizeable numbers of Middle Eastern and Indian workers to set up data systems and electronic medical records.

Immigrant professionals occupy positions at many levels of the health care workforce, bringing with them workplace norms and behaviors that may be at odds with or at least different from those usual in the US workplace. These culturally formed norms oftentimes revolve around expected manager-employee relations, managerial style, interactions with fellow workers, trust levels, and age, gender, or class relationships. As was previously pointed out, these cultural concepts are not visible but undergird attitudes and behavior. Sociologists who have studied people of different nationalities working in new corporate environments point out that they bring with them the workplace values and norms enculturated in their countries of origin, and these are not easily replaced by the norms in the new workplace cultures (Adler & Gundersen, 2008; Hofstedt, 2001). Adler and Gundersen (2008) note that managers and other employees brought up in the mores of the US workforce are often unaware that immigrant employees are following different rules for workplace relationships. This situation can interfere with the kind of teamwork that is critical in health care organizations. Understanding the concept of culture and how it can play out in the workplace is important in maintaining smoothly operating multicultural teams.

Josie, a woman from Africa, and usually a very effective lead nurse on a med-surg ward, appeared to be unable to give directions to or discipline a new, older nurse on the unit even though she had had no problems in this regard with the other nurses under her supervision, After complaints from several other nurses that the new arrival was "getting away with murder," the nursing director sat down to discuss the situation with Josie. The nurse was aware of the problem but said she found it almost painful to reprimand or firmly direct someone so much older than she.

How should the nursing director handle this situation?

Cultural differences in the way that gender and occupational position are viewed may create conflict between US-trained nurses and some physicians born and educated elsewhere because US nurses do not take well to public dressings down from doctors who feel that their gender, superior position, and education gives them this right. Cultural differences in the formality of male-female relations can cause issues: for example, modest Filipino nurses in a hospital were frightened and upset by the cheerful, seemingly flirtatious remarks directed to them by an African American mail clerk as he rolled his cart through the wards. Relationships between supervisors and employees are viewed differently across cultures, as one manager discovered after his foreign-born assistant returned from a visit to his home country with a gift of expensive stones because the manager had a lapidary hobby. Gifts to superiors were expected in the home country but this costly gift embarrassed the manager, who thought it inappropriate; he felt he had to turn it down and had a hard time explaining to his employee the nature of supervisor-employee relationships considered appropriate in the United States. Another department manager was shocked when the elderly father of the Indian lab tech she had placed on an action plan showed up in her office to let her know that he would see that his daughter "obeyed" her properly. These are very obvious differences that surfaced because they were reported to human resources departments but many cultural differences in the workplace don't become apparent at all, though they may negatively affect working relationships.

Researchers (Hofstedt, Hofstedt, & Minkov, 2005) who have examined multicultural workplaces note that problematic cultural differences in workplace values and norms are often not recognized by managers because of a phenomenon called *projected similarity*. Projected similarity is the assumption that people are more similar to you than they actually are. It involves perceiving that an action, event, or situation has the same meaning or interpretation across cultures when it actually does not. Although much cultural competence training in health care emphasizes this phenomenon as it operates between providers and patients, it is at play in the multicultural workforce as well.

In the new paradigms of patient-centered medical homes and care management models of care, there is a particularly great emphasis on cross-occupational integration and teamwork in maintaining adequate continuity in patient care. This means that members from differing cultures and occupation levels must work collaboratively in their day-to-day work lives and must overcome often conflicting work-related perspectives and values. This frequently requires that, before health care organizations can work effectively with their multicultural patients, they need to explore biases, prejudices, and differing culturally shaped work-related norms prevalent in the workplace itself (Adler, 1991).

With the intent of meeting the needs of a large contingent of Armenian-speaking persons in their service area, Health Plan XXX opened a family practice module staffed by Armenian-speaking doctors, nurses, and frontline staff. Because this group was made up of native Armenian speakers, almost all of them were immigrants. They were linguistically and culturally Armenian and unconsciously fell into patterns of Armenian interaction values and roles. This module was assigned to one department administrator after another, none of whom were of Armenian background or spoke Armenian. They always failed in managing the conflicts that arose in the module, and had difficulty implementing some of the broader organizational directives within the module. The most recent administrator admitted to the management consultant who was asked by the CEO to evaluate the situation that "I just can never figure out what is really going on!"

What recommendations could the management consultant have made to the CEO?

The multicultural health care workforce can be a significant and rich resource for cultural competence but only if a spirit of openness and collaboration prevails. Training for collaborative work in a multicultural and sometimes multilingual health care workplace often begins in new employee orientation and can be reinforced through performance evaluations. Human resource personnel, supervisors, and managers should be given training in crosscultural conflict resolution (Myers & Filner, 1997) and cultural differences in workplace attitudes and behavior. More complete treatment of workforce diversity management will be covered in Chapters Ten and Eleven of this book but it is important to underscore here that cultural competence in health care workplace relations is a basic feature of culturally competent health care systems.

SUMMARY

The need for cultural competence in health care is being driven by a confluence of factors: changes in the cultural composition of the nation's population, pervasive disparities in health status across population groups, and changes in the structure of health care delivery systems. True cultural competence requires an understanding of culture and its compelling impact on people. Though culture is universal, the content of cultures is not. Cultural competence in health care is a recognition that cultures differ in perceptions around bodily and mental health, the reality of disease, and the certainty of death. At the personal level, care providers honor a culture that guides and shapes their patients' thoughts and actions, knowing that this attitude will enhance trust and collaboration in their treatment. This is particularly important now that health care is embracing patient-centered and personalized care.

At the organizational level, shared knowledge of cultures and how people are guided by them in their health interactions with institutions make it easier to create delivery systems that are truly responsive to the needs of their patients. The best models for cultural competence in health care emphasize a prepared, willing, and collaborative staff and some very concrete actions and behaviors that enable a health care organization to serve a multicultural patient base. These models are short on theoretical formulations and long on specific actions and practices. They emphasize the need for information and data-driven planning, integrating an understanding of culture and specific group needs into outreach, treatment, and care management. Additionally, leaders of culturally competent organizations do not make the assumption that all health care workers enter the workplace with similar work-related norms, attitudes, and expectations. Culture shapes people's ideas about the value of work and the nature of workplace interactions and these may differ considerably across groups.

KEY TERMS

acculturation	cultural humility
bicultural	cultural identity
CLAS standards	cultural relevancy
cultural awareness	cultural sensitivity

epidemiological transition

ethnic group

ethnocentrism

explanatory models

internalized

national origin group

projected similarity

socialization

stereotyping

subcultures

telephonic or video interpreting
interpretation

REVIEW QUESTIONS AND ACTIVITIES

1. What is cultural competence in health care?

2. Where does culture come from? Does your culture affect the way *you* see things? How?

3. What is the difference between a racial group, a national origin group, and an ethnic group? Can a person belong to all three kinds of groups? Are there persons in the class that belong to all three?

4. What is the point of categorizing different groups of people in health care?

5. Are there persons from different subcultures in this class? Discuss how these subcultures differ from the mainstream and also what they share with the mainstream.

6. What is meant by "to have culture is human nature, but no culture is human nature"? Discuss this idea in class.

7. Discuss the differences among the terms *cultural awareness, cultural sensitivity, cultural awareness, cultural competence*, and *cultural humility*. Which ones of these do you aspire to in your work within the health system?

8. Have you seen instances of projected similarity? Discuss these.

REFERENCES

Acosta, Y. D., & de la Cruz, C. P. (2011). *The foreign born from Latin America and the Caribbean: 2010.* American Community Survey Briefs. Washington, DC: US Census Bureau.

Adler, N. (1991). *International dimensions of organizational behavior.* Boston: PWS Kent Publishing.

Adler, N. J., & Gundersen, A. (2008). *International dimensions of organizational behavior* (4th ed.). Mason, OH: Thomson South-Western.

Centers for Disease Control. (2011). *Communities at risk.* National Prevention Information Network. Retrieved from www.cdcnpin.org/scripts/population/culture.asp

Crisman, N. J., & Maretzki, T. W. (Eds.). (1982). *Clinically applied anthropology.* Dordrecht, The Netherlands: D. Reidel.

Cross, T., Bazon, D., & Isaacs, M. (1989). *Towards a culturally competent system of care* (Vol. 1). Washington, DC: Georgetown University Child Development Center.

The Cross Cultural Health Care Program. (1996). *Voices of the communities.* Seattle: Author. Retrieved from http://ethnomed.org/culture/other-groups/others/1/1/voices-of-the-communities-series-cross-cultural-health-care-program

Culhane-Pera, K. A., Vawter, D. E., Xiong, P., Babbitt, B., & Solberg, M. M. (2004). *Healing by heart. Clinical and ethical case stories of Hmong families and western providers.* Nashville: The Vanderbilt Press.

Davis, K. (1997). *Exploring the interaction between cultural competency and managed behavioral health care policy: Implications for state and county mental health agencies.* Alexandria, VA: National Technical Assistance Center for State Mental Health.

Department of Health and Human Services. (1986). *Report of the secretary's task force on black and minority health* (Vols. I and II). Washington, DC: Author. Retrieved from www.eric.ed.gov/ERICWEBPortal/search/detaining.jsp?_nfpb=true&_&ERICEvtSearch

Dionne, M., Moore, E., Armstrong, D., & Martinano, R. (2006). *The United States health workforce profile.* Rensselaer, NY: Center for Health Workforce Studies, School of Public Health, SUNY Albany.

Fadiman, A. (1997). *The spirit catches you and you fall down: A Hmong child, her American doctors, and the collision of two cultures.* New York: The Noonday Press.

Farmer, P. (2001). *Infections and inequalities: The modern plagues.* Berkeley: University of California Press.

Gilbert, M. J. (1998). *Six discussions on diversity for upper level managers.* Unpublished training program used at Kaiser Permanente, Southern California Region.

Goode, T., Dunne, C., & Bronheim, S. (2006). *The evidence base for cultural competency.* New York: The Commonwealth Fund.

Hofstedt, G. (2001). *Culture's consequences: Comparing values, behaviors, institutions and organizations across nations* (2nd ed.). Thousand Oaks, CA: Sage Publications.

Hofstedt, G., Hofstedt, G. J., & Minkov, M. (2005). *Cultures and organizations: Software of the mind* (3rd ed.). New York: McGraw-Hill.

Institute for Health Care Improvement. (2011). *Patient-centered care on medical surgical units.* Retrieved from www.ihi.org/knowledge/Pages/Changes/PatientCenteredCare.aspx

Kleinman, A. (1980). *Patients and healers in the context of culture.* Berkeley: University of California Press.

Kleinman, A., Eisenberg, L., & Good, B. (1978). Culture, illness and care. *Annals of Internal Medicine, 88*, 251–258.

Lavizzo-Mourey, L., & MacKenzie, E. R. (1996). Essential measurements of quality for managed care organizations. *Annals of Internal Medicine, 124* (10), 919–921.

Leininger, M. (1978). *Transcultural nursing concepts: Theories and practices.* Columbus, OH: Grayden Press.

Lewis, O. (1959). *Five families: Mexican case studies in the culture of poverty.* New York: Basic Books.

Meyers, S., & Filner, B. (1997). *Conflict resolution across cultures: From talking it out to third party mediation.* Amherst, MA: Amherst Educational Publishing.

National Center for Cultural Competence. (nd). *Conceptual frameworks: Models, guiding values, and principles.* Retrieved from http://www11.georgetown.edu/research/gucchd/nccc/foundations/fremeworks.html

National Institute of Medicine. (2001). *Crossing the quality chasm: A new health system for the 21st century.* Washington, DC: The National Academies Press.

National Quality Forum. (2010). *Cultural competency measures and implementation strategies.* Retrieved from www.qualityforum.org/Projects/c-d/Cultural_Competency_2010/Cultural_Competency_2010.aspx

Office of Minority Health. (2001). *National standards for culturally and linguistically appropriate services in health care: Final report.* Retrieved from http://minorityhealth.hhs.gov/assets/pdf/checked/finalreport.pdf

Omran, A. R. (1982). *Epidemiologic transition: International encyclopedia of population.* New York: Free Press.

Pedersen, P. B. (1988). *A handbook for developing multicultural awareness.* Alexandria, VA: American Counseling Association.

Smedley, B. D., Stith, A. M., & Nelson, A. R. (2002). *Unequal treatment: Confronting racial and ethnic disparities in health care.* Washington, DC: The National Academy Press.

Tervalon, M., & Murray-Garcia, J. (1998). Cultural humility vs. cultural competency: A critical distinction in defining physician training in cultural competency. *Journal of Health Care for the Poor and Underserved, 9*(2), 119–125.

Thrall, J. H. (2006). Education and cultural development of the health care workforce Part II. Opportunities for nonprofessional workers. *Radiology, 240*, 11–214.

The Western Journal of Medicine, 139(6). (1983). Special issue: Cross-cultural medicine.

The Western Journal of Medicine, 157(3). (1992). Special issue: Cross-cultural medicine a decade later.

Wilson-Stronks, A., Lee, K. K., Cordero, C. L., Kopp, M. L. & Galvez, E. (2008). *One size does not fit all: Meeting the health care needs of diverse populations.* Oakbrook Terrace, IL: The Joint Commission.

Chapter 5

HALLMARKS OF CULTURAL COMPETENCE IN HEALTH CARE PROFESSIONALS

LEARNING OBJECTIVES

- To identify challenges for health care professionals and their organizations in "walking the talk" of cultural competence

- To describe how shared values in the health care professions provide the foundation for cultural competence

- To use the Grubb Institute's transforming experiences framework to describe role development of culturally competent health care professionals

- To engage in an activity-based process of self-discovery and action planning that is grounded in the Grubb Institute's transforming experiences framework to develop and improve individual cultural competence

This chapter builds on Chapter Four by providing an opportunity to explore the **hallmarks** or distinguishing characteristics of culturally competent health care professionals and to enhance the reader's own cultural competence. We will view health care professionals in the context of their roles within a health care delivery system, consistent with the systems approach used throughout this book.

First, we explore the relationship between cultural competence and the values and ethical codes of conduct that undergird the health care professions, codes, and expectations that are at times in stark contrast to the reality of the professionals' daily working life. We examine how the contrast between expectations and reality when coupled with the human fear of differences and preference for similarity can lead to a culture of denial and de facto exclusion, even in health care organizations and on the part of health care professionals who express the best of intentions. We explain how self-development of the hallmarks of cultural competence rests on the health professional's readiness for personal growth and willingness to engage in self-reflection, including acknowledging one's own **implicit biases**, perceptual filters, and cultural blind spots.

Second, we present the Grubb Institute's transforming experience framework (http://www.grubb.org.uk/; Bazalgette, Irvine, & Quine, 2006; Reed, 2001) as a valuable reference point for self-reflection on the hallmarks of culturally competent health care professionals. The **transforming experiences framework** is grounded in the following personal and systems characteristics: (1) self-awareness, (2) desire, (3) resources, and (4) purpose and describes the relationships among four factors: person, context, system, and role. Self-awareness requires a balanced and realistic sense of one's own strengths and weaknesses as a culturally competent health care professional, and desire requires a commitment to continued learning and self-development in the context of diversity. As the Grubb Institute framework attests, personal growth also requires resources in the individual and the organization to gain and sustain cultural competence, including a systemwide commitment to the healing purpose of health care.

In the final section, we discuss the role that self-discovery plays in enabling each of us as an individual health care professional to successfully manage our self and interact with others in the context of diversity. A series of exercises provide the reader with the opportunity to engage personally in the self-discovery process. Consistent with the Grubb Institute model, specific activities focus on the person, context, and system and culminate with development of an individual action plan that, when implemented, will help to ensure that readers are able to enact their own health care professional roles as exemplars of cultural competence in action. Additional related exercises and strategies for self-development are included in other chapters, notably in Chapter Six.

PERSONAL JOURNEY OF CULTURAL COMPETENCE

It is tempting to oversimplify the journey of individual cultural competence or to assume it is unnecessary and to rely instead on the belief that one's professional status and training alone ensure cultural competence. But, are we culturally competent because we believe we are? Are we culturally competent because we want to be? Honest self-reflection, a willingness to accept feedback and to disclose the truth about our own values, beliefs, and behaviors, are essential if individual health care providers and the systems in which they deliver care are to exhibit the hallmarks of cultural competence in everyday interactions with patients, families, and with one another. Fear of being labeled as culturally incompetent is perhaps the most powerful barrier to the personal journey that is required to develop and enact the hallmarks of cultural competence as a health care professional. As discussed in the next section, it strikes at the very core of what it means to be a caring health professional. And, as described in Chapter Four, cultural competence is grounded in an **attitude** and state of mind but must be evidenced through the knowledge and skills used in clinical practice.

A Dilemma for the Health Care Professional

The compelling ethical nature of the health care professional's role demands a person to be culturally competent, yet that has not been necessarily the case in real world practice. The philosophical stance of health care creates an expectation that health care professionals will provide high-level services and care regardless of the diverse backgrounds of the patients.

Clinicians are especially trapped in this conundrum: if I am a clinician, then I am automatically held accountable to my ethical code of conduct that clearly states that I will practice without prejudice and the use of stereotypes. Given this, acknowledging the need for training to become culturally competent can be viewed as a confession of past unethical behavior by a clinician. Thus, clinicians may find it easier to just assume that in becoming a clinician, one simultaneously and automatically becomes culturally competent because working to improve one's cultural competence would first require acknowledging that one has work to do.

This dissonance between the philosophical code of conduct and reality is one of the unspoken challenges in health care. Without acknowledging that all health care professionals are human and, thus, come to their work with personal baggage packed with stereotypes and biases, there is no motivation for learning and training to acquire and maintain cultural competence. But, for any training to be effective, a gap has to be identified and a desire to close the gap must be acknowledged for the cultural competence development process to begin.

The philosophy that undergirds the values of the health professions speaks strongly to being responsive to differences by personalizing the caring and healing process and by tailoring evidence-based health care practices to the needs of individuals within the context of the patient's culture. To do so requires a strong foundation of cultural sensitivity, awareness, and competence. But the reality of interactions in the day-to-day work settings and lives of health care professionals can reveal a gap between the real and the ideal, a gap that conscious and focused effort can close. Later in this chapter, we offer the Grubb Institute framework and a series of self-development activities grounded in the framework to close the gap between the real and the ideal: culturally competent personalized care for every patient.

Readiness for Self-Development

To develop the personal hallmarks of cultural competence, health care professionals must first be ready. Avolio and Hannah (2008) identified five constructs that constitute their **model of developmental readiness:** learning goal orientation, developmental efficacy, self-concept clarity, self-complexity, and metacognitive ability. Their model indicates that readiness to develop cultural competence requires the following of health care professionals:

- *Learning goal orientation:* Seeing ourselves as works-in-progress and using positive and negative feedback about our cultural competence to develop our full potential

- *Developmental efficacy:* Having confidence in our own ability to be culturally competent

- *Self-concept clarity:* Knowing ourselves as we really are and demonstrating a balanced and realistic sense of our strengths and areas for development as culturally competent health care professionals

- *Self-complexity:* Being cognizant of our own complexity as an individual, including an awareness of how our formative life experiences and our own diverse group identities such as ethnicity, generation, and gender influence who we are in the context of diversity

- *Metacognitive ability:* Being self-aware of what we really think about diversity, engaging in honest self-reflection about how our thinking affects our emotional responses and actions in the context of diversity, and regulating our own thinking through **cognitive reframing**

How would you assess yourself against Avolio and Hannah's (2008) five criteria? Are you developmentally ready to improve your own cultural competence? The final section of this chapter includes diversity and cultural competence awareness exercises that require you to draw on your learning goal orientation, developmental efficacy, self-concept clarity, self-complexity, and metacognitive ability to identify your own areas of strength and areas for self-development as a culturally competent health care professional.

The Challenge of Implicit Bias

Implicit bias speaks to the challenge our own human nature presents to us as we strive to be culturally competent health care professionals. Biases are attitudes, that is, favorable or unfavorable dispositions. Each of us—even the most experienced and highly educated health care professionals—harbors two types of bias: **explicit biases** that we are aware we hold and implicit biases that operate outside of our conscious awareness.

An interesting approach to uncovering personal hidden biases is the Implicit Association Test (IAT), which is based on the research of Anthony Greenwald of the University of Washington and Mahzarin Banaji of Harvard University (Greenwald & Banaji, 1995). These web-based self-assessments prompt the user to link words with images that appear on the computer screen. The links reveal the user's mental associations or automatic preferences, which are indicative of the user's tendency to view one identity group more positively than another.

IATs are available on Project Implicit's website (https://implicit.harvard.edu/implicit/demo/) to self-assess your own implicit biases on the following diversity dimensions and more: black-white, gay-straight, gender-career, and old-young.

IAT results indicate (Nosek, Banaji, & Greenwald, 2002) that we collectively share common biases that favor in-groups over out-groups, such as white over black and young over old, and that these biases are evident even among out-group members such as African Americans or older people. As Dunham, Baron, and Banaji (2006) explain, preferences for society's in-groups and biases against out-groups are likely a product of our socialization, which is consistent with the social transmission theory of prejudice formation first identified by renowned psychologist and researcher Gordon Allport (1954) in his classic book, *The Nature of Prejudice*.

A recent meta-analysis of published research on the relationship between implicit bias, as measured by the IAT (Greenwald, Poehlman, Uhlmann, & Banaji, 2009) and behavior concluded that "the predictive validity of IAT measures significantly exceeded the predictive validity of self-report measures" (p. 32) for topics with high social sensitivity such as interracial and other interpersonal behavior related to group identity and diversity. So, our implicit biases are a better predictor of our behavior than are our self-reported explicit biases.

A case in point from health care demonstrates that we may harbor implicit biases that lead us to behave in a biased fashion when delivering health care even when we believe and state explicitly that we are not biased. Green and his colleagues (2007) created a clinical vignette of a patient in the emergency room with acute coronary syndrome and presented the vignette, with race randomized, to a sample of medical residents. A questionnaire to measure explicit bias and three IATs to measure implicit bias were administered to the medical residents: black-white race preference, perceptions of black-white cooperativeness with medical procedures, and perceptions of black-white cooperativeness in general.

The medical residents in the study self-reported no race preference and no race-based perceptions of differences in cooperativeness on the explicit measure. However, the IATs revealed the following:

- *Implicit* preference for whites

- *Implicit* stereotypes of blacks as less cooperative with medical procedures *and* less cooperative in general

The researchers (Green et al., 2007, p. 1231) concluded that "as physicians' pro-white implicit bias increased, so did their likelihood of treating white patients and not treating black patients with thrombolysis," which are drugs that reduce the risk of blood clots. The bottom line: being a highly educated and well-meaning health care professional does not inoculate a person from the influence of his or her own implicit bias on treatment decisions.

The impact of implicit bias is also evident in our brain functions, as evidenced by a study by Stanley, Phelps, and Banaji (2008) in which MRI brain scans of white respondents who were taking the black-white IAT evidenced greater activation of the amygdala—a region that processes alarm—when showed images of black faces than when shown white faces. However, given longer processing time, the anterior cingulate cortex and the dorsolateral prefrontal cortex—regions that temper automatic responses—were shown to moderate amygdala activation. Furthermore, the researchers found that exposure to images of friendly faces can help control the amygdala. In a *Time Magazine* article on the study (Klueger, 2008), Dr. Phelps is quoted as saying, "The more you think about people as individuals, the more the brain calms down" (p. 36). It is important, therefore, for health care professionals to acknowledge to ourselves that we do have implicit bias and consciously strive to move past those biases to see the patient in front of us as a unique individual deserving the best-quality care we can deliver. We must first surface and acknowledge our implicit biases and then consciously strive to manage their impact on our behavior as health care professionals. A way to do this through cognitive reframing is discussed later in this chapter.

In a comparative study of majority in-group implicit bias against minority out-groups in the United States and Japan (Dunham, Baron, & Banaji, 2006), white Americans were found to consistently favor white over Japanese and white over black. But, although white over Japanese explicit bias lessened as the respondents' age cohort increased from six-year-olds to ten-year-olds to adults, there was no age-related decline in the strength of the white-over-black implicit bias. As a group, white American children were significantly more likely to show explicit in-group preference than was the adult comparison group. Furthermore, in-group preference was greater when the out-group was black than when it was Japanese, irrespective of subject age. Similar results were found in Japan when the in-group was ethnic Japanese, the high-status out-group was whites, and the low-status out-group blacks.

The researchers concluded that automatic implicit attitudes are a by-product of social categorization and suggest that "fostering the creation of more inclusive in-groups that cut across the usually divisive lines of race and gender could make a virtue of what first appears a vice" (Dunham, Baron, & Banaji, 2006, p. 1280). The process of personal and health systems organizational development in this text is designed to do just that.

Previously in this text we presented a framework for the systems approach to diversity and cultural competence (Figure 1.2), reviewed how demographic and cultural diversity affect health care providers and organizations, discussed the challenges of patient and workforce diversity and disparities, and laid the foundation for cultural competence. In the discussion in this chapter, we demonstrate the challenge that building cultural competence presents to health care professionals who must confront the dissonance between role expectations and their own actual culturally competence, ensure that they are open and ready for self-development and growth as a culturally competent individual in the context of diversity, and identify, acknowledge, and address the impact of their own strengths and weakness.

Professional Values as a Foundation for Cultural Competence

Each of the health professions espouses a **value system** or a hierarchy of beliefs and convictions that guide the practitioner's conduct and choices. Consistently, the passion for healing and making a difference in the lives of others is a fundamental value expressed by health care professions and organizations. For example, the National League for Nursing (NLN) (2007) expresses its members' shared values as follows:

- *Caring:* Promoting health, healing, and hope in response to the human condition
- *Integrity:* Respecting the dignity and moral wholeness of every person without conditions or limitation
- *Diversity:* Affirming the uniqueness of and differences among persons, ideas, values, and ethnicities
- *Excellence:* Creating and implementing transformative strategies with daring ingenuity

A value-based foundation permeates the work life and career of all of the health care professions. Yet in the heat of the race, the day-to-day work settings of a clinician or administrator, these values are frequently displaced by the realities of a chaotic and complex health care environment. Perhaps this displacement occurs easily because the health care professional may not have delved into the meaning and application of each value. Practicing cultural competence in the context of diversity is about understanding one's self and each other and moving beyond simple tolerance to embracing and celebrating the richness of each individual. To do so requires self-reflection. Unless each health care professional and organization integrates and internalizes the values that drive health care delivery and develops the cultural competencies to live those values in real time, those values will be rapidly displaced in the real world.

Psychology of the Health Care Professional

Clinicians consistently rank among the Gallup poll's most trusted professionals, with nurses, pharmacists, and physicians ranking first, second, and third, respectively (Jones, 2011). The idealized conceptions of the professional role by the public and the clinician inspire trust in the patient and serve to recruit like-minded aspiring health professionals into the field. So, it is usually with the altruistic goal of helping the other that the desire for the health care professional role is conceived. The patient may also be idealized as, for example, a vulnerable, needy child or older adult who is worthy of receiving care and appreciative of the care received. Reality can be to the contrary and results in stress and disillusionment for the health care provider.

Trust can be especially challenging to establish when there is a lack of concordance between health care provider and patient on significant diversity dimensions such as race, ethnicity, gender, religion, or primary language. Although educational institutions that prepare health care professionals for practice in the field do attempt to provide experiences that highlight differences in populations served as well as differences in team members, these clinical experiences are frequently small isolated doses of the reality of differences that await the clinician-in-training in the work setting. In addition, there is often little opportunity to unpack the aspiring clinician's or administrator's own personal baggage because most curricula are not designed to explore the impact of one's self in the health care system. One's self is simply the black box through which all the clinical experience is filtered, translated, and acted on with the other. It's dangerous not to have identified the contents of the black box and can intensify the difference between the ideal and the reality of one's cultural competence.

Imagine the following situation: The white female nursing student was taking the patient's pulse to determine his heart rate. The patient, a very dark-skinned African man, described his experience of being touched by the white female nursing student as if his skin were dirty and expressed feeling that her desire was to make the least amount of physical contact possible. What if you were the white female nursing student in this patient encounter? How would you respond to the patient's feedback? How would you explain the patient's perception? Whether he did indeed experience bias or prejudice or simply the nervousness that may accompany learning a new skill is not knowable. But in the end, the patient felt dehumanized and devalued by the experience. If the nursing student had greater awareness of racial dynamics and training in managing the interaction in a way that minimizes negative potential while enhancing positive potential, her approach and the patient's experience may have been different.

Human Fear of Difference and the Culture of Exclusion

Another contributing factor that can result in a gap between ideal and real in health care is the very human fear of differences. Health care professionals, like the rest of society, are challenged by human fears of differences and, thus, are susceptible to unconsciously operating from a model of exclusion rather than inclusion. The ideals of inclusion that are valued and promulgated by the profession and espoused by the clinician are often selectively applied in daily interactions (Malone, 1993).

There is a comfort level of security, perhaps false security, which comes with homogeneity and the lack of differentiation. According to Klein (1984), it begins early and presents itself in the baby's fear of separating from the mother in the early years of child development. Gutmann (2003) discusses this fear of separation and its relationship to the human fear of the "other." Underrepresented minority groups can be readily available targets of fear of the other. Gutmann (2003) concludes that without engaging with the other, there is no personal transformation. Self-righteousness and the belief in one's own "purity" can be facades that bind health professionals and others into unrealistic role expectations and self-concepts that prevent engagement with the reality of the need to build higher levels of cultural competence in ourselves and our organizations. The perfect and the flawed, the black and the white, the gentle and the tough are threads of the fabric of life that we yearn to simplify through distinguishing ourselves and those we perceive to be like us from the "other."

FRAMEWORK FOR ROLE DEVELOPMENT

Bazalgette, Irvine, and Quine (2006) of the Grubb Institute state clearly that taking a role cannot be simply an automatic, semiconscious reflex; it must be a process that takes into account one's gifts and limitations as well as an understanding of the context and system in which one plays the role. As the Grubb Institute's transforming experience framework (Figure 5.1) illustrates, action that serves the purpose of the organization results from the health care professional's enactment of his or her role. And how we enact our roles reflects the following:

FIGURE 5.1 Grubb Institute's Transforming Experience Framework

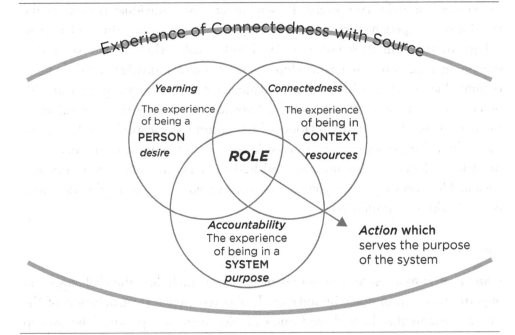

Source: Reprinted with permission of the Grubb Institute.

- Who we are and aspire to be as a person

- The contexts in which we were socialized as a person and a health care professional as well as the organizational context, including the community and society

- The system or the health care organization in which we enact our role with accountability to serve its purpose or mission

Following is an overview of each of the four aspects of the transforming experience framework as applied to role enactment of the culturally competent health care professional. Person, context, system, and role are all affected by the health care professional's broader life philosophy, which the model refers to as "experience of connectedness with source." Thus, our life philosophy is an overarching influence on how we enact our professional roles, which in turn reflect our understanding of person, context, and system.

Person

Person is described as the locus of desire, a desire for transformation, and a desire to become culturally competent. Person rather than individual is used in the transforming experience framework to emphasize the connectedness of human beings, to view ourselves not as isolated individuals, when it may seem that everything exists only in relationship to our isolated individual needs, but as persons able to engage with others, interconnected and seeking engagement with others for affirmation, affection, and acknowledgment. It is the core values of the person that form the foundation of a transformative experience. It is these core values that attract others to invest loyalty in and support of the person in the role as clinician, administrator, and leader. What are your core values as a person? How do they affect your desire to enact your role as a culturally competent health care professional?

Context

Context refers to a reservoir of abundant resources, including the challenges and opportunities within one's boundaries. It also represents a constellation of the various systems that have shaped one's development as a person. The overlap identified in Figure 5.1 points to the effect that context has on person and, of course, a person has on context. For example, an African American person growing up in rural Kentucky during the fifties before integration experienced a different context in his or her formative years than an African American person growing up in the seventies in an integrated ethnically diverse urban community. Both contexts provide resources but different ones. As with any resource, there is always a resisting force, that is, a challenge that can obscure the person's ability to see and use the resources internally and externally available. Progress, growth, and success, all characteristics of excellent leadership, are earned and measured against obstacles, challenges, and resistances.

The context of the health care system itself also affects enactment of the role of a culturally competent health care professional. Take, for example, a southern university hospital steeped in tradition and respected as a great care-giving institution, but with a context that includes a history of discrimination and enforcing Jim Crow laws during the days of segregation when hospital, schools, water fountains, and lodging were separate. This context provided daunting challenges for its clinicians and leaders to be perceived as culturally competent, even if engaging in best practices. Many in the external African American community may continue to fear the hospital and distrust its leadership. Acknowledging the truth and the impact of this historical context while striving to build a new context of inclusion are all essential parts of the cultural competence process.

System

System is the structure for achieving shared purpose. Balzagette, Irvine, and Quine (2006) define a system as a web of human activities within a boundary, which differentiates that system from other systems in their context. The authors further emphasize that every activity within the system boundary is reflected in the system as a whole; therefore, changing a system in part has an effect on the whole of the system.

The legitimate primary purpose of a health care organization is to provide safe quality care to all patients, irrespective of gender, race, ethnicity, primary language, sexual orientation, or other diversity dimensions. To achieve this purpose requires leadership commitment. However, some health care systems may not have been designed for their legitimate and ideal purpose but rather for the convenience and well-being of the staff, the reputation of its physicians, the accomplishment of its financial goals, or another less lofty purpose. When a misshapen purpose is the guiding framework, the likelihood of culturally competent clinicians and leaders is diminished. The concept of a person with desire as the stimulus for action seeking to engage with others using and managing the context is achieved through a systems framework with a supportive purpose, as illustrated in Figure 1.2.

Role

Role is the resultant manifestation (behavior) of integrating person (desire), context (resources), and system (purpose). Taking up the role requires disciplined behavior to serve the purpose of the system. Role does not exist without person, context, or system. The role of clinician requires extensive academic and experiential preparation with usually some ritualistic boundary that is crossed before taking on one's professional identity, for example, an academic credential or licensure. Health care educators speak of socializing their students into the professional role. This alludes to a shared mental representation of how a nurse, doctor, physical therapist, or health care administrator behaves in clinical and nonclinical settings. Taking a health care role demands not only academic preparation but also mental and emotional work to consciously shape one's behavior to confom with the mental representation espoused by teachers, leaders, and mentors, and then integrate into one's own picture of a clinician or leader. The more the person is aware of role taking and makes conscious choices about how to manifest that role, the more opportunity there is to learn and practice cultural competence. This shaping and integration is not done in a vacuum but must be tailored to the particular system within which the clinician or administrator is working. If a system values diversity, then there is more pressure on persons in health care professional roles to exhibit behavior that reflects value for diversity.

JOURNEY OF SELF-DISCOVERY

This section contains a series of self-exploration exercises that are organized around the Grubb Institute's transforming experiences framework. Insights gained through the personal journey provide a strong foundation for the development of cultural and linguistic competence in the health professional, which is reflected in how we communicate with patients and colleagues and the decisions we make in health care organizations.

Person: Who Am I?

The following exercises encourage the reader to self-reflect and consider how group identities and implicit bias affect interactions among patients and health care professionals. Then, the reader is introduced to cognitive reframing as a tool to manage the impact of his or her own group identities and implicit biases.

Group Identity Circle

Draw a circle. Think of the groups you personally identify with and divide your circle into pie slices, each representing one of your identity groups with the size of the pie slice representing how important that group is to your own identity. Choose one of your identity groups and recall a positive experience that made you proud to be a member of that group. For the same or another group, recall a negative experience that caused pain because of your group membership. How do your group identities influence your values, beliefs, or behaviors? Who you are as a person results not only from your individual temperament or personality but also from the groups you identify with and how you experience your group identities. For example, you and your colleague may share the same ethnic or gender identity group but you may experience that identity differently. What personal strengths and challenges does this activity reveal to you in the role of culturally competent health care professional? How will you build on the strengths and address the challenges?

1. *Group identity and personal experience.* Exploring how we experience our group affiliations can provide us with more insight into the roles that racial, ethnic, gender, and other group identities play in our personal interactions within health care organizations. This section leads the reader through a series of interviews designed to increase awareness of the power and impact of group identities on our individual experiences and responses.

   Interview three individuals: a person of color, a woman, and a person with a disability. Ask each one the following question: What does it mean to be (blank)? Fill in the blank with only one characteristic, that is, the person's race, gender, or physical ability. Jot down their responses. Interview three other individuals: a white person of either gender, a male of any race, and an able-bodied person of any race or gender. Ask each one the same question: What does it mean to be (blank)? Keep the question focused only on the specific group-identity characteristic under discussion. If the interviewee starts talking about another group-identity characteristic—for example, if the individual addresses the question, What does it mean to be white? and begins to discuss what it means to be a woman or to be Jewish—take steps to bring the discussion back to being white. Jot down the responses of each interviewee.

Then, ask a colleague or friend to interview you. Be aware of your responses and your feelings during the interview process. Compare the interviews. Was it easier for minority group members to talk about the meaning of their race or gender than it was for majority group members? Did majority group members seem to be aware of any privileges and entitlements they may have experienced as a consequence of their group identity? Did minority group members discuss discrimination, prejudice, or stereotypes they may have experienced as a result of their group identity? Does group identity carry the same meaning with the same intensity of feeling for majority and minority group members? What personal strengths and challenges does this activity reveal to you in the role of a culturally competent health care professional? How will you build on the strengths and address the challenges?

2. *Implicit bias assessment.* Go to the Harvard Implicit website and take at least three implicit attitude tests (https://implicit.harvard.edu). What did you think, feel, and do when you received your results? Are they the results you expected? Do you believe the results are valid? Why or why not? What do you think the results mean? What personal strengths and challenges does this activity reveal to you in your role as a culturally competent health care professional? How will you build on your strengths and address your challenges?

3. *Cognitive reframing.* Cognitive reframing is a technique for intervening in the chain of what we think, feel, and do by changing the thought that starts the chain. Imagine, for example that you're a nurse providing discharge instructions to an obese patient with type 2 diabetes and the IAT revealed that you have an implicit bias in favor of thin over fat. Your think, feel, do chain might go like this:

Think: "Fat people are lazy and unmotivated; no matter what I tell her she'll just go home and eat whatever she feels like and get even fatter. We'll see her in here again soon with more diabetic complications."

Feel: Disgusted and unmotivated to communicate with the patient

Do: Go through the motions of describing lifestyle changes to reduce weight and manage diabetes but without feeling.

How might this health care encounter change if instead you reframed your thought?

Think: "It's hard to lose weight but some patients do succeed. Perhaps this patient will be a success story!"

Feel: Empathetic with the patient and willing to communicate

Do: Talk about the challenges of weight loss, listen to the patient's feedback, and refer the patient to community-based support services for weight loss and diabetes management.

Our thoughts structure our experiences and thus frame what we feel and what we do. When we change our thoughts, we change our feeling and thus act differently. We can also change our actions, which over time can change our thoughts. For example, imagine you're a Gen X health care administrator trying to get your baby boomer nurses to buy into the electronic medical record (EMR) system, which was just adopted at great expense to the organization:

Think: "Those baby boomer nurses are so set in their ways and ignorant of technology; I wish those dinosaurs would just retire!"

Feel: Anger and frustration

Do: Work around the problem by hiring Gen Y support staff to shadow the nurses and do data entry at a high cost to the organization and to the quality of bedside care.

Perhaps you aren't quite ready to reframe your thought but taking a different course of action might get you to that point. Alternative actions might include incentives for participating in EMR training, rewards for nurses who use the EMR most effectively, peer mentoring for nurses who are not tech savvy, providing case examples of how the EMR saves lives, and listening to the nurses' rationale for their resistance. Over time, acting as if you believe the baby boomer nurses will begin to use the EMR effectively will in turn change your thought because what you used to believe ("Those baby boomer nurses are so set in their ways and ignorant of technology") no longer fits your experience.

Consider your own experiences with diversity as a health care professional. Identify a time when your think, feel, do chain resulted in an action that did not reflect cultural competence. Jot down what you thought, felt, and did. Then reframe your thought and try it out. What feeling would result from this reframed thought? What action? How would cognitive reframing change the outcome? Alternatively, think of actions you could take to change your thinking. Consider your IAT results. If they revealed, for example, an implicit bias in favor of white over black, what actions could you take to address your bias? Cognitive reframing is a powerful tool and its effective use is a hallmark of the culturally competent health care professional.

Context: What Influences Me?

Our beliefs about our own and others' group identities, our implicit attitudes, and our cognitive, affective, and behavioral processes are shaped through experience. The following exercises encourage the reader to self-reflect and consider how his or her own formative life experiences, images in the media, and group identities shape experiences and influence actions and reactions in the context of diversity.

Lifeline Graph

Cultural programming is subtle but extremely powerful in shaping how we see ourselves, members of our own identity groups, and members of other identity groups. We learn about our own and other identity groups in a variety of ways. Our earliest attitudes usually are shaped by our experiences with family members, school relationships, peer group influence, and media exposure.

The lifeline activity can be used to uncover the milestone experiences that helped to shape our current attitudes, beliefs, and behaviors about key aspect of identity such as race, ethnicity, gender, age, religion, sexual orientation, and physical ability. To use the lifeline most effectively, create separate lifeline graphs for each dimension of diversity. For purposes of illustration, let's use race. On the lifeline graph shown in Figure 5.2, plot the earliest memory you have of an experience that affected you on a personal level that involved race. Try to recall the event that marks your first awareness of race as a significant diversity dimension. The event can be an experience in which you participated directly or an event in the larger society that you became aware of through the media. Events in which you personally participated can be either intra- or inter-group, that is, either with others from your own racial or ethnic identity group or with people from another racial or ethnic identity group. On the horizontal axis, locate your age at the time that the event occurred. On the vertical axis locate the degree of emotional intensity, either positive or negative, that you felt when the event occurred. Plot the event at the intersection on the lifeline graph. Recall what happened at the time. What did you think, feel, and do? Jot down the key emotions you felt.

FIGURE 5.2 Lifeline Graph

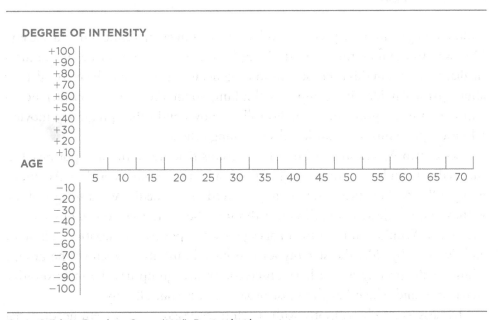

Source: © Eclipse Consultant Group. (2004). Reprinted with permission.

Now move to a later age and event and repeat the process. Continue the lifeline activity until you reach your current age. Reflect on how the events you plotted on the lifeline graph influence your attitudes, beliefs, and behaviors about race or ethnicity today. Did the emotional intensity of events increase or decrease as you grew older? What pattern of emotionally positive or emotionally negative events do you see on your lifeline graph? If the event involved racial or ethnic discrimination, were you a perpetrator, victim, bystander, or intervener? Which events would you feel most comfortable sharing with others? Why?

Share the exercise with someone you trust from a racial or ethnic identity group that is different from your own. Ask him or her to also complete the lifeline graph. Afterward, discuss both of your lifeline graphs as well as the conclusions you each drew from the events plotted on your graphs. Discuss what you learned and how you felt while undertaking the lifeline activity. Were your experiences and reactions similar or different? Do the lifeline graphs of individuals who are members of racial or ethnic identity groups that have been the target of discrimination or negative stereotyping differ from the lifeline graphs of individuals who identify with a group that has not been targeted? How might different lifelines affect inter- and intra-group relationships in health care organizations?

Images in the Media

Cultural programming is pervasive and occurs within every segment of our society. One way to examine this is by studying how groups are portrayed in the mass media. Your task in this exercise is to study general messages that the media deliver about particular identity groups. In thinking about the media, consider newspapers and other print media, radio call-in shows and other programs, movies, television programs, and music videos, among others.

Select two American racial or ethnic groups that are commonly portrayed in the media. Include a white ethnic group and a Latino, Asian, or African American group. Observe how these groups are portrayed in the media. What images of the groups you've selected are reinforced through the portrayals you've observed in the media? Would you label the images you see as positive or negative? Think of and list, side by side, the stereotypes you have heard about each of the groups whose media portrayals you have observed. Which group has the most positive stereotypes and which has the most negative? Ask yourself why.

Discuss your observations with a white colleague and an ethnic or racial minority colleague to ascertain if your conclusions about how minority ethnic and racial identity groups are handled by the media are the same or different. Do your white and ethnic or racial minority colleagues share the same point of view?

Thinking About Multiple Dimensions of Diversity

This exercise explores three dimensions of diversity and requires the reader to imagine a scenario in which one of their group identities might serve as a professional liability or a barrier to receiving high-quality health care.

What if you worked in another country where language, religion, and gender role relationships between men and women are strictly defined and regulated? The customs are very different from your own and the people in the host country view your country as inferior to theirs. What would you have to do to stay connected to the organization in which you work?

What if your age was thought to be a liability? Imagine that your seniority as a manager is not viewed as an asset by executive leadership and that your supervisor is younger than your youngest child. You've proposed workable solutions that would correct several major problems that are adversely affecting the bottom line, but your younger supervisor routinely dismisses your input. What barriers would you have to overcome to be recognized as a valuable employee? Now reverse this situation. What would you have to do to have your skills and talents noticed if your supervisor was considerably older than you and, in your estimation, lacked the technical skills to advance the department and remain current in the job?

What if your sexual orientation could cost you a promotion? Imagine you are a manager who is gay. Suppose also that one of the ways middle managers tend to succeed in your organization is by frequently attending social functions to raise money and develop corporate donors. You have been in a stable relationship for ten years, yet at many of the social functions you find your colleagues introducing you as an eligible bachelor. Suppose your boss is homophobic and doesn't acknowledge it. What do you do to advance your career and maintain your sense of self?

System: What Structure Do I Operate In?

Careful observation of the health care organization itself will provide the health care professional with important insights into how the system contributes or detracts from the health care professional's ability to enact his or her role with cultural competence. To truly make a difference, self-exploration of person, context, and system must result in an action plan. An action plan template rounds out this section, which concludes with observations about the value and challenges of self-exploration for culturally competent health care professionals.

The Power of Observation

Observe management and staff in the health care organization where you work. If you are not yet employed as a health care professional, select a local health care organization. Begin the journey by taking a walk around the health care facility. Pay close attention to the racial, gender, and other visible group identities of employees at varying levels and in different roles in the organization. Who occupies the management, professional staff, skilled, and semi-skilled positions? Note your reactions to what you see. How do you explain the gender and racial and ethnic distribution in the organizational hierarchy? Do you find yourself justifying why certain racial and gender groups tend to occupy certain roles? What assumptions do you make about identity groups that are clustered in particular positions?

Observe the patients now. What are the characteristics of patients by gender, race, age, or other visible group identities? Is there similarity between the overall mix of employees and the mix of patients being served? When patients enter a health care organization do you think it is important for them to see service providers who are members of their identity groups? Is staff composition at certain levels in any way related to patient cooperation, patient disclosure of information, or the amount of information physicians, nurses, and other clinicians give to patients about their condition? Have you any evidence relating older patients' feeling valued and respected to the ages of the staff that provide care to them? Do you observe physically challenged patients being treated with dignity and respect? Do you think the quality of patient care would be different if care providers were more diverse?

Observe patient and staff interactions. What are the skills that caregivers need to be effective in serving the patient base? How do staff attitudes and behavior affect patient cooperation? Do clinicians need to know about patients' belief systems to influence their cooperation in taking medication, recognizing and reporting physical problems and symptoms, and seeking information about their condition? Do you think the quality of patient care would improve if physical therapists, pharmacists, and other clinicians knew more about patients' identity groups?

Observe staff interactions and teamwork. How well do staff from different racial or other identity groups work together? Do identity groups cluster in the cafeteria or in the hallways of the health care organization? What successes and failures have you observed among staff in planning? How do nurses and service workers such as nurses' aides or patient transporters communicate? How do administrators relate to support staff? How would you describe the quality and effectiveness of communication between doctors and nurses, between administrators and staff, between service workers and supervisors? Do you observe any patterns in communication styles and group identities?

Observe the environment. Does the physical plant reflect the life experiences of patients and staff? Do artwork, magazines, and the style of interpersonal etiquette and greetings communicate acceptance and understanding of patients' varying identity groups? Are the magazines in the hospital waiting rooms reflective of the many cultures of patients? If there is a large Latino or Asian patient base, does the hospital purchase magazines and newspapers in Spanish and different Asian languages? Does the artwork reflect the images of all of the identity groups served by the health care organization?

Role: How Do I Want to Operate?

What did you learn about your strengths and areas for development as a culturally competent health care professional? What actions can you take to improve your performance? Use Table 5.1 to record your personal action plan.

Observations

Personal journeys like the one outlined in this section can often lead to insights such as the following:

- Behavior is more easily changed than are attitudes and beliefs about group identity.
- Clinical and administrative staff and patients as well bring preconceived attitudes and beliefs about their own and other identity groups into the daily interactions in the health care organization.

TABLE 5.1   Journey of Self-Discovery: Action Plan

What are the personal strengths I discovered through the self-exploration exercises?	What actions can I take to build on these strengths?	What are personal shortcomings I learned about through the self-exploration exercises?	What actions can I take to address these shortcomings?
Example: I have friends from many different ethnic groups.	*Example: I can talk openly to my friends about our cultural similarities and differences.*	*Example: I have an implicit bias that favors straight over gay.*	*Example: I can attend diversity training seminars to learn more about sexual orientation.*

- Managers' styles result, in part, from their group identities and influence the ways in which they recognize and reward employees.

- Cultural styles are deeply embedded in social behavior and influence the ways in which health care is delivered and received.

The personal journey exercises presented here are first steps on the road to discovering that managing people and delivering care in a multicultural context pose unique challenges for the health care professional. In every health care professional role, self-awareness is critical as one engages with others, especially in situations when the power differential between patient and provider is usually weighted in favor of the provider. Self-awareness includes desire for greater cultural competence and an appreciation for one's baggage of stereotypes and prejudicial feelings frequently collected early in life but added to and enhanced throughout life. Self-awareness guides one's understanding of one's hidden and exposed gifts and challenges. It is self-awareness of how the person captures and effectively uses the context of resources and resistances to become more culturally competent. This is all accomplished on behalf of maximizing the purpose of the health care system: providing safe and quality care to all people while acknowledging the uniqueness and difference of those served.

SUMMARY

The hallmarks or distinguishing characteristics of culturally competent health care professionals cannot be meaningfully summarized in a checklist. However, the shared values of the health professions, which emphasize high-quality personalized care and respect for each person, make cultural competence a requirement, not an option, for the health care professional. Health care professionals must surmount many challenges on the journey of cultural competence, including facing the contradiction between reality on the ground and the ideals of the profession and, most important, acknowledging the need for self-development and personal growth to build their own cultural competence.

The Grubb framework and the self-development exercises presented in this chapter are valuable tools in the process of self-assessment from which insights into key aspects of cultural competence can be gleaned, including one's own readiness for self-development as well as the ability to identify and manage implicit bias and successfully enact one's role as a culturally competent health care professional in a health care organization. Ultimately, the hallmark or distinguishing characteristic of a culturally competent health care professional is active engagement in an ongoing process of self-discovery through which strengths and areas for development are identified and acted on as the health care provider strives to continuously improve the process and outcome of care for each patient. Chapter Six focuses on training for knowledge and skills in cultural competence, an organizational practice that reflects a commitment to the systems approach through assisting health care professionals in self-development of the hallmarks of cultural competence and in walking the talk of culturally and linguistically appropriate heath care.

KEY TERMS

attitude	implicit biases
cognitive reframing	model of developmental readiness
explicit biases	transforming experiences framework
hallmarks	value system

REVIEW QUESTIONS AND ACTIVITIES

1. Look up your professional association's value statement. Are diversity and cultural competence mentioned? What does the value statement tell you about your organization's commitment to developing culturally competent health care professionals? What actions are being taken by your professional association to build cultural competence within its members?

2. Interview three colleagues from your class. Ask each one to complete this statement: My role as a culturally competent _____ (nurse, doctor, manager, speech therapist, etc.) is to _____. Ask them to explain their answers. Using the concepts of person, context, and system, present a rationale for the similarities and differences in their answers.

3. Complete this statement: My role as a culturally competent _____ (nurse, doctor, manager, speech therapist, etc.) is to_____. Using the Grubb Institute's transforming experience framework, explain how the system (the organization itself), the context of the organization (for example, the community's diversity, human and financial resources, health risks, and indicators), and your personal values influenced your answer. If you are not currently employed as a health care professional, answer this question with reference to the system and context you want to work in.

4. Complete a separate lifeline graph for each of the following diversity dimensions: race or ethnicity, gender, sexual orientation. For each graph, answer the following questions: What lessons did I learn from my lifeline experiences? How do those lessons affect my beliefs and behaviors today? How would my beliefs and behaviors have changed had my experiences been different?

5. List the five groups that are most significant to your individual identity. List at least three things you believe and three things you do that you attribute to each group membership. Remember a time when you have had a positive experience due to one of these group identities. Then, remember a time when you have had a negative experience due to one of these group identities. Do you believe your own group identities affect how you relate to others, even in the workplace? Why or why not?

6. Go to the IAT website, https://implicit.harvard.edu, and take three IAT tests that are relevant to your workplace relationships. Then, check the FAQs

(frequently asked questions) posted on the website. Now, what do you think the results mean? Assume you want to take action to reduce or eliminate a bias that you have. What actions could you take?

7. Complete your personal action plan for self-development using the template provided in Table 5.1. Compare actions plans with a colleague and together agree on a timetable for taking the actions you have identified to develop your personal cultural competence.

REFERENCES

Allport, G. (1954). *The nature of prejudice.* Reading, MA: Addison-Wesley.

Avolio, B. J., & Hannah, S. T. (2008). Developmental readiness: Accelerating leader development. *Counseling Psychology Journal, 60*(4), 331–347.

Bazalgette, J., Irvine, B., & Quine, C. (2006). The absolute in the present: Role—the hopeful road to transformation. In A. N. Mathur (Ed.), *Dare to think the unthought known?* Tempere, Finland: Aivoairut Publishing.

Dunham, Y., Baron, A. S., & Banaji, M. R. (2006). From American city to Japanese village: A cross-cultural investigation of implicit race attitudes. *Child Development, 77*(5), 1268–1281.

Green, A. R., Carney, D. R., Palin, D. J., Ngo, L. H., Raymond, K. L., Iezzoni, L. I., & Banaji, M. R. (2007). Implicit bias among physicians and its prediction of thrombolysis decisions for black and white patients. *Journal of General Internal Medicine, 22*(9), 1231–1238.

Greenwald, A. J., & Banaji, M. R. (1995). Implicit social cognition: Attitudes, self-esteem, and stereotypes. *Psychological Review, 102*(1), 4–27.

Greenwald, A. G., Poehlman, T. A., Uhlmann, E. L., & Banaji, M. R. (2009). Understanding and using the implicit association test: III. Meta-analysis of predictive validity. *Journal of Personality and Social Psychology, 97*(1), 17–41.

Gutmann, D. (2003). *Psychoanalysis and management: The transformation.* New York: Karnac Books.

Jones, J. M. (2011). *Record 64% rate honesty, ethics of members of Congress low.* Washington, DC: Gallup. Retrieved from http://www.gallup.com/poll/151460/Record-Rate-Honesty-Ethics-Members-Congress-Low.aspx

Klein, M. (1984). *Psychoanalysis of children.* New York: Free Press.

Kluger, J. (2008, October 20). Race and the brain. *Time,* p. 36.

Malone, B. L. (1993). Caring for culturally diverse racial groups: An administrative matter. *Nursing Administrator Quarterly, 17*(2), 21–29.

National League for Nursing. (2007). *The NLN Report,* Summer, 1.

Nosek, B. A., Banaji, M. R., & Greenwald, A. G. (2002). Harvesting implicit group attitudes and beliefs from a demonstration web site. *Group Dynamics, 6*(1), 101–115.

Reed, B. D. (2001). An exploration of role as used by the Grubb Institute. London: The Grubb Institute.

Stanley, D., Phelps, E., & Banaji, M. R. (2008). The neural basis of implicit attitudes. *Current Directions in Psychological Science, 17*(2), 164–170.

Chapter 6

TRAINING FOR KNOWLEDGE AND SKILLS IN CULTURALLY COMPETENT CARE FOR DIVERSE POPULATIONS

LEARNING OBJECTIVES

- To distinguish between cultural competence training focused on attitudes and training focused on knowledge and skills

- To clarify principles that support knowledge and skills training in health care

- To examine the essential knowledge and skills training for health care management

- To examine the essential knowledge and skills training for persons involved in direct patient care

(Continued)

- To describe how cultural competence knowledge and skills can enhance the therapeutic encounter

- To describe how support service employees in health care can benefit from skills and knowledge training

- To examine factors involved in assessing cultural competence training

- To list some of the cultural competence training resources available

Prior chapters have presented a rationale for cultural competence in health care: an increasingly diverse national population that is reflected in the patient populations and workforces of health care organizations, disparities in health access and status across population groups, and cultural differences that affect patient care and service delivery. In Chapter Five we considered the theory, perspectives, and activities that promote culturally sensitive attitudes and values in health care organizations and professionals. The emphasis there was on the way health care workers *think* about and *respond emotionally* to diverse patient populations and the need for cultural competence in health care. In this chapter, we examine the kinds of training needed to develop the knowledge and skills necessary to create culturally competent health care delivery. The emphasis here is on what people working at different levels in health care need to *know* and *do* in order to promote culturally competent care.

The chapter begins with a set of eight overarching principles that we believe are useful in organizing all trainings that are focused on building cultural competence knowledge and skills. These principles are useful in organizing cultural competence training in academic institutions and in health care organizations, although the emphasis is on the latter. The reasoning behind each of these principles is explained. Then the focus of the chapter turns to the special information and skills needed by health care managers and administrators. Clinicians and direct care providers need another and different skill set and knowledge base, which are discussed in the following section of the chapter. Health care practice disciplines and associations have endorsed cultural competence education and training; a sample of these will illustrate the perspectives of different professional groups. The support and service personnel that keep a health care organization running smoothly also need cultural competence skills, and some of these will be touched on. To improve training and to give feedback to the organization, the trainings received by the various segments of the workforce need to be assessed in terms of their worth to the organization and the individual. As will be discussed, evaluation of cultural competence training takes various forms, depending on the recipients of the training and the goals.

Finally, a wealth of resources to be used in developing the knowledge and skills base for cultural competence has evolved. The available toolkits, online training courses, websites, webinars, and listservs can be extremely helpful in an ongoing and developmental approach to cultural competence knowledge and skill building. Some of the most useful of these will be presented throughout the chapter and in the resources section at the end.

EIGHT PRINCIPLES FOR KNOWLEDGE AND SKILLS TRAINING

The goals of cultural competence skills and knowledge training should be (1) increased quality of care to diverse populations, (2) clinical excellence and strong therapeutic alliances with patients, (3) reduction of health care disparities among the populations served, and (4) a workforce that performs effectively within a diverse service community. With these goals in mind the following principles can structure knowledge and skills training.

Principle one: In the training, there should be a broad and inclusive definition of cultural and population diversity, including consideration of races, ethnic groups, social classes, age cohorts, genders, and sexual orientation.

We have seen that groups of people differ on a number of dimensions and that these dimensions affect their worldviews, their health care needs, and their interactions with the health care systems. Many of these groups have been shown to receive a lower quality of care than others, and several have experienced discriminatory treatment through lack of understanding and prejudiced attitudes. Some groups have important cultural or religious practices that are ignored or discounted, causing them to distrust or have conflicts with their providers.

Poverty and lack of education precludes access to good health care for many, as does an inability to conform to the expectations of the providers to whom they do have access. Health care organizations in different locations serve different mixes of these populations so their delivery of services will be affected in variant ways. If cultural competence training is to be useful to health care systems, it needs to address the different characteristics and needs of all these variant groups within their service populations. A broad definition of population diversity draws attention to these different needs.

Principle two: Training should not be a one-time undertaking but should be developmental and ongoing, moving from general information to the more specific.

Unfortunately, some organizations feel that they have "covered" cultural competence knowledge and skills training by having managers, clinicians, and support staff at every level of the organization participate in a single prestructured educational program or brief course, ignoring the fact that workers and professionals at different levels of the organization interact with diverse groups in completely different ways and ignoring the reality that the cultural composition of each community may differ from others. Similarly, even a well-thought-out one-day program focused on important general facts about patient and community characteristics, with participation by workers at all levels of the organization, will be just enough, it is hoped, to raise cultural awareness and whet appetites for more specific trainings that follow. Cultural awareness and sensitivity, as was noted in prior chapters, reflect appropriate attitudes, necessary but not sufficient for the action taking required of cultural competence. Action taking requires a broad array of specific knowledge and skills tailored to different sets of recipients.

Principle three: Knowledge and skills training should not be one-size-fits-all but should be focused on specific job-related functions and health care disciplines.

One-size-fits-all trainings are useful and usually appropriate at the beginning stages of cultural competence knowledge and skills training in which general, contextual information useful to all segments of the workforce is covered. Information on the demographic characteristics of the local communities such as the kinds of cultural groups that make up the community, the balance of immigrant and nonimmigrants, the languages spoken, and the socioeconomic class mix of the surrounding population are important facts for everyone to know. Which of these segments of the community and how many are actually served by the health care organization are also critical pieces of general information for the entire workforce. A brief description of important epidemiological issues that characterize the populations in the service area would be useful information for everyone. An organization might even clarify the characteristics of its own work force as compared to and contrasted with that of the communities it serves. This information might be somewhat sensitive but, carefully presented, it is likely to raise awareness and foster discussion of the need for training throughout the organization.

However, people's jobs and positions within a health care organization are extremely different by function, that is to say, how they influence and carry out the overall mission, goals, and work of the organization, how and to what extent they interact with patients, and what knowledge and skills they already use in everyday practice. Consequently, the knowledge and skills added through cultural competence training will need to be job related so that they can be practically integrated into the different functional areas. Hospice nurses need different cultural competence skills and information than obstetrical nurses, for example. Cooks need different information than receptionists. Psychiatrists need information on cross-cultural differences in mental health and surgeons need still other types of information. One size definitely does not fit all.

Principle four: Knowledge and skill training should be focused on factual information and how-tos with practical application rather than theory or didactics. The training should be viewed as augmenting existing skills and knowledge bases.

The goal of cultural competence training is to provide higher-quality care to diverse populations by helping health care professionals and staff to be more effective at their jobs when they work with multicultural patients. For this, they may need to learn how-to skills for successful use of a telephonic or remote interpreter in order to talk with patients or information about the dietary practices of a local population in order to teach a health education class on diet and type 2 diabetes. Even if health care providers of many kinds are assumed to have been given general education on the needs of different populations during their career preparation, targeted information in the context of everyday practice is very useful. However, health care practitioners are proud of their knowledge and skills, and cultural competence training should be viewed as augmenting or strengthening these recognized preexisting capacities. Giving health care personnel specific information and tools that inform their practices is directed toward increasing their confidence and skill in working with diverse groups.

Principle five: Cultural competence knowledge and skills training should be integrated into as many other types of training as possible.

Integrating cultural competence knowledge and skills into other training that is not specifically focused on cultural issues is an effective strategy. For example, if a training program for care managers of renal patients is undertaken, a small segment of that training can provide information on the demographics of the organization's renal patients and cultural issues around family involvement in care giving can be discussed. Perhaps some skills for eliciting patients' and families' understanding of the long-term prognosis can be taught. Many health care disciplines require **continuing education**; therefore training programs that integrate cultural knowledge and skills can be sought out or the inclusion of such materials can be requested of continuing education trainers.

Principle six: Knowledge and skill training should be buttressed by ongoing self-assessment as well as feedback to the trainers and organization.

Cultural competence training can be followed up by self-assessments over time that examine the usefulness of information and skills that have been taught. Training can be improved through feedback on the value of the information and skills in actual practice. Many times skills learned in cultural competence training prove to be useful in working with all patients, and this can be part of an assessment as well. Care providers are often creative in integrating cultural competence skills into preexisting skills, and opportunities should be made available for them to share their innovations. Assessments need to be expressly tailored to the target audiences of the training as well as its specific content.

Principle seven: Wherever possible, there should be an attempt to build an evidence base for the training by looking at health outcomes, costs, and patient, provider, and consumer satisfaction data following implementation of training.

Building an evidence base for cultural competence training is not easy to implement. However, as with all health care practices and interventions, training has to be subject to the efficacy test: Did it improve the quality of care in some measurable way? Did it make care more efficient or cost effective? Did it improve patient satisfaction or trust? Provider satisfaction? Did the use of a competency-based tool or strategy result in better adherence to a treatment regimen? Prevent hospital readmissions? Or, the ultimate measure, did it improve health outcomes such as better blood pressure control or more immunizations or more smoking cessation among patients? In the long run, cultural competence training in health care will be considered valuable only if it is seen to be effective in improving patient care or reducing the cost of care.

Principle eight: No cultural competence trainings should take place until and unless the sponsoring health care organization or institution is ready and able to support the knowledge and skills that are taught in the training.

If an organization undertakes cultural competence training, management must be ready to support the skills and practices that the employees and health professionals have learned. This may mean a greater or lesser degree of organizational change and budgetary support. It is frustrating, for example, for physicians and nurses to learn how to use interpreters effectively in health care encounters with patients who can't speak English, only to learn that no interpreters are available or few speaker phones for telephonic interpreting have been bought and placed in convenient locations. It is daunting for care managers to learn that no fields for entering patients' race, ethnicity, or language have been entered on the organization's data system so they have no way to quickly find out and plan for the language needs of specific patients when they come in for service. Health educators, having been trained in the dietary customs of ethnic groups in their service areas, need to have translated materials that address the pros, cons, and suggestions for changes that are relevant to the diets of those groups; therefore, funds for translated materials should be budgeted.

In accord with the recommendation that specific types of knowledge and skills are required for different positions within a health care organization, we will first look at what managers need to know.

CULTURAL COMPETENCE KNOWLEDGE AND SKILLS FOR ADMINISTRATORS AND DIRECTORS

The cultural competence of health care organizations ultimately rests on the policy making, planning, and oversight of the top-level administrators and directors (Nashimi, 2006). These may include chief executive officers (CEO), chief operations officers (COOs), presidents and vice presidents, hospital administrators, medical directors, nursing directors, and chiefs of service, to name some of the leadership positions in health care organizations. In terms of delivery systems, the organizations may be large, networked health plans; staff-model health management organizations; public, private, or teaching hospitals; community clinics or independent practitioner medical groups. Health care organizations run in size from national health plans to local community hospitals and clinics.

However, the preponderance of health care is delivered locally, in hospitals, clinics, and independent medical groups, and it is the local-level administrators and managers who will oversee care to specific communities even within national health care organizations. If they are uninformed about cultural competence in health care services, they will be unable to make appropriate policy, do strategic planning around care to diverse populations, or support the cultural competence of the professionals and employees they manage. Although there is extensive literature on management of a diverse workforce as examined in Chapters Ten and Eleven of this book, there is very little specific training for administrators of health care organizations who must plan and oversee culturally competent care delivery. It seems to be assumed that administrators, most of whom have training in business administration or health care administration, have had cultural competence training, but that is a dangerous assumption because few health care administration courses are offered on the subject of actually structuring a culturally competent health care organization. As the leader's attitudes toward cultural competence frequently shape the way the organization as a whole embraces it, the leader's knowledge base is important, and he, she, or they often need to build a knowledge base from scratch for themselves. Here are some sources that can be tapped to help build the requisite knowledge base.

ACHIEVING ORGANIZATIONAL CULTURAL COMPETENCE: RESOURCES FOR MANAGERS AND ADMINISTRATORS

One Size Does Not Fit All: Meeting the Health Needs of Diverse Populations. The Joint Commission. http://www.jointcommission.org/assets/1/6/HLCOneSizeFinal

Encouraging More Culturally and Linguistically Competent Practices in Mainstream Health Care Organizations: A Survival Guide for Change Agents. The California Endowment. http://www.compasspoint.org/sites/default/files/docs/research/494_lonnerfull.pdf

Multicultural Health Care: A Quality Improvement Guide. National Committee on Quality Assurance. http://www.ncqa.org/Portals/0/HEDISQM/CLAS/CLAS_toolkit.pdf

Implementing Multicultural Health Care Standards: Ideas and Examples. National Committee on Quality Assurance. http://www.ncqa.org/Portals/0/Publications/Implementing%20MHC%20Standards%20Ideas%20and%20Examples%2004%2029%2010.pdf

A Manager's Guide to Cultural Competence Education for Health Care Professionals. The California Endowment. http://www.calendow.org/uploadedfiles/managers_guide_cultural_competence%281%29.pdf

A Comprehensive Framework and Preferred Practices for Measuring and Reporting Cultural Competency: A Consensus Report. National Quality Forum. http://www.qualityforum.org/Publications/2009/04/A_Comprehensive_Framework_and_Preferred_Practices_for_Measuring_and_Reporting_Cultural_Competency.aspx

Cultural competence training for administrators is complex, and trainers should consider what administrators need to know to oversee culturally competent care delivery. The very first thing that administrators must be familiar with is the diversity that exists in the communities and service areas in which their organizations are located. Census data will give them the statistics but these statistics can be fleshed out with personal experience (Lonner, 2007) through **community-based training**. For example, one CEO of a California health plan took his fellow administrators to meet with local advocacy groups, to a farm labor camp, and they also participated together in community health fairs. They took the opportunity to meet with community groups representing the different cultures in their community. Another administrator met regularly with the heads of community clinics that were located in the ethnic neighborhoods his hospital served and became familiar with the language needs and social determinants that affected health in these areas. It is useful to compare the demographics of their organization's patient base with the demographics in the overall community and to examine why they serve more or less of the **market share** of specific groups. There may be excellent reasons for these differences but they should know the reasons.

Managers need to know enough diversity epidemiology to be able to plan to meet the health care needs of specific groups within their population bases. A medical director in a county-organized health plan reported, for example, that they were giving their doctors actionable data about the disparities among the patients they serve, not just nationwide epidemiological data (Lonner, Gilbert, Quan, Roat, & Kuramoto, 2008). Such leadership knows about the linkage between quality of care, disparities, and cultural competence, and also needs to know how to set goals and track disparities within their patient population though HEDIS measures or other metrics that can measure health care outcomes by ethnic and racial groups and other diversity dimensions.

Culturally competent managers need to be aware of national and state legislation around linguistic access and cultural competence training for health care providers. If they serve Medicaid, SCHIPS, or Medicare patients, they need to be familiar with the cultural and linguistic requirements of the Centers for Medicaid and Medicare Services (CMS), based on the CLAS standards. They need to be acquainted with the accreditation requirements around cultural competence that are being used in the assessments of the Joint Commission (2012), the National Quality Forum (2009), and the National Committee on Quality Assurance (NCQA, 2010). These assessments have now become items in health care evaluations that are examined by employers who contract for health care insurance for their diverse employees and are important in marketing to diverse population groups (Rose, 2011).

Because top-level management usually will not be involved in the actual implementation of cultural and linguistic competence activities, they will need to know enough about culturally competent health care to make sure that they hire and appoint human resource directors, quality assurance managers, department administrators, chiefs of service, nursing directors, and others who do have cultural competence planning capacity. A guide prepared by the Industry Collaborate Effort (2006) on how to assess a potential employee's knowledge of cultural competence has a series of questions to ask potential employees. One of the most useful questions is, "In the health care field we come across patients of different ages, language preference, sexual orientation, religion, culture, gender, and immigration status, all with different needs. What skills from your past employment or education do you think are relevant to the diversity you will find in this job?"

This question should allow a better understanding of the interviewee's approach to customer service across the spectrum of diversity, previous experience in serving a diverse population, and also indicate whether his or her skills are transferable to the position in question.

An administrator will want a workforce and team of health care professionals who are trained in cultural competence and so will need to be knowledgeable enough to oversee human resource personnel in appropriate selection of trainers. Two resources are readily available on the Internet to brief managers on this issue: *A Guide to Incorporating Cultural Competency into Health Professional Education and Training* (Beamon, Divisitty, Forcina-Hill, Huang, & Shumate, 2006) and *A Manager's Guide to Cultural Competence Education for Health Care Professionals* (Gilbert, 2003a). The former contains a checklist of subjects to be covered in cultural competence trainings, including rationale, key aspects of cultural competence, health disparities, factors influencing health, and crosscultural clinical skills. The latter differentiates between cultural competence training and workforce diversity training, gives a checklist for choosing a cultural competence trainer, and makes clear the need for organizational support following training. The NCCC maintains a consultant bank, archived by US geographical areas and training specialty, and a cultural and linguistic competence resource database. Additional NCCC resources include *A Guide to Planning and Implementing Cultural Competence Organizational Self-Assessment* and *A Planner's Guide for Infusing Principles, Content and Themes Related to Cultural and Linguistic Competence into Meetings and Conferences*, all of which are available on the NCCC website.

Administrators must not only have the knowledge and skills to build the infrastructure to support culturally and linguistically appropriate care, but they must also be skilled intercultural communicators in their own right. From mediating a dispute between a Gen X female nurse manager and a baby boomer male MD to explaining to the board the rationale behind the organization's recent adoption of domestic partner benefits or the need to offer flexible benefits, administrators must model the cultural competence they want staff to exhibit with one another and with patients.

Moreover, although training for health care providers and support staff involved in direct patient interaction is focused on responding effectively to patient diversity, training for administrators emphasizes responding to staff diversity. In fact, such training for administrators is often referred to as diversity or diversity management training rather than cultural competence training. Knowledge and skills training in diversity management commonly includes areas such as generational and gender differences in communication styles, LGBT employee concerns, mediating disputes between disciplines such as nurses and physicians, or managing the effect of staff religious diversity in the organization.

Consistent with the eight principles that also apply here, the most effective training experiences for administrators will include case examples and emphasize interaction and engagement rather than **didactic** presentations. **Executive coaches** often work individually with administrative leadership to provide the confidentiality and personal support that cannot be offered in a group training session. Although diversity training for administrators is sometimes offered within the health care organization, often such training is done at conferences with peers from other organizations who can share challenges, solutions, knowledge, skills, and best practices. Of course, when cultural competence training occurs in a setting that involves the entire staff of an organization, it is important that administrators participate in order to show the staff that they embrace and stand behind the training. Only administrators who model cultural competence themselves can create a culture, climate, and infrastructure for culturally competent patient care and develop and lead a culturally competent health care organization.

It may certainly seem as though this is a lot of information for busy, high-level administrators and managers to access and absorb. It is. However, it may be possible to have assistants access and summarize the information for the management team, even though it will be critical for the team to review, discuss, and consider all of the cultural competence issues that relate to their health care organization and decide how they are to be managed. Such discussion can be facilitated by a knowledgeable management consultant. The resources on organizational cultural competence cited in the box entitled "Achieving Organizational Cultural Competence" can be a good start.

When senior leadership is truly informed about the role of culture and linguistics in health care, they tend to be well aware of the implications of these factors on the work of the many departments that they oversee. They are also aware of the cultural competence activities that occur in and across the organization's departments and can encourage collaboration when appropriate. Most critical, if the leadership of an organization is visible and vocal in support of cultural and linguistic issues, it is easier for staff to acknowledge the importance of cultural competence in the work they do.

CULTURAL COMPETENCE TRAINING FOR HEALTH CARE PROFESSIONALS IN DIRECT PATIENT CARE

Although there is little explicit or long-established training in how to deliver culturally competent health care services for senior and middle health care managers, there are a vast array of resources and training strategies focused on clinicians, nurses, and other health care professionals who work in direct patient care. Cultural competence education and training has received its most complete theoretical and practical development among physicians, nurses, and medical anthropologists. Beginning with Arthur Kleinman in the early 1980s and continuing through the present, a number of physician leaders, for example, Joseph Betancourt, Alex Green, Emilio Carrillo, Francis Lu, and others who also had anthropology degrees, such as Robert Like and Kathleen Culhane-Pera, began developing practical and pedagogically sound ways to bring cultural competence education to physicians. In nursing, trainers such as Josie Campina Bacote and Marjorie Kagawa-Singer, building on the foundation laid by Noel Chrisman and Madeleine Leininger, developed cultural competence training for nurses. Surprisingly, though many of the allied health professions endorse cultural competence in their mission statements, there has not been intensive development of cultural competence professional education and training outside medicine and nursing.

Support from the Clinical Professions

Many of the agencies in charge of accrediting schools that educate health professionals endorse the need for cultural and linguistic competence education. Statements from these bodies help make the case for cultural and linguistic competence education as an accepted aspect of professional knowledge. Some of these are reviewed in the following lists.

- Accreditation Council for Graduate Medical Education (Stewart, 2001): As a component of systems-based practice, in order to best serve a patient population a student must be familiar with the natural history and epidemiology of major health problems in the community. A background in understanding cultural norms and health beliefs is also of critical importance.

- Liaison Committee on Medical Education (2000), *Standard on Cultural Diversity*: Faculty members and students must demonstrate an understanding of the manner in which people of diverse cultures and belief systems perceive health and illness and respond to various symptoms, diseases, and treatments. Medical students should learn to recognize and appropriately address gender and cultural biases in health care delivery, while considering first the health of the patient.

- American Association of Colleges of Nursing (2008): The rationale for proposing the integration of cultural competence in nursing education is to support the development of patient-centered care that identifies, respects, and addresses differences in patients' values, preferences, and expressed needs. Further rationale includes the mandate to eliminate health disparities, for which nurses need to be prepared to address in a global environment and in partnership with other health care disciplines. The AACN (2011) has developed curricular guides for cultural competence training of baccalaureate- and graduate-level nursing students, which may be accessed on their website.

- The Association of American Medical Colleges (2007), in a good effort to standardize cultural competence training for medical students, has created the *Tool for Assessing Cultural Competence Training (TACCT)*, a self-assessment tool for use by medical colleges in examining their curricula for inclusion of attitudes, knowledge, and skills related to cultural competence. The tool, accompanied by a guide for its use and relevant resources, is available on the website of the AAMC. The AAMC (2005) also published *Cultural Competence Education*, which outlines cultural competence curricula for medical schools.

It is also encouraging that there is very strong support from many practice associations in the health care field that fosters cultural competence among their members. A very small sample follows.

- The American College of Emergency Physicians: This organization believes that quality health care depends on the cultural competence as well as the scientific competence of physicians. It also believes that cultural competence is an essential element of the training of health care professionals.

- American Nurses Association: Knowledge of cultural diversity is vital at all levels of nursing practice. Knowledge about cultures and their impact on interactions with health care is essential for nurses, whether they are practicing in a clinical setting, education, research, or administration.

- The Society for Public Health Education (SOPHE): By acknowledging the value of diversity in society and embracing a crosscultural approach, SOPHE supports the worth, dignity, potential, and uniqueness of all people.

- The American Dentistry Association (ADA): As part of its core values or guiding lights, the ADA embraces diversity and cultural competence in its programs, partnerships, and coalition activities.

- The National League for Nursing: The core value diversity is defined as affirming the uniqueness of and differences among persons, ideas, values, and ethnicities. Although diversity can be about individual differences, it also encompasses institutional and systemwide behavior patterns. The National League for Nursing has created a toolkit for nursing educators that can be accessed on their website.

For a more complete list of practice endorsements, see Gilbert and Soto-Greene (2003).

The professional literature of medicine and nursing contains much information on the care of culturally and linguistically diverse populations. For example, beginning with the *Western Journal of Medicine* in 1983 and the *Journal of Transcultural Nursing* in 1989 and continuing into the present, several medical and nursing journals have devoted theme or supplemental issues to the topic of cultural competence (e.g., *Academic Medicine, 77,* 2002; *78,* 2003; *Journal of General Internal Medicine, 19,* 204; *Journal of Transcultural Nursing, 18,* supplement, 2007). *The Journal of Transcultural Nursing* has crosscultural health care as its major focus.

New Jersey added impetus to the development of cultural competence training for physicians when it became the first state to pass legislation requiring cultural competence in education for physicians and medical students as part of licensure. In 2005 California also adopted legislation requiring cultural competence in continuing medical education (CME) training for physicians; in 2006, Washington State followed suit. New York, Arizona, and Ohio have proposed similar legislation (Graves, Like, Kelly, & Hohensee, 2007). As a result, cultural competence training is increasingly offered in web-based programs and webinars and by training consultants, usually for continuing education credits.

The essential focus of cultural competence training in the health professions is on the care-giving relationship between providers and patients and on how to deliver specific services to diverse patient populations (American Institutes for Research, 2002; Gilbert, 2003b). Cultural competence training takes place in multiple venues and at many levels of professional education. An underlying motivation for all hands-on health care providers is that they want to be confident that the care they give their patients is high quality and has good outcomes. They also value information and skills that make their work with patients easier and more efficient.

Cultural Competence Training in Clinical Education

A number of medical and nursing schools include cultural competence training (see Crandall, George, Marion, & Davis, 2003; Gilbert & Soto-Greene, 2004), either as stand-alone courses or, more often, integrated throughout courses, rotations, and preceptorships. The medical discipline of family practice, in particular, early on sought to include cultural competence training integrated into medical school education with detailed and well-developed curricula (Culhane-Pera, Reif, Engli, Baker, & Kasselkert, 1997; Like, Steiner, & Rubel, 1996). An excellent example of the institutionalization of cultural competence throughout medical education is shown in the activities of Harvard Medical School, which include faculty development, case-based education, and the increase of a variety of strategies and resources for learning about disparities and patient culture (Harvard Medical School, 2006a, 2006b). Recognizing that diversity in faculty and students promotes inclusion and culturally competent nursing practice, a resource for nursing educators has been developed by the National League for Nursing. Their diversity toolkit focuses on the lack of diversity in nursing educators and students, directly addressing the pipeline issue described in Chapter Three of this book. Directed to administrators and faculty members, the toolkit provides strategies and resources for recruitment and retention of nurse administrators, faculty members, and students in nursing schools throughout the nation (Task Group on Expanding Diversity in the Nurse Education Workforce, 2009).

Some residency programs also include a focus on cultural competence skills. They can be devoted to medical specialties, such as psychiatry (Lu et al., 2010), or can be more broadly focused. An outstanding example of such a residency program is the family practice residency program at White Memorial Medical Center in Los Angeles (Ring, Nyquist, & Mitchell, 2008). The program is overseen by an ethnically diverse faculty and attracts ethnically diverse residents. The White, as it is called in the community, is located in central Los Angeles and its patients are drawn from Korean, Mexican American, Japanese, Chinese, Mexican Indian, and other ethnic communities. Cultural competence training is integrated into the program for all residents and at every year of the residency and has been designed by physicians and a behavioral health specialist.

However, despite these excellent examples, it has been pointed out that in undergraduate and graduate medical education, cultural competence as a comprehensive curricular thread is unevenly applied (Crandall, George, Marion, & Davis, 2003). As a consequence of the uneven or minimal inclusion of cultural competence teachings in professional education, many practicing health care professionals are confronting diverse patient populations with little knowledge and few culturally focused skills. Additionally, many health care professionals entered the workforce prior to the advent of cultural competence training in professional schools of any kind.

For physicians, nurses, and allied health professionals already in practice, continuing education in cultural competence is often offered in-house by staff model and networked health plans. Some staff model health plans, such as Kaiser Permanente, have developed ongoing training and educational materials for their clinical staff, such as their physician handbooks on culturally competent care, each one focused on a different population group among the patients Kaiser serves. Cultural competence training is also integrated into many specialty-based conferences and seminars and into Area Health Education Center programs.

There are frequently opportunities to integrate cultural competence training into other training that is being offered at off sites, seminars, conferences, and other developmental programs. For example, in one Southern California area, seminars on type 2 diabetes for clinicians included information on how Mexican and Vietnamese immigrants each understood diabetes and the methods each traditionally used to treat it. Similarly, a two-day conference on hospice and palliative care that drew practitioners from all of California included a daily session on issues in crosscultural pain management and another on crosscultural mourning and bereavement practices. One independent practice association in Southern California mounted six one-hour lunchtime CME training sessions for its networked physicians, each one on a different medical subject. The final twenty minutes of each session was devoted to knowledge and skills in cultural competence integrated into the topical focus of the day. Using this approach, the trainer was able to show that cultural issues were involved in a wide number of clinical areas: cardiology, HIV/AIDS, kidney failure, depression, and childhood asthma. Integrating cultural competence training in this way emphasizes the relevance and usefulness of cultural information in specific aspects of health care.

Strategies for Training Health Care Professionals in Culturally Competent Care: A Knowledge Base and Skills Development

In considering the training of hands-on providers, we would do well to revisit the definition of cultural competence in health care, given by Lavizzo-Moury and MacKenxie (1996) because it succinctly encompasses all the elements that need to be addressed in training: "Cultural competence is the demonstrated awareness and integration of three population-specific issues: health-related beliefs and cultural values, disease incidence and prevalence, and treatment efficacy. But perhaps the most significant aspect of this concept is the inclusion and integration of the three areas that are usually considered separately" (p. 919). Translated into training terms, this implies that cultural competence training should focus on learning about the impact of a patient's culture on health and disease, the disparities and epidemiological characteristics of specific populations, and evaluating treatment and health delivery for its effectiveness in meeting the needs of diverse patients (Gilbert, 2003b).

In teaching health professionals about the beliefs and values of people with different cultural backgrounds, there was initially an emphasis on lists of traits and norms identified with specific cultural groups. This approach had numerous drawbacks, as noted in Chapter Four, because within each culture there are many individuals and subgroups that vary in their internalization of normative cultural traits. Cultural lists tend to promote stereotypes (Kleinman & Bensen, 2006) and are problematic when it comes to interacting with individual patients who may deviate from the trait list in many ways. Learning about the cultural beliefs, norms, roles, and behaviors typical of a cultural group is useful in raising awareness of possibilities to investigate further, but no more than that. Fortunately, more sophisticated techniques are currently being taught that are useful for exploring patients' understanding of health conditions and the context for their illnesses and health. The knowledge and process approaches to cultural competence discussed in the following section can be used with students or practicing physicians and nurses.

Considering the Universal Aspects of Culture That Affect Health Care

One approach that fits into the repertoire of different kinds of health providers is to encourage providers to consider the aspects of *any* culture that might be expected to affect an individual's health and health care. Knowing that there are universal factors that are found in *all* cultures, but understanding that these universals are quite differently expressed in *each* culture, can give clinicians a direction in exploring cultural concepts that isn't trait based but still allows for the influence of cultural beliefs, norms, and values to surface. Following is a list of factors that can affect health and health care, are present in every culture, and that may differ significantly between patients and providers from different cultures. Moreover, these factors are important to consider in giving personalized patient care to any patient. Using a simple list such as this one as a springboard for discussions can facilitate learning about different cultures without resorting to a trait list. Of course, the trainer or facilitator needs to be familiar with numerous cultures in order to use such a list effectively. A brief discussion will demonstrate how this might be so.

CULTURAL FACTORS THAT AFFECT HEALTH CARE

- The meaning of symptoms

- Perceptions of anatomy and bodily functions

- Perceptions of appropriate treatment

- Autonomy and self-efficacy

- Gender roles

- Childbirth and reproduction

- Family involvement and inclusion

- Orientation to prevention

- Pain expression and management

- Diets and dietary practices

- Concepts of death and dying
- Expectations of health professionals

Symptoms are not necessarily simple! Most of us have experienced headaches, upset stomachs, respiratory problems, and body aches. What these symptoms mean can be differently interpreted. Maybe they are God's punishment for a broken rule or commandment, maybe the work of an evil eye, maybe we just drank too much alcohol last night and we'll know better next time. What causes these symptoms (their **etiology**) and others more severe in nature are explained differently across cultures. Pain in the area of the kidneys may mean one thing to one cultural group and another to a different group. Stomach pain, bowel problems, and trouble breathing may be seen as the result of anything from the work of a spirit to bacteria and viruses. Even the functions of the bodily organs and the interaction of elements of the body's systems can be construed differently, as easily can be seen when looking at, for example, traditional Chinese medicine's organization of the body into meridians, the categorizing of the bodies organs into warm and cold, and the effect of the flow of chi, the life force, though the system.

Medical anthropologists doing research in cultures across the world and among immigrants to the United States report a phenomenon termed *culture bound* or **ethnomedical syndromes** (Winkelman, 2009). This term refers to a recognition of symptoms and an understanding of physiological processes that differ from biomedical diagnostic criteria. Such syndromes are most commonly encountered in immigrant populations from rural areas of their native countries. An example of an ethnomedical syndrome commonly found among Mexican immigrants is that of *mollera caida* or fallen fontanel in an infant. The folk medical explanation of the depressed fontanel in an infant's scull is that it is the result of a fall or sudden withdrawal from the nipple but it is also a medically recognized symptom of dehydration resulting from diarrhea. Similarly, some Korean elders, most often women, suffer from a syndrome of diffuse, usually gastrointestinal, symptoms, aches in the chest area, fatigue, and headache called *hwabyung*, sometimes called *fire sickness*. The symptom syndrome is a somatic response to very sad or traumatic life circumstances, often culturally treated by family support and care (Pang, 1990), but sometimes is presented to doctors for medical treatment. In both of these cases, the provider needs to elicit from the patients their understanding of their condition before working toward a treatment plan that will be accepted by the patients.

The experience of symptoms, their severity, and perceptions about their meaning are what usually bring people into health care encounters. These ideations may already have shaped their expectations about what should constitute appropriate treatment. The provider cannot always assume that symptoms mean the same thing to the patient as they do in allopathic medicine. The meanings and causes a patient ascribes to symptoms, their thresholds for seeking care, and their ideas about treatment and cures are called the patient's *explanatory model* (Kleinman, Eisenberg, & Good, 1978). This model may be derived from traditional health concepts learned in another culture, it might simply be the result of little education or low health literacy, or it may be a very scientifically oriented model. In any case, before providers can confidently do a diagnosis and recommend treatment plans, they will need to determine how and to what extent the patient's explanatory model differs from their own and respectfully negotiate the differences. A bit later in this chapter we will discuss a tool, the Eight Questions, designed to do just that.

The level of a patient's **self-efficacy** in the face of physical and mental problems differs individually and crossculturally and may critically affect the patient's willingness to undertake treatment and prevention activities that involve behavior change. Self-efficacy is an individual's belief in his or her own ability to carry out a task or to cope with the challenges of life. Levels of self-efficacy may be culturally shaped, as in the case of some cultures in which women are not expected to have any control over their household finances, food preferences, social lives, or dealings with the world. Low self-efficacy may also be the result of long-term poverty or the bewilderment of an immigrant in a new environment. Individual self-efficacy may be affected by a culturally derived fatalism in which resignation to fate or the will of God is seen as a virtue or a coping strategy. In some cases, aging erodes an individual's sense of self-efficacy. An inability to prevent health problems in their country of origin may reduce a patient's belief in his or her ability to carry out new prevention activities. Lack of proficiency in English may cause a patient to be unsure about following instructions or understanding treatment plans. Providers will need to determine if any of these factors influence a patient's ability or willingness to accept and adhere to treatment plans or to carry out prevention activities.

Another major aspect of most cultures that can affect health care is conformance to behaviors and norms associated with gender roles. Ideations associated with male roles may cause underreporting of severe symptoms or pain, reluctance to depend on others, or unwillingness to disclose emotional response to diagnosis and prognosis. Women may be unwilling to consider their own health needs if it means inconveniencing others. Many cultures have specific ideas about the care of mothers before and after childbirth, including the use of cultural midwives and dietary restrictions and prescriptions that may or may not be compatible with current obstetrical practices and practices on obstetrical wards. Gender norms may make it difficult for women and men to speak openly about bodily functions or sexual relations to opposite-sex providers or even to same-sex providers An extreme example of conflicting concepts of gender norms is the practice of female circumcision, also known as female genital mutilation (FGM), which is still practiced in some cultures, though outlawed in the United States, and is still valued by women as a sign of female purity, presenting medical and ethical problems to obstetricians and nurses who are called on to provide care to immigrant patients who have been circumcised. The following case study illustrates how gender roles can affect health care treatment.

GENDER ROLES AND FAMILY INVOLVEMENT

Gloria, twenty-three, a Mexican immigrant in her seventh month of pregnancy, is feeling embarrassed about the subject the physician assistant (PA) has broached. Though treated once before during this pregnancy, she has been re-inflected with chlamydia, a sexually transmitted infection.

Gloria is afraid to discuss this problem with the man she lives with, the father of her two-year-old daughter, though she knows he has re-infected her. Both he and Gloria are in the United States without papers. They live with Jose's married brother and wife, Juana, who are legal residents. Jose works construction with his brother, who is also his boss. Juana has accompanied Gloria to this visit to help interpret and is shocked and angry at Jose. She is going to "make sure my husband tells Jose a thing or two."

- *Why is Gloria feeling embarrassed, afraid, and vulnerable?*

- *Do you think Juana's solution is promising?*

- *Is she overstepping her role as interpreter?*

- *What does all this have to do with gender roles?*

- *What is the best thing for the PA to do?*

The influence of families can never be overestimated ether in their absence or their presence. The social context of the patient will be different depending on whether the family is a single, female-headed household, a nuclear family, a multigenerational household, or a familial network that extends across national borders. Family relations and reciprocal obligations and responsibilities and family strengths and weaknesses often will shape a patient's experience of illness and health. Immigrants may be isolated from their families of origin due to migration or they may be embedded in an extended family who joined them at various times in migration. The absence of family may mean a dearth of supportive relations and limits on care-taking resources. However, the strong influence of the family may affect such things as the reporting of family medical histories (some families are reluctant to reveal family information), the ability of the patient to make autonomous decisions, or to carry out treatment recommendations such as dietary changes. How will a chronic illness affect family functioning? Family resources? In the context of the patient's culture, how is a sick person supposed to act? To bear illness and pain stoically with forbearance or can he or she express discomfort openly and expect to be cared for with close and ongoing attention from relatives?

Usually family or a significant other is involved in and may shape a patient's decisions around health care. Sometimes it is difficult to know precisely who the important family decision makers are but this information is important to health care providers. Death and dying often present problems with family communication about prognosis to the dying member, which may be culturally derived (Brotzman & Butler, 1991). Ritual care of the body by relatives is prescribed by some religions and attendance to dying persons by appropriate holy men, priests, or monks is often requested by family. Crosscultural definitions of what constitutes death often vary and need to be considered in death-related conversations with patients and families about life-prolonging methods and organ donation so this information will be critical to physicians and hospital ethics consultants (Klessig, 1992).

Dietary recommendations, so common in treating chronic conditions such as high blood pressure and diabetes, may run counter to customary eating habits, and if the patient is not the one who chooses the family menus, that person will need to be identified and involved in dietary planning. Similarly, religious proscriptions and dietary laws, ongoing or related to specific religious days of observance, need to be considered in treatment plans that involve changes in diet or hospital dietary planning.

Expectations about the role of the health care provider differ across cultures and socioeconomic classes. People immigrating from cultures with a historically strong authoritarian bent may expect physicians and nurses to be the experts and highly directive. In some areas of the United States, where there are large concentrations of immigrant populations, there are many folk healers, such as *parteras* (midwives) and *curanderas* (healers) among large groups of Mexicans or *shamans* among settlements of Hmong. Many immigrants are accustomed to getting diagnoses and medications from *yerberos*, or folk pharmacists. Having become accustomed to relationships with these types of care providers, which are usually highly individualized, patients may be uncomfortable or confused in a busy clinic or hospital where many people are being treated. People from impoverished circumstances and battles with bureaucracies may not believe health care providers are interested in their care. It may take some time before individuals who have had these experiences feel comfortable in participating in medical decision making with their providers.

Many of the items listed in "Cultural Factors That Affect Health Care" affect aspects of diagnosis, expectations about treatment, and the ability to carry out treatment that will constitute important information to every member of the caregiving team, from physicians and nurses to care managers to physical therapists, psychologists, and health educators. Additionally, they will be useful in any practice arena, from primary care to specialty practices.

However, cultural competence training is much more effective with clinicians if the trainer is also able to zero in on more narrowly defined sets of information during ongoing **developmental training** that focuses on specific areas of service delivery and, whenever possible, the population groups that are found in the communities in which the health care organization is located. Thus, obstetrical and gynecological physicians and nurses will value information on the birth and reproduction practices of, say, Somalis and Hispanics who live in the area but will find their mental health concepts somewhat less valuable than will psychiatric social workers, psychiatric nurses, psychiatrists, and other behavioral health specialists. The former will find informative the cultural basis and appropriate responses to, say, the frequent Somali practice of female circumcision. The latter will find special relevance, for example, in concepts from the DSM-IV outline for cultural formulation in consideration of cultural factors affecting diagnoses of depression and somatoform disorders (Lu, 2006; Messich et al., 1999).

Cultural concepts around death and dying pertinent to local community groups will be especially salient to intensive care nurses and hospitalists as well as hospice professionals. Internists working with HIV and AIDS patients will want to have information on the attitudes toward gay men in local population groups and culture-related sexual practices among gay and straight members of those groups. All this is not to say that information on cultural orientations and practices of local population groups should always be siloed in developmental training going forward, but in order to be practical and thus effective, trainers need to consider what is meaningful and helpful in the everyday practice of different health care professionals. Good continuing education courses developed for different disciplines can shape specific foci to meet different needs.

Finally, information about genetic, cultural, and social determinants that affect the epidemiological patterns across population groups is another set of information that is critical for health professionals to have. This will necessarily include health care disparities in access, treatment, and health statuses across diverse groups as described in Chapter Two. In this context, the role of **cultural epidemiology** can be discussed. This term refers to the study of the way in which cultural norms, values, and behavior affect the onset, course, and outcome of disease as well as its incidence and prevalence (Trostle, 2005). Here again, the epidemiological generalizations describing the health issues and risks of specific groups are useful starting points and should be used to heighten awareness and prompt inquiry in caring for individuals from those groups. A developmental process of going from the general to the specific is useful. Information about epidemiological patterns and disparities at the national level is important to all health care workers, and may well have been covered in professional schools, but perhaps more important is knowing how these patterns and disparities are reflected in the social, economic, and health conditions in local communities. In discipline-focused seminars and CME, local disparities data that are especially salient to the different medical disciplines will warrant a close look.

Some Tools Useful in Teaching Cultural Competence to Health Care Professionals

Understanding these cultural concepts is at the core of a patient-centered care philosophy that explores and responds to patient's needs, values, and preferences. Learning about the cultural and social context of a patient's health in enough depth that patient and providers can build a trusting, workable **therapeutic alliance** usually doesn't occur in a single encounter. The goals of sensitively eliciting information about the patient's explanatory model are twofold: first, to develop an understanding of how the patient sees his or her health needs in such a way that it shows respect for the patient and, second, to negotiate a basis of trust in the therapeutic alliance between patient and health care provider even when patient and provider perspectives differ. Dr. Francis Peabody, in a famous lecture given to Harvard medical students in 1926, remarked, "The significance of the intimate personal relationship between physician and patient cannot be too strongly emphasized, for in an extraordinary number of cases, both diagnosis and treatment are dependent on it" (Peabody, 1927, p. 878). That remark was directed to doctors but is applicable to the role of any health care professional who works closely with patients. Increasing understanding between patient and health care professionals who differ by class, culture, gender, sexual orientation, or any other diversity criteria is a major objective of cultural competence training.

A number of tools have been developed that can help a clinician or other provider to elicit information leading to an understanding of the cultural factors discussed in the foregoing section of this chapter. One of them is the well-known group of eight questions that Arthur Kleinman and his colleagues published in 1978. These questions appear in almost every cultural competence curriculum designed for clinicians, probably because they can't be improved on, and because, with a few word changes, they can be readily adapted to meet the needs of different practices and the communication style of the individual practitioner.

THE EIGHT QUESTIONS

- What do you think caused your sickness or problem?

- Why do you think it started when it did?

- What do you think the sickness does to you? How does it work?

- How severe is your sickness? Do you think it will last a short time or a long time?

- What are the chief problems the sickness has caused you?

- What do you fear most about this sickness?

- What kind of treatment do you think you need?

- What are the most important results you hope to gain from the treatment?

Source: Adapted from Kleinman, Eisenberg, and Good (1978).

These eight questions serve as a strategic communication approach to obtaining in-depth and necessary information about how patients understand their health problems, and they also can serve as an important training tool to engage health care providers in discussing their experiences with patients of different cultural backgrounds. The questions not only yield insight into the patient's explanatory model, but also provide an understanding of the patient's subjective experience of his or her condition. Clinicians may want to discuss techniques for integrating or adapting the questions into the subjective aspect of patient assessment.

On gaining an understanding of the patient's explanatory model, the next step is for the provider to respectfully acknowledge any differences between the patient's model and the provider's, first by explaining his or her own (without using medical jargon), then pointing out areas of similarity and disagreement between the two perspectives. From that base, a negotiated agreement about treatment may be reached. This may be possible through including many of the patient's ideas in the plan as long as they do not conflict with the provider's plan and do not pose any harm to the patient. A widely used **mnemonic** in cultural competence training—LEARN—developed by Berlin and Fowkes (1983) condenses these strategies: L = listen with sympathy and understanding to the patient's problem; E = explain your perception of the problem; A= acknowledge and discuss the differences and similarities; R = recommend treatment; and N = negotiate treatment when necessary. Mnemonics are a time-honored method that health care professionals use to organize and memorize all manner of data (Mnemosyne was the Greek goddess of memory). A number of other mnemonics that are intended to shape cultural interactions between patients and providers are available in the Association of American Medical Colleges' publication, *Cultural Competence Education for Medical Students* (2005).

A mnemonic approach was used to guide culturally competent interactions between patient and provider when dealing with genetics data in primary care (Reynolds et al., 2005). This is a sensitive subject because risk factors for some diseases are associated with genetic mutations found in specific ethnic and racial populations. Genetics-based medicine is a new and complex domain of health care. The authors exemplify use of the mnemonic PRACTICE in skillfully diagnosing and discussing consent and potential parental genetic testing in the case of an anemic Cambodian infant boy discovered to have hemoglobin E/beta thalassemia, an inherited disease that occurs more frequently in Southeast Asians than in other Asian groups. In the mnemonic, the P = prevalence reminds clinicians that disease burden is multifactorial in all populations and includes environmental as well as genetic factors; R = risk, a reminder to the clinician to consider the possibility of a genetic etiology; A = attitude, a reminder that patients and providers bring their cultures into the clinic, and that there may be differences to understand and negotiate; C = communication of new and complex concepts across cultural and language barriers is difficult but critically important; T = test, a reminder that the clinician must fully understand the level of effectiveness of a genetic test and its predictive value in order to convey this information to patients prior to testing; I = investigation of family history of diseases through patient report and records will be sensitive and time consuming; C = consent for genetic testing is required and the patient must be informed of the implications of testing in a manner that is understandable within his or her cultural context; E = empowerment, which reminds the clinician that each patient should be encouraged to weigh the risks and benefits of genetic testing and be empowered to make the decision for themselves. The authors make the point that such complex and delicate discussions require the help of appropriate and skilled interpreters. They further point out that going forward such discussions with patients will become more common as more genetic information related to disease and health risks is uncovered in genome studies. Their anticipation of the role of cultural competence in such discussions and their modeling of a culturally sensitive approach is innovative and a good example of how mnemonics can be useful.

Case studies are another familiar learning tool used throughout the health care provider community and providers are usually already skilled in dissecting case material. Case studies are excellent inasmuch as they can render cultural perspectives concrete in the actions and situations of specific patients (Clark & DeLisser, 2009). If constructed with in-depth cultural knowledge, cases can provide context for what may otherwise be seen as unreasonable actions and ideas on the part of patients as well as skillful or inept responses of care providers. In discussing cases, providers can bring into play their analytic prowess and can enrich discussions by describing their experiences with similar cases. This is important because it is always respectful, whenever possible, to build cultural competence discussions on existing provider strengths and skills.

Case studies should contain enough clinical detail so that they are interesting to students with specific professional backgrounds, for example, medical details for doctors and advance practice nurses, counseling-related details for health educators, and so on. If the training is directed to providers in a single practice discipline, the case studies should be consistent with that practice; if the training encompasses a wide variety of health providers, the case studies used for discussion should reflect that diversity. Some case studies should reveal patients' family, social, or economic contexts that affect their care. Described locations of case-based interactions should be realistic and clinically accurate, whether they portray hospital floors, clinic, home, or class surroundings (see Galanti, 2008, for examples of case studies in hospital settings). Case studies also provide the opportunity for interprofessional learning among health care providers collaborating with a focus on patient care.

Case study materials lend themselves to video presentations, which can be very effective with good facilitation and sufficient time for discussion. Fortunately, there is a variety of video case material dealing with clinical issues that is excellent for cultural competence training. For example, The California Endowment teamed with Kaiser Permanente to create ten case-based video vignettes, *The Multicultural Health Series*, which used on-site clinic and hospital locations and professional actors. The cases cover a wide range of issues from phone interpretation to religious practices, elder care, venereal disease, childbirth, and death. The extensive facilitator's guide can be downloaded from The California Endowment website, and the videos can be ordered from the foundation free of charge as well. Additionally, The Commonwealth Fund has made several cultural competence trigger case-based videos available on YouTube. It cannot be emphasized enough that giving health care professionals ample opportunity to discuss case materials, mnemonics, and patient encounters is critically important. Professionals respect and learn from the experiences, successes, and failures of their peers. Talking very often becomes the teaching tool and a very good one. The following case can be used to encourage discussion of end-of-life issues with patients and families from different cultures.

A DIFFICULT VISIT

You are a primary care physician and Mr. Kim is a seventy-year-old Korean immigrant with a history of abdominal pain. He has lived in the United States for seven years. Earlier this year he was diagnosed with gastric cancer and underwent a gastrectomy six months ago. He has been readmitted to the hospital for nausea, vomiting, dehydration, and weight loss. His son, who owns and runs a 7-Eleven, has asked to talk to you about further curative surgeries or chemotherapy, and you were told by the oncologist that no treatment is available for cure. He has a liver metastasis on the CT scan of his abdomen and you will need to tell the sons and daughters about this. They have insisted that you do *not* tell the patient about the spread of cancer. Mr. Lee's wife has accompanied her son on this visit; she speaks little English and appears nervous and confused. How would cultural competence training help you handle this visit?

Cultural Competence

Epidemiology: Gastric cancer is the most common malignant neoplasm among Asians in China, Japan, and Korea, with the highest rate in Japan and Korea.

Culture: In traditional Korean culture, when the father of the family is disabled or dead, the eldest son is the decision maker, not the wife.

Communication: You need an interpreter outside the family and physician skills in using interpreters.

A number of excellent interactive and case-based cultural competence–training courses for clinical care are available on the Internet. Among the best are free courses for physicians and nurses offered by the Office of Minority Health on its Think Cultural Health website.

WEB-BASED TRAINING FOR PHYSICIANS

A Physician's Practical Guide to Culturally Competent Care. Case-based. No cost. Nine hours. AMA/PRA category 1 credits. https://www.thinkculturalhealth.hhs.gov/

Physician Update: Physician Update Cultural Competency Self-Study Program. No cost. Six hours. Continuing medical education (CME). http://culturalmeded.stanford.edu/pdf%20docs/INFORMED%20NJCC-Final.pdf

Quality Interactions for Physicians. Case-based. $99 2.5 hours CME and $139 6 hours CME. Also prices for up to fifty clinical staff with one-year access. http://www.qualityinteractions.org/index.new.html

An excellent book for cultural competence training is by family practice physician Kathleen Culhane-Pera and her colleagues (2003). It presents clinical and ethical case studies (called case *stories* in the book) of interactions between the local Hmong community and health care professionals. The cultural and clinical analyses in the book give many illustrations of how culturally responsive health care is and is not enacted, covering such subjects as childbirth, reproductive health, pediatric care, chronic disease, mental illness, and end-of-life situations. The book is organized as a teaching tool with many thought-provoking questions for discussion following each case story.

Critically, the book deals sensitively with crosscultural conflict issues between patients and clinician in the understanding of symptoms, diagnosis, and treatment. It takes up knotty issues relating to some of the challenges to professional ethics encountered in providing multicultural health, such as when it is appropriate for a physician to override or comply with a patient's or a family's wishes. Following is a portion of the authors' analysis of this subject.

ETHICAL DILEMMAS IN CULTURALLY RESPONSIVE CARE

Delivering culturally responsive health care requires attention to the "routine" (for US practitioners) ethical questions and some special ethical questions that arise in cross-cultural health care relationships. When serving patients with different cultural perspectives on illness and healing, and with different moral commitments and practices, which aspects of their health care ethics are providers willing to modify or forgo? . . . Each provider must decide how he or she will determine the best interests of patients with diverse health beliefs . . . We recommend that practitioners make a commitment to respect patients' and families' wishes—except when a treatment decision poses a significant and disproportionate ethical challenge to professional integrity. This intermediate criterion commits neither the error of radical cultural relativism nor the error of radical ethnocentrism (Culhane-Pera et al., 2003, pp. 317–318).

Can you think of situations in which a provider would have to override a patient's or family's wishes given these criteria? Before doing so, what efforts should be made to reach agreement? What do you think is meant by radical cultural relativism *and* radical ethnocentrism?

A comprehensive model for culturally responsive care, based on the recommendations of community members and health care providers, is outlined in good detail in this book. Figure 6.1 is perhaps the most thorough-going example of culturally competent care philosophy available in the literature on cross-cultural health care. It is accompanied by many thought-provoking questions and recommendations for each section of the model. For example, to amplify section three of the model, which deals with learning about the prevailing health beliefs, practices, and values of the groups served, it asks the provider to consider such issues as what historical or cultural barriers interfere with trust of US health care practitioners; what behaviors demonstrate respect for persons, patients, and families; and what are the privacy needs and expectations of patients from this group? Although Culhane-Pera and colleagues primarily address clinicians, their book's contents will be helpful to a wide range of providers engaged in direct patient care.

Health care providers should be given the opportunity to hear the views of and interact with community leaders, religious leaders, and even some of the folk

FIGURE 6.1 The Healing-by-Heart Model for Culturally Responsive Health Care

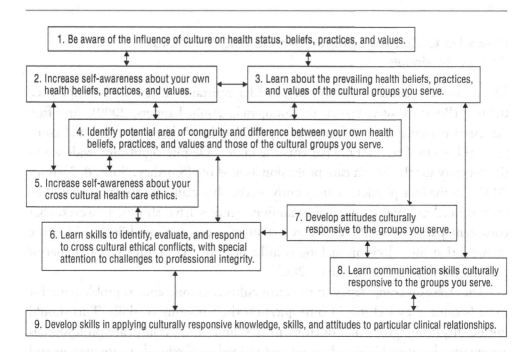

Source: Culhane-Pera, K. A., Vawter, D. E., Xiong, P., Babbett, B., & Solberg, M. M. (2003). Reprinted with permission.

practitioners, such as shamans, *curanderas*, and *parteras*, if these people play an important role in the local communities. An interesting example of close interaction between shaman and allopathic health care providers is ongoing in Merced, California (Udesky, 2003), where there is a very large Hmong population whose clashes with the medical community were made famous by Fadiman (1997) in her book *The Spirit Catches You and You Fall Down*. The community hospital and a clinic decided to give the many shamans in the community a course in allopathic medicine and in turn the shamans educated the doctors about their beliefs and work. Trained shamans, wearing badges, are now allowed to perform quiet curing rites in the hospital. Though unusual, the size of the immigrant community and ongoing culture clashes with the medical establishment warranted the program, which has been a success. Similarly, the family practice residency program run by the White Memorial Hospital in Los Angeles, has had local *curanderos* familiarize residents with the beliefs surrounding the treatments they perform and has on rare occasion made a referral to a *curandero* from the city's huge Latino population (Brown, 2009). The book by Culhane-Pera et al. described previously (2003) grew out of a collaboration between Minnesota health care providers and members of the Hmong community.

Obstacles to Cultural Competence Training for Health Care Professionals

There has been some discussion of provider resistance to cultural competence training (Boutin-Foster, Foster, & Konopasek, 2008; Landers, 2009). An often expressed perspective from health care providers is, "I don't need cultural competence because I treat all my patients the same." Despite significant evidence to the contrary for the health care profession as a whole (Smedley, Stith, & Nelson, 2003), individual physicians frequently make this claim in asserting that they do not need cultural competence training. Studies have shown, however, that consistent patterns of differential treatment take place even while providers are unaware that their decision making is influenced by race, ethnicity, or gender of patients (Embinnder & Shulman, 2003).

The stress on competency in the term cultural competence is problematic for some because they feel it calls into question their training or skills. This should not be surprising, given that doctors, nurses, and other health care professionals are among the most highly educated and trained professionals in the nation and are extremely proud of their hard-earned educational achievements. It is felt by some that by stressing competence, there is somehow an implication of *in*competence. However, as Joseph Betancourt, a physician with extensive experience in cultural competence training, succinctly stated, "The goal of this set of teachings is not about making anybody feel they are incompetent or racist in any way. It is about professional development. It is about learning the latest science in communications and communicating across cultures" (Landers, 2009, p. 1).

Care should be taken when discussing health care disparity statistics that the trainees are not made to feel individually responsible for these disparities. In this regard it is helpful for training focused on bias, self-reflection, and discrimination to be conducted separately from training centered on knowledge and skills. Experienced trainers have found that it is usually easier for health care professionals to accept cultural competence training that is directed to acquisition of information and skills rather than didactics (Betancourt, 2003). As they acquire competence in applying information and skills in the care of diverse patients, the experiential learning that results will most probably feed into the self-reflection that is involved in attitude change and can facilitate discussion of bias and ethnocentric perspectives.

One group of physicians who addressed the subject of physician resistance to cultural competence training (Boutin-Foster, Foster, & Konopasek, 2008) suggested that rather than delving right into the cultures of others who might differ from physicians, medical students and providers should first be taught to explore medicine as a culture, reflecting on its biases, language, and worldview: "In the context of cultural competence education, in order for students to develop a new perspective on the importance of culture, they must first appreciate the processes that frame their own attitudes about health and illness and then question their prior assumptions" (p. 108). In other words, in order for doctors to appreciate the impact of culture on others, they must first be made fully aware that their perspectives, too, are a product of enculturation and that medicine itself is a unique culture.

Resistance is sometimes based on the idea that cultural competence, exclusive of genetic and disparities epidemiological data, is "soft" and not scientific. Since about 2000, there has been a strong emphasis on **evidenced-based medicine**. What this means, of course, is that all aspects of medical care must be based on clear and well-supported facts supporting efficacy or some other desired outcome. Carefully designed tests and examinations must support diagnosis; medications have to show measurable efficacy and so must treatment procedures. So far, a strong evidence base linking culturally competent care to desired outcomes has not been created. However, a negative argument can be made: the high level of disparities in health status and outcomes for minorities does seem to indicate that in the care of patients who differ in culture from most of their providers something is amiss. It is also possible to make the case that many medical processes commonly used in their practices by providers also do not have an evidence base relative to patient outcomes or cost-effective, efficient care, for example, the pervasive fifteen-minute appointment or the use of SOAP notes (S = subjective, O = objective, A = assessment, P = plan) to organize patient visits, to name just a couple. What evidence do we have that fifteen minutes is the most effective amount of time for a routine medical visit or that SOAP notes are the best way to structure a visit?

Health care providers are only too aware that much that affects the health and well-being of their patients is far out of the provider's control, and they feel powerless to affect or change many of the conditions that result in poor health for some of their patients. Because that is the case, this real or perceived lack of control has been a rationale for ignoring many of the social and cultural determinants of health. This is clearly not an unreasonable stance: it is shared by many professionals, including educators, who recognize their limited capacity to deal with outside factors affecting the lives of students they teach. However, the movement to patient-centered care with its recognition of the social determinants of care, patient and family decision making, and patient values is an attempt to change that perspective. The knowledge and skills taught in cultural competence training are helpful in taking care of *all* patients. Bringing at least some of the patient's world into the exam room and acknowledging its effect on the patient *with* the patient and family is a humanizing and empowering process and may well add to providers' confidence that they can work with patients struggling with adverse economic circumstances or from cultures very different from their own.

Unfortunately, some resistance to cultural competence training can be laid at the door of poorly prepared trainers who have little experience in working within the culture of medicine and health care. Cultural competence training should take into consideration the level of education and professional backgrounds of health care providers, and training materials and perspectives should be attuned to those levels. Ways to integrate cultural competence concepts into the many preexisting skills of health care professionals can be developed, such as encouraging the entering of cultural or life-context information about patients into the medical record keeping, which is already a well-developed skill. In all training, enough time always should be allowed for providers to bring in their own experiences and techniques they have used successfully with diverse patients.

If outside trainers are brought into an organization or invited to seminars and conferences to do cultural competence training, it is important that they be familiar with clinical operations, the exigencies of patient care, and at least the relevant vocabulary of the targeted trainees. It is very helpful for trainers to have a good understanding of the specific communities that are served locally and be prepared to develop and select training materials accordingly. Nothing renders a workshop for physicians and nurses, for example, more dead in the water than for a trainer to be unfamiliar with the vocabulary, work environment, and demands of the workplace. One poorly prepared cultural competence trainer can do great damage and actually promote resistance.

CULTURAL COMPETENCE TRAINING FOR SUPPORT STAFF

A different set of skills is needed for support staff, which includes a broad spectrum of jobs such as parking attendants, receptionists, admissions clerks, transporters, and assistants of various kinds. Other kinds of service workers, such as security, food, and environmental service workers, can benefit from training. Frequently, support staff and service workers are left out of education and development trainings that focus on cultural competence even though they can be very important in patients' overall experience with the health care organization. Recognizing that these important personnel are often the first and last contacts a patient has on a visit, a number of health care organizations have taken pains to train them in how to work effectively with persons who have limited English proficiency, accents, or a style of communication that is unfamiliar. The National Center for Cultural Competency (nd) has an excellent short document, *Cultural Competence: It All Starts at the Front Desk*, which outlines what an organization needs to do to make sure that employees meet the multicultural public in a courteous and effective manner. Among the recommendations it contains are the following:

- Policies and procedures on how to serve individuals who speak little English or have other communication needs are written and well known to staff at all levels of the organization.

- Staff is aware of the language access services of the organization and can use them effectively.

- Starting with new employee orientation, staff is included in professional development and training on cultural and linguistic competence and appropriate communication and courtesy.

- Supervisors understand the behaviors, attitudes, and skill sets required by their supervisees for meeting diverse patient populations.

- Supervisors are trained to support their staff in culturally sensitive performance and include that aspect of their performance in evaluations.

- Mechanisms should be in place so that patients can lodge complaints anonymously.

- Organization policies include efforts to recruit and retain staff that reflect the cultural and linguistic diversities of the communities served.

- All support staff and service workers need to be aware of the cultural and linguistic characteristics of the communities served. Health care organizations can supply and teach service personnel how to use "I speak" cards for helping limited English speakers and distribute cultural phrase books and pictures to help facilitate communication when no interpreters are available. Personnel at key points of contact can be taught how to use telephonic interpreters or how to access on-site interpreters.

The quality interactions program at Massachusetts General Hospital has produced a one-hour, web-based module for nonclinical staff. The module teaches concepts and skills for understanding and interacting with persons from culturally diverse backgrounds, including patients, customers, and coworkers.

THE ROLE OF ASSESSMENT IN CULTURAL COMPETENCE TRAINING

Assessment of cultural competence training is the final step in a systematic approach to training because it feeds back into the training loop, either by demonstrating that the training was effective or that further training may be needed. Assessments may be at the organizational level or the individual level, depending on the nature of the training. In the final analysis, however, the effects of the training should be realized in the health outcomes of the patients served.

We began our discussion of training with management. The effective test of cultural competence at the management level will be in the policies and structuring of health care delivery that reflect a commitment to the diverse communities served. The National Quality Forum (2009) has specified a number of items in its leadership domain that are indicators of upper management mastery of cultural competence knowledge and skills. They include evidence of community engagement, workforce diversity, written policies supporting cultural competence and reduction of disparities in the organization's mission and goals, fiscal support and appropriate allocations for ongoing cultural competence training of the workforce, and data gathering and quality analysis of health processes and outcomes by race and ethnicity of patients. In other words, the cultural competence of the health care organization is itself a reflection and test of the knowledge and skills of its executive-level managers.

Assessment of cultural competence knowledge and skills among health care professionals is a somewhat more complex matter (Betancourt, 2003). At least one group of researchers noted that a scan of studies evaluating cultural competence training of health professionals showed that most lacked sufficient scientific rigor to determine the impact of training on actual health care practices (Lie et al., 2010; Price et al., 2005). Another review of training evaluations (Goode, Dunne, & Bronheim, 2006) also came to a similar conclusion although they were more optimistic about the few positive effects they uncovered.

Betancourt and Green (2010) point out that one test of knowledge is whether the clinician has acquired an understanding of the characteristics of the community in which he or she practices or trains. This would include cultural groups, their historical relationship to the locale, and their associated epidemiology. It would also include health care disparities across local groups, socioeconomic levels, the presence of immigrant groups in the service area, predominant languages, folk healers, traditional medical beliefs, and ethnopharmacology. Knowledge of this kind can be assessed on a paper-and-pencil test, and often is, in professional education and continuing medical education courses. A frequently used method is the pre- or posttest. A study examining the effectiveness of a program designed to improve the cultural competence skills of health care providers and administrators through pre- and posttesting reported statistically significant improvements in trainees' self-reported knowledge and skills (Khanna, Cheyney, & Engle, 2009). Clinicians themselves also can give feedback on how useful they think this information is to them and how it may be helpful in practice. Usually evaluation of knowledge and skills training ends there. However, it would certainly be possible and feasible to ask about the value of training after some time had elapsed in order to determine if health care providers felt that the training had an impact on their practice or their comfort level in working with diverse patients. This approach would certainly be useful if a developmental approach to training is being used for it would give trainees an opportunity to discuss refinements, caveats, and innovations to skills and strategies taught in training.

Assessment of cultural competence skills, that is, elicitation of the patient's explanatory model, the listening and negotiating skills, and the ability to ferret out a potential area of conflict between the patient's and the clinician's per-spectives are far more difficult to assess. In professional schools this can be done by having students analyze cases and through videotapes or observation of stu-dents in interaction with patients. However, among practicing health care pro-viders, assessing cultural competence skills is not easy. Patient satisfaction questionnaires, broken down by patient ethnicity and translated into appropriate languages as part of an ongoing patient satisfaction assessment of individual providers, has been done by some health organizations but this is not a common practice, requires substantial buy-in from providers, and is an indirect measure of provider skills. Most such surveys probe the patient's perceptions on whether their needs were met and whether the clinician listened carefully to them and answered all of their questions. No attempt is usually made to link the levels of satisfaction so measured with whether or not the physician has received cultural competence training, although it clearly could be. The assumption is that if the patient is satisfied, patient-provider communication has also been satisfactory. Ngo-Metzger and colleagues (2006) advocate for incorporating patients' evalu-ations of provider cultural competence in five domains: communication, respect for patient preferences, shared decision making, experiences related to trust and distrust, and experiences of discrimination and linguistic competency. Betancourt and Green (2010) suggest that patient and provider satisfaction with health care encounters may be one measure of the effects of training. There are a variety of self-assessments such as the National Center for Cultural Competence's (nd) *Cultural Competence Health Practitioner Assessment*, which may be useful to health care providers in assessing their own cultural competence and which also could be helpful to trainers as they design training courses.

SUMMARY

Cultural competence training focused on knowledge and skills spotlights the acquisition of useful knowledge and the development of usable skills, which, it is hoped, will lead to higher-quality care for diverse populations. This training is best conducted developmentally, that is, over time, rather than in a single session or two. Although there is information that is helpful to all health care workers, practical cultural competence training addresses the specific and different needs of management, hands-on care providers, and support staff because they perform different functions within a health care organization.

Cultural competence training for management helps organizational leaders understand the communities their institutions serve and guides them in setting policies that support cultural competence in health care delivery as well as modeling cultural competence in their own interactions. Cultural competence training for health care professionals, such as clinicians and nurses, focuses on information and skills needed in direct patient care. These involve understanding of epidemiological data for the populations they serve and knowledge of health care disparities as part of those data (Gilbert, 2003b). Health care providers also need information on universal aspects of culture that affect the life and health of patients and make up the context for patients' differing explanatory models of their health and illness. They need to acquire the trust-building communication skills that will allow patients to disclose cultural concepts and give the provider insight into the social determinants that affect their health. Clinicians, nurses, and other health professionals are particularly interested in information that will increase the quality of care they personally can give their patients. Support staff and service personnel who have frequent but brief and often impersonal contact with patients are typically the "face" the organization shows to the community. These workers need skills that help them interact with diverse patients and their families in ways that make them feel welcome, comfortable, and respected when they come to the organization for care.

KEY TERMS

case studies

community-based training

continuing education

cultural epidemiology

developmental training

didactic

ethnomedical syndromes

etiology

evidence-based medicine

executive coaches

job function

market share

mnemonic

self-efficacy

symptoms

therapeutic alliance

REVIEW QUESTIONS AND ACTIVITIES

1. What is the point of separating the cultural competence training of managers and clinicians? On what kinds of cultural competence topics would it be good to engage them together?

2. Imagine that you are setting up a cultural competence training for doctors and nurses that would include knowledge and skill training, developmental training, integrated training, community-based training, and didactic training. How would you plan the overall training agenda? What sort of elements would you include? Leave out?

3. What might be some of the obstacles encountered in cultural competence training for health care administrators? How could they be overcome?

4. Several resources for managers were listed in "Achieving Organizational Cultural Competence." Assign members of the class to download and review the resources for discussion in class. What are the similarities? Differences? Pick the one you think would be most valuable to managers hoping to learn about cultural competence.

5. Think about the last illness or health problem that you experienced. Examine your own explanatory model. Did you put a name to your health problem? What caused you to give it this name? How would you have responded to the Eight Questions? Before this class did you know you had an explanatory model for any of your health problems?

6. Imagine that you are a CME instructor and you are giving a day-long training on breastfeeding to a group of obstetrical nurses. How would you go about integrating cultural competence information and skills into the training? What kinds of information would you include? What kinds of preparation do you need to do in order to teach the course?

REFERENCES

American Association of Colleges of Nursing. (2008). *Cultural competency in baccalaureate nursing*. Retrieved from http://www.aacn.nche.edu/leading-initiatives/education-resources/competency.pdf

American Association of Colleges of Nursing. (2011). *Cultural competency in baccalaureate nursing*. Retrieved from http://www.aacn.nche.edu

American Association of Colleges of Nursing. (2011). *Toolkit for cultural competence in masters and doctoral education nursing education*. Retrieved from http://www.aacn.nche.edu/education-resources/Cultural_Competency_Toolkit_Grad.pdf

American Institutes for Research. (2002). *Teaching cultural competence in health care: A review of current concepts, policies, and practices*. A report prepared for the Office of Minority Health. Washington, DC: Author.

Association of American Medical Colleges. (2005). *Cultural competence education for medical students*. Retrieved from http://www.aamc.org/download/54338/data/culturalcomped.pdf

Association of American Medical Colleges. (2007). *A tool for assessing cultural competence training (TACCT)*. Retrieved from http://www.aamc.org/download/54344/data/tacct_pdf.pdf

Beamon, C. J., Divisitty, V., Forcina-Hill, J. M., Huang, W., & Shumate, J. A. (2006). *A guide to incorporating cultural competency into health professionals' education and training*. Prepared for the national Health Law Program. Retrieved from www.healthlaw.org/images/stories/issues/CulturalCompetency.052306.pdf

Berlin, E. A., & Fowkes, W. C. (1983). A teaching framework for cross cultural health care. Application in family practice. *Western Journal of Medicine, 12*(139), 93–98.

Betancourt, J. R. (2003). Cross-cultural medical education: Conceptual approaches and frameworks for evaluation. *Academic Medicine, 78*(6), 560–568.

Betancourt, J. R., & Green, A. R. (2010). Linking cultural competence training to improved health outcomes: Perspectives from the field. *Academic Medicine, 85*(4), 583–585.

Boutin-Foster, C., Foster, J. C., & Konopasek, L. (2008). Viewpoint: Physician, know thyself: The professional culture of medicine as a framework for teaching cultural competency. *Academic Medicine, 83*, 106–111.

Bronheim, S. (nd). *It all starts at the front desk*. Washington, DC: National Center on Cultural Competence, Georgetown University. Retrieved from http://gucchd.georgetown.edu/products/NCCC_FrontDesk.pdf

Brotzman, G. L., & Butler, D. J. (1991). Cross-cultural issues in the disclosure of a terminal diagnosis. *The Journal of Family Practice, 32*(4), 426–427.

Brown, P. L. (2009, September 20). A doctor for disease, a shaman for the soul. *New York Times*, p. A20.

Crandall, S. J., George, G., Marion, G. S., & Davis, S. (2003). Applying theory to the design of cultural competence training for medical students: A case study. *Academic Medicine, 78*(6), 588–594.

Culhane-Pera, K., Reif, C., Engli, E., Baker, N., & Kasselkert, R. (1997). A curriculum for multicultural education in family medicine. *Family Medicine, 29*(10), 719–723.

Culhane-Pera, K. A., Vawter, D. E., Xiong, P., Babbett, B., & Solberg, M. M. (2003). *Healing by heart: Clinical and ethical case stories of Hmong families and western providers.* Nashville: Vanderbilt University Press.

Culture & Linguistic Workgroup. (2006). *Better communication, better care: tools to care for diverse populations.* Industry Collaborative Effort. Retrieved from http://www.iceforhealth.org/library/documents/ICE_C&L_Provider_Toolkit_7.10.pdf

Embinnder, L. C., & Shulman, K. A. (2000). The effect of race on the referral process for invasive cardiac procedures. *Medical Care Research Review, 1,* 162–177.

Fadiman, A. (1997). *The spirit catches you and you fall down: A Hmong child, her American doctors, and the collision of two cultures.* New York: The Noonday Press.

Galanti, G.-A. (2008). *Caring for patients from different cultures: Case studies from American hospitals* (4th ed.). Philadelphia: University of Pennsylvania Press.

Gilbert, M. J. (Ed.). (2003a). *A manager's guide for cultural competence education of health care professionals.* Retrieved from www.calendow.org/uploadedfiles/managers_guide_cultural_competence(1).pdf

Gilbert, M. J. (2003b). *Principles and recommended standards for cultural competence education of health care professionals.* Los Angeles: The California Endowment. Retrieved from www.calendow.org/uploadedFiles/principles_standards_cultural_competence.pdf

Gilbert, M. J., & Soto-Greene, M. L. (Eds.). (2003). *Transforming the face of health professions through cultural and linguistic competence education: The role of the HRSA centers of excellence.* Retrieved from http://www.hwic.org/resources/details.php?id=1965

Goode, M. A., Dunne, C., & Bronheim, S. M. (2006). *The evidence base for cultural and linguistic competence in health care.* A Commonwealth Fund Report. Retrieved from http://www.commonwealthfund.org/Publications/Fund-Reports/2006/Oct/The-Evidence-Base-for-Cultural-and-Linguistic-Competency-in-Health-Care.aspx

Graves, D. L., Like, R. C., Kelly, N., & Hohensee, A. (2007). Legislation as intervention: A Survey of cultural competence policy in health care. *Journal of Health Care Law and Policy, 10,* 339–361.

Hark, L., & DeLisser, H. (2009). *A case-based approach to training health professionals.* Malden, MA: Wiley-Blackwell.

Harvard Medical School. (2006a). *Cross-cultural education primer.* Retrieved from www.hms.harvard.edu/cccec/teaching/primer/index.htm

Harvard Medical School. (2006b). *Culturally competent care education at Harvard Medical School.* Retrieved from www.hms.harvard.edu/cccec

Joint Commission. (2012). *Advancing effective communication, cultural competence and family centered care.* Retrieved from www.jointcommission.org/Advancing_Effective_Communication/

Journal of General Internal Medicine. (2004). 19(2). [Issue on racial and ethnic disparities.]

Khanna, S. K., Cheyney, M., & Engle, M. (2009). Cultural competency in health care: Evaluating outcomes of a cultural competency training among health care professionals. *Journal of the National Medical Association, 101*(9), 886–892.

Kleinman, A., & Benson, P. (2006). Anthropology in the clinic: The problem of cultural competency and how to fix it. *PLoS Medicine, 3*(10), 1673–1676.

Kleinman, A., Eisenberg, L., & Good, B. (1978). Culture, illness, and care: Clinical lessons from anthropologic and cross-cultural research. *Annals of Internal Medicine, 88*(2), 251–258.

Klessig, J. (1992). The effect of values and culture on life support discussions. *Western Journal of Medicine, 157*(3), 316–322.

Landers, S. J. (2009, October). Mandated cultural competency: Should physicians be required to take courses in cultural competency? *American Medical News.* Retrieved from www.ama-assn.org/amednews/2009/10/19prsa1019.htm

Lavizzo-Moury, R., & MacKenzie, E. R. (1996). Essential measurements of quality for managed care organizations. *Annals of Internal Medicine, 12*(10), 919–921.

Liaison Committee on Medical Education (LCME). (nd). *LCME accreditation standards.* Retrieved from http://www.lcme.org/standard.htm

Lie, D. A., Lee-Rey, E., Gomez, A., Bereknyei, M. S., & Braddock, C. H. (2010). Does cultural competency training of professionals improve patient outcomes? A systematic review and proposed algorithm for future research. *Journal of General Internal Medicine, 26*(3), 317–325.

Like, R. C., Steiner, R. P., & Rubel, A. J. (1996). Recommended core curriculum guidelines on culturally sensitive and competent care. *Family Medicine, 27,* 291–297.

Lonner, T. (2007). *Encouraging more culturally and linguistically competent practices in mainstream health organizations: A survival guide for change agents.* The California Endowment. Retrieved from http://compasspoint.clientrabbit.com/sites/default/files/docs/research/494_lonnerfull.pdf

Lonner, T., Gilbert, M. J., Quan, K., Roat, C., & Kuramoto, F. (2008). *Scan of cultural and linguistic services at local initiatives and county organized systems.* Final report to The California Endowment. Unpublished.

Lu, F. G. (2006). DSM-V outline for cultural formulation: Bringing culture into the clinical encounter. *Focus, 4*(1), 9–10.

Lu, F., Lim, R., & Mezzich, J. (1995). Issues in the assessment and diagnosis of culturally diverse individuals. *American Psychiatric Press Review of Psychiatry* (Vol. 12). Washington, DC: American Psychiatric Press.

Lu, R. F., Koike, A., Gelleman, D., Seretan, A., Servis, M. E., & Lu, F. (2010). *A four-year model curriculum on culture, gender, LGBT, religion, and spirituality for general psychiatry residency training programs in the U. S.* Retrieved from http://www.psych.org/Share/OMNA/Minority-Council/Cultural-Competence-Curriculum.aspx?FT=.pdf

Messich, J. E., Kirmayer, L. J., Fabrega, H., Parron, D. L., Good, B. J., Lin, K.-M., & Manson, S. M. (1999). The place of culture in DSM-IV. *Journal of Nervous and Mental Disorders, 187*, 457–464.

Nashimi, R. (2006). *A framework for cultural competency measurement and accountability.* The Commonwealth Fund. Retrieved from http://www.commonwealthfund.org/Publications/ Commentaries/2006/Oct/A-Framework-for-Cultural-Competency—Measurement-and-Accountability.aspx

National Center for Cultural Competence. (nd). *Cultural competence health practitioner assessment.* Retrieved from http://nccc.georgetown.edu/features/CCHPA.html

National Committee on Quality Assurance. (2010). *Implementing multicultural health care standards: Ideas and examples.* National Committee on Quality Assurance. Retrieved from http://www.ncqa.org/Portals/0/Publications/Implementing%20MHC%20Standards% 20Ideas%20and%20Examples%2004%2029%2010.pdf

National Quality Forum. (2009). *A comprehensive framework and preferred practices for measuring and reporting cultural competency.* Retrieved from http://www.qualityforum.org/Publications/ 2009/04/A_Comprehensive_Framework_and_Preferred_Practices_for_Measuring_and_ Reporting_Cultural_Competency.aspx

National Quality Forum. (2011). *Healthcare disparities and cultural competency consensus standards.* Retrieved from http://www.qualityforum.org/Projects/h/Healthcare_Disparities_ and_Cultural_Competency/Healthcare_Disparities_and_Cultural_Competency.aspx?section= CallforCandidateStandards2011–10–182012–01–18#e=1&s=&t=2&p=

Ngo-Metzger, Q., Telfair, J., Sorkin, D. H., Weidmer, B., Weech-Maldonado, R., Hurtado, M., & Hays, R. D. (2006). *Cultural competency and quality of care: Obtaining the patient's perspective.* Report prepared for The Commonwealth Fund. Retrieved from http://www.commonwealth-fund.org/usr_doc/Ngo-Metzger_cultcompqualitycareobtainpatientperspect_963.pdf

Pang, K. Y. (1990). Hwabyung, the construction of a Korean popular illness among elderly Korean women in the United States. *Culture, Medicine and Psychiatry, 14*(4), 495–512.

Peabody, F. (1927). The care of the patient. *Journal of the American Medical Association, 88,* 877–882.

Price, E. G., Beach, M. C., Robinson, K. A., Green, A., Palacio, A., Smarth, C., Jenckes, M., Feurstein, C., Bass, E. B., Powe, N. R., & Cooper, L. A. (2005). A systematic review of the methodological rigor of studies evaluating cultural competence training of health care professionals. *Academic Medicine, 80*(6), 578–586.

Reynolds, P. P., Kamei, R. K., Sunquist, J., Khanna, N., Palmer, E. J., & Palmer, T. (2005). Using practice mnemonic to apply cultural competency to genetics in medical education and patient care. *Academic Medicine, 80*(12), 1107–1113.

Ring, J., Nyquist, J. G., & Mitchell, S. (2008). *Curriculum guide for culturally responsive health care: The step by step guide for cultural competence training.* Oxford, UK: Radcliffe Publishing.

Rose, P. (2011). *Cultural competency for health administrators and public health.* Sudbury, MA: Jones and Bartlett.

Smedley, B. D., Stith, A. Y., & Nelson, A. R. (Eds.). (2003). *Unequal treatment: Confronting racial and ethnic disparities in health care.* Washington, DC: National Academies Press.

Task Group on Expanding Diversity in the Nurse Education Workforce. (2009). *National League of Nursing toolkit.* National League of Nursing. Retrieved from www.nln.org

Trostle, J. A. (2005). *Epidemiology and culture.* New York: Cambridge University Press.

Udesky, L. (2006, June 4). Training Hmong shaman in the ways of western medicine is saving lives in Merced. *San Francisco Chronicle.*

Wilson-Stronks, A., Lee, K. K., Cordero, C. L., Kopp, M. L., & Galvez, E. (2008). *One size does not fit all: Meeting the health care needs of diverse populations.* Oakbrook Terrace, IL: The Joint Commission. Retrieved from www.joint.commission.org/assets/1/6/HLConeSize.Rinal.pdf

Winkelman, M. (2009). *Culture and health: Applying medical anthropology.* San Francisco: Jossey-Bass.

PART THREE

CULTURAL COMPETENCE

AND HEALTH CARE

DELIVERY

The ultimate goal of cultural competence is to ameliorate disparities. Self-awareness and development of requisite skills and knowledge lay the foundation but ultimately cultural competence must be put into practice in everyday interactions in the health care organization. The patient experience with care is shaped by each encounter or interaction with a provider of health care or related services from the receptionist and the admissions clerk to the phleboto-mist, nurse, physician, or allied health professional. In each of these health care encounters it is important to put cultural competence awareness, knowledge, and skills into practice, which is the focus of Chapter Seven, "Cultural Competence in Health Care Encounters."

Cultural competence in the context of health care delivery can be a delicate balancing act. Providers of health care and related services must be responsive to the cultural and language needs of patients and their families, and at the same time they must represent the perspective of the culture of medicine in order to ensure that each patient has access to the best evidence-based treatment available. Thus, cultural competence in the context of the health care encounter can be viewed as a negotiation. Sometimes the patient's perspective should prevail, sometimes the provider's, and sometimes collaboration or compromise will result in the optimal outcome. A rich history of research and practice from the fields of transcultural nursing and medicine provide valuable information about how to interact with patients in a manner that reflects cultural competence. Care that is safe, high quality, and patient-centered cannot otherwise be delivered.

As Chapter Eight, "Language Access Services and Crosscultural Communication," emphasizes, patients and families with limited English proficiency (LEP) add another layer to the challenge of cultural competence. Language and communication barriers are especially important to address in interactions with LEP patients and their families. Providers must be aware of legislative, regulatory, and accreditation requirements that guide the provision of language access services (LAS) and the myriad resources available to assist with implementation because the provision of LAS is an important quality of care and safety issue. Pitfalls abound from common but mistaken practices such as using untrained interpreters and translators or failing to demonstrate awareness of important aspects of nonverbal communication and other cultural perspectives that can derail the effectiveness of the health care encounter, thus contributing to disparities.

In the final chapter of Part Three, Chapter Nine, "Group Identity Development and Health Care Delivery," we explain that cultural competence in the context of health care delivery is even more complex than communication style and language differences would indicate on the surface. That is because all members of an identity group such as race, ethnicity, gender, or sexual orientation do not experience their membership in that group in the same way. The constellation of attitudes and beliefs that shape how we experience and enact our group affiliation is referred to as group identity status, and frameworks for minority and majority group identities are available to assist the health care professionals in delivering culturally competent care to patients irrespective of the patient's group identity status and to understand how their own group identity status influences their encounters with patients and others in the health care organization.

No group identity status is right or wrong; each is simply a different constellation of attitudes and beliefs that shape how we experience and enact our group affiliation. Because group identity status is not immutable, it can be changed through experiences, self-reflection, and conscious decisions on the part of the health care provider, thus contributing to cultural competence in health care delivery. Cultural competence in health care delivery depends on health care professionals who exhibit the skills discussed in Part Three in their everyday interactions with patients, their families, and one another.

Chapter 7

CULTURAL COMPETENCE IN
HEALTH CARE ENCOUNTERS

LEARNING OBJECTIVES

- To define the health care encounter and its role in the systems approach to cultural competence

- To review and discuss the practical application of six widely used cultural competence models from the transcultural nursing field

- To relate the six cultural phenomena identified in the GDTAM to the culturally responsive health care encounter: communication, space, social organization, time, environmental control, and biological variations

- To describe how to use the LEARN mnemonic to improve cultural responsiveness in the health care encounter

As attention to patient-centered culturally and linguistically appropriate care has grown, several models and frameworks to assess and build cultural responsiveness in the health care encounter have emerged. This chapter will review and discuss the practical application of the following six widely used models:

- Leininger's Sunrise Model

- Purnell's Model for Cultural Competence

- Campinha-Bacote's Process of Cultural Competence in the Delivery of Health Care Services

- Jeffreys' Cultural Competence and Confidence (CCC) Model

- Andrews and Boyle's Transcultural Concepts in Nursing Practice

- The Giger-Davidhizar Transcultural Assessment Model (GDTAM)

In Chapter Four, we described the evolving understanding of cultural competence from an initial emphasis on cultural awareness, sensitivity, and relevancy, all of which focused on provider attitude rather than provider knowledge and skills, to a new emphasis on cultural competence and cultural responsiveness. These are action-oriented terms that stress the need to concentrate on what providers do, not simply what they think or know. This chapter builds on this groundwork by moving our focus to the **health care encounter** itself, defined broadly as *a planned or unplanned interaction between a provider of health care or related services and a recipient of care or information* such as a patient, client, family member, or community member. For ease of expression and clarity, we will generally refer to participants in a health care encounter as providers and patients but we encourage the reader to remember that the definition of a recipient of care or information is broader. Given this broad definition of a health care encounter, each visit to a health care organization consists of numerous encounters with many representatives of the health care organization: the receptionist who schedules the appointment, the emergency room clerk inquiring about insurance, the volunteer providing directions, the nurse checking vital signs, the intern or resident on grand rounds, the phlebotomist drawing a blood sample, the speech therapist conducting a diagnostic exam, the physician providing cognitive services, and the nurse educator providing postdischarge instruction, among others. Each of these health care encounters influences the patient's experience with the health care organization and the process and outcome of care, which is why the systems approach (see Figure 1.2) is essential.

The true test of cultural responsiveness is in the health care encounter, which represents center stage where the reality of the theories, training, assumptions, and social and cultural challenges are interwoven and enacted by individual providers, resulting in positive or negative health care experiences and outcomes. Preparation to become culturally responsive unfolds in the reality of the interaction because it is when we are with the "other" that our ability to embrace the uniqueness of and differences among individuals becomes visible and expresses itself through action (National League for Nursing, 2007).

Even though any encounter in the context of diversity requires cultural responsiveness to be successful, missteps in communication during a health care encounter can be especially damaging due in large part to the **power** differential between the provider and the recipient of care. Those seeking care and their loved ones may find themselves in a dependent role, vulnerable due to illness and the anxiety it may produce, or simply because of the need for information, medical intervention, or expertise they cannot provide for themselves. In contrast, the health care provider may rest in the seat of perceived healer, savior, or expert; the power differential tends to favor the provider. Because power is most fundamentally the ability to change others without having to change yourself, providers may find power sharing challenging because it necessitates rethinking their own role and that of their patients.

Of course, a power differential that generally favors the provider also operates in health care encounters between individuals of the same culture, race, ethnicity, gender, sexual orientation, socioeconomic status, language, or other diversity dimension. But the power differential can feel enormous to the recipient in an encounter with a provider when a difference in a significant diversity dimension is added to the mix. And culturally competent providers will recognize this and the concomitant need to be culturally responsive in health care encounters with diverse patients. From the physician communicating results of a surgical procedure to an LGBT patient's life partner to the nurse educator giving discharge instructions to a patient whose primary language is not English, to a white physical therapist providing rehabilitation services to an African American hip replacement patient who has not completed high school, cultural responsiveness is essential to establishing the trust that is the foundation of a successful health care encounter.

A culturally responsive health care encounter requires that the provider takes action to moderate the power differential in order to form a partnership or therapeutic alliance with the patient that is more balanced. Of course, diverse patients also play a role in the health care encounter and, as is the case with the provider, come to the encounter with their own "baggage." In the health care encounter, however, the onus is on the provider to be culturally responsive irrespective of whether the patient is or not because cultural responsiveness and patient-centered care is about meeting the patient where he or she is and, thus, contributing to a successful therapeutic relationship.

Cultural responsiveness does not, however, mean that anything goes and does not require the provider to accommodate everything the patient wants. There are, for instance, ethical and legal limits to the acceptance of cultural differences, for example, crosscultural clinical encounters that surface ritualistic behavior relating to female genital cutting, circumcision, genital mutilation, or early marriages of children. However, the cultural differences that challenge the health care provider's ethical and legal limits tend to be exceptions compared to those that need to be acknowledged and appreciated. When these cultural barriers in the health care encounter negatively affect access, communication, or trust and lead to patient dissatisfaction and lack of adherence with prescribed treatment, the result is too often poorer health outcomes. Health care encounters, like all other encounters between individuals, involve negotiation: the participants must establish common ground and shared purpose and agree to express themselves in ways that are mutually understood and accepted for a health care encounter to be experienced by both parties as successful.

Nunez and Robertson (2006) summarize the required transformation in the following way: "Healthcare providers must be able to shift from a problem- or disease-focused perspective to the human and contextual perspective of the patients who present to them. They must also be able to recognize their own biases, prejudices and stereotypes. This change of perspective includes considering how patients' concerns might influence communication and clinical assessments. To succeed in this more patient-centered approach, providers must enhance the communication skills necessary to negotiate effectively and collaboratively with patients to optimize outcomes that work within the patients' world" (p. 371). The models presented in the following sections are designed to help the provider do just this in the context of the health care encounter.

MODELS FROM TRANSCULTURAL NURSING

The models discussed in this as well as the subsequent section will help the reader unbundle aspects of the health care encounter that can make or break cultural responsiveness as experienced by the patient. Used appropriately, these models can empower health care providers to identify their own areas of strength and areas in need of development, building on the self-assessment activities included in Chapter Five. Each of these models can also be used to frame the cultural health assessment, which surfaces aspects of the patient's values, beliefs, behaviors, and genetic or biological make-up that may have an impact on the health care encounter.

The theoretical foundation for cultural competence in the health care encounter was built for the most part by the nursing profession through the discipline known as *transcultural nursing*. Over forty years of published literature, including academic journal articles and books, have resulted from this groundbreaking work (Murphy, 2006). This foundational work is relied on by myriad other health professions to frame academic research, education and training curricula, and culturally responsive professional practice.

Madeline M. Leininger is the founder of the **transcultural nursing** discipline, which she characterizes as a "substantive area of study and practice focused on comparative cultural care (caring) values, beliefs, and practices of individuals or groups of similar or different cultures. Transcultural nursing's goal is to provide culture specific and universal nursing care practices for the health and well-being of people or to help them face unfavorable human conditions, illness or death in culturally meaningful ways" (Leininger & McFarland, 2002, p. 46).

Leininger (1987) identifies three stages in the historical evolution of the transcultural nursing discipline:

- 1955–1975: Establishment of the field

- 1975–1983: Expansion of transcultural nursing programs and research

- 1983–present: Worldwide establishment of the transcultural nursing field

The Transcultural Nursing Society (TNS) (www.tcns.org), founded by Leininger in 1974, began offering a certified transcultural nursing (CTN) program in 1988 and published the inaugural issue of the well-regarded *Journal of Transcultural Nursing* in 1989. TNS welcomes members from across the health professions who share its goal of providing culturally competent care.

In the following section, we provide an overview of six prominent models of culturally competent care that have emerged from the transcultural nursing literature, are widely referenced and used by other health professions, and are especially relevant to the focus of this chapter, cultural responsiveness in the health care encounter.

Each of the six models (Table 7.1) emphasizes a different essential lesson for the culturally responsive health care encounter. Which model do you find most personally useful? Which lessons will you focus on at this stage of your personal development as a culturally responsive health care provider? Consider these questions as you read about the six models.

TABLE 7.1   Six Prominent Models from Transcultural Nursing

Model	Essential Lesson for the Culturally Responsive Health Care Encounter
Leininger's Sunrise Model	To be culturally congruent, providers must collaborate with the patient by sharing power and respecting the patient's culture as well as their own.
Purnell Model for Cultural Competence	To be consciously competent, a provider must acquire relevant culture-specific information about the patient.
Campinha-Bacote's Process of Cultural Competence in the Delivery of Health Care Services	To be culturally responsive, the provider must begin with cultural desire, that is, have the attitude that reflects I "want to" not I "have to" do so.
Jeffreys' Cultural Competence and Confidence (CCC) Model	To continue to develop cultural responsiveness, providers should exhibit moderate levels of self-efficacy, defined as a balance between confidence and concern about their skill set, which is most likely to motivate further learning.
Andrews and Boyle's Transcultural Concepts in Nursing Practice	Culturally responsive care is dependent on the strength of the provider's verbal and nonverbal crosscultural communication skills.
Giger-Davidhizar Transcultural Assessment Model (GDTAM)	Culturally responsive care requires that the provider evaluate how the following six cultural phenomena may affect cultural responsiveness in the health care encounter: communication, space, social organization, time, environmental control, and biological variations.

Leininger's Sunrise Model

Leininger's Sunrise Model, also referred to in the literature as the Sunrise Enabler, depicts factors influencing care as specified in culture care theory (Leininger, 2002). Leininger recommends using the Sunrise Model with culture care theory to "discover factors related to cultural stresses, pain, racial biases, and even destructive acts as nontherapeutic to clients" (Leininger, 2002, p. 190) and "to provide culturally congruent nursing care in order to improve or offer a different kind of nursing care service to people of diverse or similar cultures" (Leininger, 1996, p. 72). Culturally congruent nursing care is defined as "those cognitively based assistive, supportive, facilitative, or enabling acts or decisions that are tailor-made to fit with an individual's, group's, or institution's cultural values, beliefs, and lifeways in order to provide meaningful, beneficial, and satisfying health care, or well-being services" (Leininger, 1991, p. 49). As such, the Sunrise Model is especially useful to the health care provider in identifying and addressing aspects of the health care encounter that contribute to or distract from culturally responsive care delivery and is consistent with the systems approach to patient-centered care described in Figure 1.2.

The Sunrise Model views the delivery of culturally responsive care as the provider's ultimate goal. The model unbundles the factors that support or detract from the provider's success in doing so and serves as a visual representation of the process itself. To meet the goal of culturally congruent care delivery, the provider must make transcultural care decisions and actions in collaboration with the patient, resulting in culture care preservation and maintenance, culture care accommodation and negotiation, or culture care restructuring and repatterning, as appropriate. But to collaborate with the patient in making transcultural care decisions, providers must understand their own as well as the patient's worldview and its cultural and social structure dimensions, especially as they influence care expressions, patterns, and practices and beliefs about health, illness, and death.

Providers who wish to apply Leininger's Sunrise Model to self-evaluation and development in the context of the health care encounter can begin by considering the following questions:

- What do I believe about health, illness, and death? How do my identity group memberships, such as gender, ethnicity, socioeconomic status, profession, and so on, influence my beliefs?

- How open am I to seeing value and truth in worldviews and beliefs that differ from my own?

- What do I know about the similarities and differences between my worldview and beliefs and those of the patient I am interacting with?

- What knowledge do I need to acquire about the culture, worldview, health beliefs, and practices of my patient before the health care encounter?

- How can I interact in the health care encounter to acquire knowledge during the encounter and test my assumptions about the patient's culture, worldview, health beliefs, and practices?

- How successful am I in negotiating with my patient in the health care encounter? How will I know if the patient perceived the encounter as successful?

Now read the following scenario and address the associated questions. Consider how Leininger's Sunrise Model could be used to design training to improve cultural responsiveness in this scenario and others like it.

CULTURAL RESPONSIVENESS SCENARIO ONE

Two young physical therapy trainees, James and Kenneth, are discussing their assignment outside the patient's room. James says to Kenneth, "This should be a piece of cake. I just need to tell him that he's got to follow up on out-patient services. He's from the Islands and you're from the Islands so I thought if you went in with me, together we could make sure that he understood everything. In fact, because you're from the same place he is, why don't you explain to him about following up?"

"Well," responds Kenneth, "I'm not really from the Islands; my parents are, but I'm sure I know enough about my people to be able to help you out." They enter into sixty-five-year-old Joseph Sampson's room and James says, "Hey, Joe, we're here to explain the next steps after you're discharged from the hospital today. Kenneth, my partner, he's going to give you the run down. His parents are from Jamaica, you know, the Caribbean, just like you. Trinidad and Jamaica are about the same, right?" Mr. Sampson turns his back on the two young men and refuses to speak with them.

What assumptions did James make about ethnicity and culture?

How did his assumption affect the health care encounter?

Why did Mr. Sampson react the way he did?

What could James and Kenneth do to develop their cultural competence?

Is there anything the health care organization or the supervisor should do to apologize and ensure that future health care encounters are more culturally responsive?

As the Sunrise Model depicts, culturally congruent care cannot be delivered without knowledge and respect for not only your own but also your patient's worldview, culture, and preferred care expressions, patterns, and practices. The health care encounter is best viewed as a negotiation in which the patient and the provider learn about one another's perspectives and agree on common ground and shared purpose. When this happens, the health care encounter is culturally responsive and therefore beneficial to patient and provider.

Purnell Model for Cultural Competence

Larry Purnell first developed the Purnell Model for Cultural Competence as a clinical assessment tool for student nurses. Since then, the model has been translated into French, Spanish, Flemish, and Korean and is widely applied across the health professions (Purnell, 2002). The model is especially useful to providers in determining exactly what cultural information about the patient will be needed to engage in a culturally competent health care encounter with that person.

The Purnell Model, initially published in 1998, is a visual depiction of twelve domains of patient culture that the provider may need knowledge of as a precondition for the delivery of culturally responsive care. The model, which consists of concentric circles, depicts the twelve domains as wedges of an inner circle contained within the outer circles that represent the context of global society, community, family, and person. The innermost circle is empty, representing that which is unknown about a cultural group. The twelve domains include general and specific cultural characteristics. Although detailed knowledge about all of the specific cultural domains and cultural characteristics is not needed for every health care encounter, the provider does need general information about the culture of the patient and must also acquire the specific cultural knowledge that is pertinent to the encounter. Following are the twelve domains:

- Overview and heritage
- Communication
- Family roles and organization
- Workforce issues
- Biocultural ecology
- High-risk behaviors
- Nutrition
- Pregnancy and childbearing practices
- Death rituals
- Spirituality
- Health care practice
- Health care practitioner

At the foot of the model, providers are seen to reside along a continuum that ranges from unconsciously incompetent, consciously incompetent, consciously competent, and unconsciously competent. Providers who "don't know that they don't know" are viewed as incompetent but unconsciously so, whereas providers who "know that they don't know" or discover that they don't know in the course of the health care encounter are also viewed as incompetent but consciously so. When a provider becomes aware that he or she needs the general and specific cultural knowledge about the patient as specified in the Purnell Model for Cultural Competence *and* acquires that knowledge, the provider has now evolved to conscious competence. When the provider's knowledge base and facility in its application during the patient encounter is well established, the provider is characterized in the model as unconsciously competent.

Providers who wish to apply this model to self-evaluation and development in the context of the health care encounter can begin by considering the following questions:

- Which of the twelve domains define knowledge I already have about my patient's culture?

- Which of the twelve domains define knowledge I need to acquire about my patient's culture?

- How can I acquire vital knowledge about my patient's culture?

- How will I know where I reside along the continuum of unconscious incompetence to unconscious competence? Does where I reside on the continuum differ by cultural group?

The Purnell Model emphasizes the need for information about a patient's culture and assists the provider in identifying exactly what information is needed, given the nature and purpose of the health care encounter. Valid general and specific information about cultural beliefs and practices of diverse groups is now widely available on the web as well as in journal articles, practice guides, and books. The web resources that accompany this book include links to such information. Of course, it is important not to overgeneralize about cultures. Not every member of a group shares the worldview or displays the values, beliefs, and behaviors that may be commonly associated with that group. Furthermore, as discussed in Chapter One and referenced throughout this book, each person is a member of many identity groups and individuals differ in how they experience their identity group memberships. Consequently, the health care provider must not use cultural knowledge to stereotype patients. Otherwise, the result will be unconscious incompetence.

Campinha-Bacote's Process of Cultural Competence in the Delivery of Health Care Services

Josepha Campinha-Bacote, president of Transcultural CARE Associates, developed the Process of Cultural Competence in the Delivery of Health Care Services Model, which emphasizes the important role that a key affective characteristic—cultural desire—plays in the process of cultural competence.

Campinha-Bacote (2008) defines **cultural desire** as "the motivation of the nurse to 'want to' engage in the process of becoming culturally competent; not to 'have to.'" She further states that cultural desire "includes a genuine passion and commitment to be open and flexible with others; a respect and understanding of differences, yet a commitment to build upon similarities; a willingness to learn from patients and others as cultural informants; and a sense of humility" (pp. 142–143). Her model depicts cultural desire as the base of a volcano, which erupts with cultural awareness, cultural knowledge, cultural skill, and cultural encounters.

Campinha-Bacote (1999, pp. 204–205) defines the other constructs in her model as follows:

- *Cultural awareness:* A "deliberate cognitive process" through which health care providers become aware of, appreciative of, and sensitive to the patient's culture as well as to their own culture and personal biases

- *Cultural knowledge:* The "process of seeking and obtaining" valid and relevant information about the patient's culture

- *Cultural skill:* The process of applying awareness and knowledge in the health care encounter to obtain cultural information about the patient that is relevant to the encounter and to perform a "culturally based physical assessment," taking into account "physical, biological, and physiological" variations that can be associated with ethnicity, as discussed in Chapter Two of this book and later in this chapter

- *Cultural encounters:* The process of engaging in direct crosscultural interactions to build cultural awareness, knowledge, and skill and counter the tendency to stereotype that can result when providers lack sufficient personal experience with diverse group members to see variation within cultural groups and consequently stereotype patients

Campinha-Bacote also developed a self-assessment instrument—Inventory for Assessing the Process of Cultural Competence Among Health Professionals Revised (IAPCC-R)—that students and providers can use to evaluate their proficiency on each of the five constructs in her model. The IAPCC-R is available for purchase on the Transcultural CARE Associates website and in her 2007 book, *The Process of Cultural Competence in the Delivery of Healthcare Services: The Journey Continues*, which describes in detail the five constructs in her model and their application in the health care encounter.

Providers who wish to apply Campinha-Bacote's model to self-evaluation and development in the context of the health care encounter can begin by considering the following questions:

- How strong is my cultural desire? What actions can I take to make it stronger?

- Am I aware of the impact of culture on the health care encounter? What evidence supports my self-assessment? How can I build greater awareness?

- What are my cultural skills in the health care encounter? What are my areas for development? What evidence supports my self-assessment?

- What are the sources of my cultural knowledge? Are these sources valid? Do I use my cultural knowledge appropriately? How can I obtain more valid cultural knowledge that is relevant to the health care encounter?

- Do I approach or avoid cultural encounters with people I perceive to be different from myself? How can I create opportunities in my life for more frequent professional and personal crosscultural encounters?

Campinha-Bacote's Process of Cultural Competence in the Delivery of Health Services Model emphasizes the need for cultural desire to generate cultural awareness, skills, knowledge, and encounters. Campinha-Bacote's model stresses the importance of the health care provider's heart-felt personal commitment through depicting the affective construct—cultural desire—as the base of the volcano of cultural competence in the delivery of health care services. It's considered important that her model also emphasizes cultural competence as a process, not a destination. By continually stoking cultural desire; building cultural awareness, skills, and knowledge; and engaging in cultural encounters, the health care provider strengthens his or her ability to be increasingly responsive to diverse patients' needs.

Jeffreys' Cultural Competence and Confidence (CCC) Model

Marianne Jeffreys developed the Cultural Competence and Confidence (CCC) Model to serve as a comprehensive framework for teaching and learning about cultural competence. The CCC Model was introduced in Jeffreys' book (2006) entitled *Teaching Cultural Competence in Nursing and Health Care: Inquiry, Action, and Innovation*, which is now in its second edition (2010). As with Campinha-Bacote's model, the CCC Model is paired with a self-assessment instrument.

Jeffreys' model emphasizes the role of **transcultural self-efficacy**, defined as confidence in one's own ability to develop and apply cognitive, practical, and affective transcultural nursing skills. Self-appraisal is an essential component of the model and Jeffreys observes that those with self-reported levels of self-efficacy that are either very high or very low will be less likely to deliver culturally appropriate care than those with moderate levels of transcultural self-efficacy. This is because over-confident providers will not pursue development of transcultural skills because they believe they already possess them and those with low transcultural self-efficacy will avoid opportunities to develop transcultural skills due to their lack of confidence. However, providers with moderate levels of transcultural self-efficacy exhibit a balance between confidence and concern about their skill set, which is most likely to motivate further learning. Training, therefore, should focus on reducing the self-efficacy of providers who are overconfident and building the self-efficacy of those who are underconfident while providing the opportunity for those with moderate levels of self-efficacy to continue to develop their affective, cognitive, and practical transcultural nursing skills, which the CCC Model defines as follows (Jeffreys, 2006, 2010):

- Affective skill development builds self-awareness about the provider's own culture and personal biases and their effect on the health care encounter.

- Cognitive skill development builds general and specific knowledge about patient culture and its effect on the health care encounter.

- Practical skill development builds the provider's capacity to exhibit cultural competence through communication and interaction with patients in order to develop and implement a valid patient-specific cultural needs assessment.

Providers who wish to apply Jeffreys' CCC Model to self-evaluation and development in the context of the health care encounter can begin by considering the following questions:

- How do I rate my own transcultural self-efficacy? How does my rating affect my motivation to develop my affective, cognitive, and practical transcultural skills?

- Am I self-aware about my own culturally based values, beliefs, and behaviors, especially as they pertain to the health care encounter? Am I committed to continually developing my self-awareness? What am I doing to build my *affective* transcultural skills?

- What knowledge do I have about the culture, worldview, health beliefs, and practices of my patients? What additional knowledge do I need? What am I doing to build my *cognitive* transcultural skills?

- Does my style of communication with the patient in the health care encounter enable me to deliver patient-centered care that is culturally responsive? What am I doing to build my *practical* transcultural skills?

Jeffreys' CCC Model emphasizes the importance of transcultural self-efficacy and explains how not only a lack of confidence but also an overabundance of confidence can lessen motivation to develop affective, cognitive, and practical transcultural nursing skills. Realistic self-appraisal, formal education, role models, mentors, and professional experiences are all part and parcel of building and continually developing our performance as culturally competent providers in the health care encounter.

Andrews and Boyle's Transcultural Concepts in Nursing Practice

Margaret M. Andrews and Joyceen S. Boyle developed the Transcultural Concepts in Nursing Practice Model, which posits crosscultural communication as a bridge between provider and patient. The model identifies specific aspects of communication that the provider must be aware of and respond to in order to communicate effectively with diverse patients and is the theoretical framework for their textbook, *Transcultural Concepts in Nursing Care*, first published in 1989, and now in its fifth edition (2007).

As the model depicts, communication has verbal and nonverbal dimensions, occurs in an environmental context, and reflects the similarities and differences in the provider's and patient's cultural values, beliefs, and behaviors, especially as they relate to health care. Important aspects of verbal communication include language and the culturally appropriate use of titles and exchange of greetings and key aspects of nonverbal communication include time, space, distance, modesty, and touch. The reader is encouraged to read Chapter Eight and the next section of this chapter for a detailed discussion of specific aspects of crosscultural communication that can enhance or detract from culturally competent health care delivery. Andrews and Boyle (2007) emphasize that, instead of concentrating on "simply memorizing the esoteric health beliefs and practices of a litany of different groups," the focus must be on enhancement of the health care providers' cultural assessment skills and their application in the health care encounter. In this fashion, providers can "assess and care for clients from virtually any and all cultural groups that they might encounter in their professional careers" (p. xii).

Now read the following scenario and address the associated questions. Consider how the CCC Model could be used to design training to improve cultural responsiveness in this scenario and others like it.

CULTURAL RESPONSIVENESS SCENARIO TWO

A nineteen-year-old Latino male was admitted to the hospital with a gunshot wound to the back of his leg. His injury was the result of an encounter with the police who had randomly stopped his car and were performing a search when he fled the scene. He was placed on the orthopedics floor in an empty four-bed room at the end of the corridor and the staff seemed anxious and wary of his presence. Although his leg was immobilized in traction, his loud rap music, girlfriend's visits throughout the day, and use of profanity to demand service were building a wall of distance between the young man and the staff. No one wanted the patient in 454 D as an assignment and most staff avoided the room during their shifts. The nurse manager requested consultation from a psychiatric clinical nurse specialist that worked with the staff throughout the hospital. The consultant interviewed staff members to assess the situation and to determine what interventions had been made. The staff explained that nothing worked and that they had just given up and stayed away, describing the patient as "Latino, loud, and dangerous." Except on admission to the unit, no one had actually had a conversation with Manuel. The consultant sat down by Manuel's bedside and asked him how he was experiencing his hospitalization. Manuel explained that he felt isolated and was sure that he could die in this large empty room and that no one would know and no one would help. He described how infrequently he saw staff or anyone except his girlfriend and family and how angry he was with the staff for treating him as if he were contagious. The consultant acknowledged Manuel's sense of isolation but also his responsibility in helping to create and sustain the situation. He told the consultant that he knew he frightened the staff and found a small level of satisfaction from this. The consultant recommended compromise that required behavioral change on the part of Manuel and the staff. For Manuel: turn the music down, stop the profanity, and speak politely with the staff. For the staff: move Manuel to a room closer to the center of activity and reengage with him through their physical presence and conversation. And, with the assistance of the consultant, explore the role that bias and cultural style differences may have played in this scenario.

What is your reaction to the consultant's recommendations?

Do you think the consultant's suggested compromise will resolve the conflict? Why or why not?

Are there other recommendations that you would make?

Providers who wish to apply Andrews and Boyle's Transcultural Concepts in Nursing Practice Model to self-evaluation and development in the context of the health care encounter can begin by considering the following questions:

• What aspects of verbal and nonverbal communication do I use effectively in health care encounters with diverse patients? Which aspects do I need to develop?

- What do I know about similarities and differences in verbal and nonverbal communication norms among cultural groups? What else do I need to learn?

- Do I focus on memorizing the health beliefs and practices of different groups or on developing my crosscultural communication skills? Which approach do I believe is more important to cultural competence in the health care encounter and why?

Andrews and Boyle's Transcultural Concepts in Nursing Practice Model emphasizes the role of effective crosscultural communication in the culturally competent health care encounter. By staying focused on self-development, providers can learn to communicate effectively in the health care encounter and apply transcultural concepts to professional practice.

GIGER-DAVIDHIZAR TRANSCULTURAL ASSESSMENT MODEL (GDTAM)

Joyce Newman Giger and Ruth Davidhizar developed the Giger-Davidhizar Transcultural Assessment Model (GDTAM) in 1988 for use with nursing students (Giger & Davidhizar, 2002). The GDTAM is the sixth and final model discussed in this chapter and will be used to frame a broader discussion of the six cultural phenomena identified in the GDTAM (Giger & Davidhizar, 2008) that shape health care encounters in the context of diversity. The six phenomena are as follows:

- Communication
- Space
- Social organization
- Time
- Environmental control
- Biological variations

The GDTAM serves as the organizing framework for Giger and Davidhizar's textbook, *Transcultural Nursing: Assessment and Intervention*, first published in

1990 and now in its fifth edition (2008). The model provides a framework for the provider's cultural assessment and thus can be used to enhance cultural responsiveness in the health care encounter.

Communication

The first cultural phenomenon in the GDTAM, communication, is the bridge to connecting with the other and therefore is the pathway to mutual trust, understanding, and respect between patient and provider in the health care encounter. Without communication we are alone in the world, unable to negotiate with one another to identify the common ground and shared purpose essential to a health care encounter that is perceived as effective by patient and provider. In fact, communication is so important to diversity and cultural competence in health care that Chapter Eight of this book is dedicated to the topic and builds on the concepts introduced in this section.

Effective crosscultural communication between providers and patients requires attention to the cultural dimensions of not only verbal and nonverbal communication in a face-to-face setting but also written communication, including discharge instructions and informational brochures pertinent to the patient's diagnosis and treatment plan. LEP (limited English proficient) patients as well as patients with limited literacy will require special attention that can be effectively provided only through the systems approach (see Figure 1.2).

Culture and communication style are inseparable. One's culture is transmitted and preserved through communication. Children exhibit learned cultural patterns, including aspects of communication style, by age five (Anderson, 2003). Culture affects, reflects, and at times determines communication style and preferences and communication can affect, reflect, and mold culture.

In the health care encounter, it is critical to know that the intended message is received and understood. In the 1950s, decades before the diversity and cultural competence movements, Dr. Harry Stack Sullivan, the psychiatrist whose work provided a foundation for interpersonal psychoanalysis, emphasized the importance of **consensual validation** in the therapeutic relationship between provider and patient. Consensual validation is the process of ascertaining whether the receiver grasped and comprehended the intended message of the sender. In the context of diversity, this simple tool of confirming and disconfirming the receipt and understanding of information exchanged in the health care encounter is essential.

Projection is a psychodynamic process that can have an adverse impact on effective communication in the health care encounter, especially in the context of diversity. Projected similarity occurs when providers attribute their own feelings, thoughts, desires, expectations, and even behavior to the patient, assuming that their own beliefs, values, and cultural behavioral patterns are shared and valued by the patient. Sondra Thiederman (1986) suggests that projected similarity may lead not only to the inadequate provision of care, but also to patient non-adherence with the recommended treatment plan. Even problems such as pain management, which has not only physiological but also cultural and psychological aspects, may not be addressed to the patient's satisfaction when the provider falls prey to projected similarity (Davidhizar & Hart, 2005).

As discussed further in the next chapter, in oral communication, meaning is transmitted verbally and nonverbally. Body movements, intonation, facial expressions, and physical distance are all important aspects of nonverbal communication. Knapp and Hall (1992) identified five important aspects of nonverbal communication as follows:

- Emblems or nonverbal symbols that can be translated into a word, phrase, or symbol. Sign language used in the operating room is an example. Another is the thumbs-up signal that can indicate success or agreement but, with a slight modification, in Brazil, could indicate an obscenity (Giger & Davidhizar, 2008).

- Affect displays, including facial expressions that convey feelings such as smiles or frowns.

- Illustrations, including nonverbal acts such as pointing toward an object or trying to describe a situation without using words.

- Adapters, defined as nonverbal behaviors that modify what is being said. For instance, folded arms may indicate disagreement and a wave may be used to welcome someone or to dismiss the other's comment.

- Regulators, which are nonverbal movements that act as bridges in continuing the interaction and providing feedback. Head nodding or changing one's gaze or moving the body forward are examples of regulators.

Effective communication is key to a successful health care encounter. Culturally competent providers are aware of the verbal and nonverbal aspects of communication and their relationship to key diversity dimensions such as ethnicity and gender. Most important, culturally competent providers are able to **self-monitor** and adapt their style to communicate effectively with each individual patient.

Space

Space is the second cultural phenomenon in the GDTAM's organizing framework. The provider's ability to manage spatial distance in culturally responsive ways is important to the health care encounter. **Proxemics** is a field of study that focuses on the cultural meaning of interpersonal distance in communication. An individual's personal space is in part culturally determined. Within personal space, there is outer space, or the physical area that surrounds one's body, and there is inner space, which can best be described as the medium that filters the incoming stimuli that a person receives (Scott & Dumas, 1995). Scott (1988) describes inner personal space as dynamic, invisible lines of demarcation (boundaries) consisting of four layered areas: (1) the inner spirit core, (2) an area of thoughts and feelings perceived as unacceptable, (3) an area of thoughts and feelings perceived as acceptable, and (4) an area of superficial public image. If patients feel the provider has invaded or violated their defined outer or inner personal space, the health care encounter will be adversely affected. The culturally competent health care provider must navigate inner and outer space effectively in the health care encounter.

Space can also be seen as tactile and visual; tactile and visual spatial experiences are so entwined that it's difficult at times to separate the two. Infants and young children clearly demonstrate this as they reach across space to grasp, fondle, hold, and mouth everything in their visual space. Giger and Davidhizar (2008) make the following distinction: "Tactile space separates the viewer from the object while visual space separates the objects from one another" (p. 53).

Frequently, touch is a tool used in the health care encounter. It is the most personal of all the sensations and has been described as confirmation for the reality perceived through other senses (Montague, 1986). Touch can convey the most intimate caress or the most violent attack. Touch has the ability to penetrate the layers of personal inner space to evoke unacceptable thoughts and feelings or threaten one's public image of one's self. For example, a female nurse from a nontactile family culture may experience discomfort when a male client from a tactile family culture stands close enough to touch in the health care encounter. Interestingly, close enough to touch is frequently determined according to the situation, individually and culturally. Clients who step back or pull their chairs back in the health care encounter are sending the message that they require additional space. Due to the nature of the health care encounter, touching is an essential part of the interaction, but, depending on the culture, it may have unexpected meaning. For example in the Thai and Vietnamese cultures, the head is traditionally viewed as sacred; it is the seat of life. The belief is that when the head is touched, the spirit leaves through this passage (Carson, 2000).

For the health care provider touch is a major part of the healing process and the health care encounter. There is often heightened sensitivity when primary and secondary sexual features are considered, such as mammograms, vaginal, and prostate exams. However, certain patients may also experience heightened sensitivity with taking blood, giving injections, and receiving bed baths.

An appropriate strategy to address space is the use of effective communication so that the patient understands the procedure and intent and the provider understands the cultural concerns related to touch. Once again, the provider must make every effort to tailor the care to the individual because to do so is the essence of patient-centered care.

Spatial behavior can also be explored through the concept of territoriality. According to Davidhizar and Giger (1998), territoriality is related to the need for control, authority, and legitimate power over an area of defined physical space. Hayter (1981) identifies three significant aspects of territoriality that must be addressed by the provider in a culturally responsive health care encounter:

- A definable physical space such as one's assigned room or area

- A personal space such as one's own bed

- The territory of expertise or role

Hayter (1981) explains that these three aspects of territoriality provide security, privacy, autonomy, and self-identity. In the health care encounter, patients often experience loss of control over one or more of these aspects of territoriality to the detriment of the healing process. The remedy is to partner with the patient to restore autonomy and control. Hayter (1981) recommends that the provider ask the patient's permission to enter his or her space as a way of acknowledging that the patient, not the provider, controls the space.

Structural boundaries that clearly identify personal territory such as closed doors are also of significance in managing the health care encounter. In addition, in health care settings, there are usually some identified patient-free zones, such as the nursing station or staff lounge. Providers and patients must navigate these territorial boundaries and establish a shared understanding so that conflict does not derail the culturally responsive health care encounter.

Appropriate physical distancing from others is determined culturally and situationally (Murray & Huelskoetter, 1991) and involves the concepts of space and territoriality. The renowned anthropologist Edward T. Hall (1966) explains that, in Western culture, three dimensions of space or territory are defined as follows: the intimate zone (0 to 18 inches), the personal zone (18 inches to 3 feet), and the social or public zone (3 to 6 feet). The intimate zone is reserved for people who are closely connected, the personal zone for friends, and the social zone for business and professional associates. The health care encounter is complex because it often involves the closeness of the intimate zone while still being a professional interaction. This paradox challenges patient and provider and, because the dimensions of intimate, personal, and public zones vary considerably across cultures, it is important for the provider to have knowledge of cultural variations in spatial requirements.

Watson (1980) analyzed the dimensions of personal space by country and found that individuals in the United States, Canada, and Britain required the most personal space whereas Latin American, Japanese, and Arabic persons needed the least. And, for some Asian countries, maintaining distance is a sign of respect, with the definition of respectful distance changing in relationship to status in the group. As residents of the United States become increasingly culturally diverse, health care providers will need to interact skillfully with patients who have widely varying definitions of personal space and settle on mutually acceptable norms and boundaries with the patient.

Ethnic groups may use shared space differently from one another, which can cause conflict in the context of diversity. People from group-oriented cultures may be perceived by people from individual-oriented cultures as crowding the emergency room or the hospitalized patient's room during visiting hours. Although European American cultures tend to be more individual oriented,

Asian, Latino, African American, and Mediterranean American cultures are more group oriented. Twenty relatives at the patient's bedside is not unusual when viewed through the group-oriented lens of collectivity, but may be perceived as strange, inappropriate, or not conducive to health care by those who subscribe to the biomedical model, which is based on individual patient autonomy (Kaegi, 2004). Providers or other patients and their visitors may experience a feeling of being overwhelmed and react from a defensive position and struggle to manage the space to meet the clinical and emotional support needs of themselves and their patients. Emotional support is critical and very difficult to give if the provider is drowning in his or her own reactive behavior. Navigating these conflicts is not simple and is more easily done in an organization that takes a systems approach to diversity and cultural competence (see Figure 1.2) because organizational supports for the provider struggling to meet the cultural demands of diverse patients in a shared space are in place.

When an illness requires hospitalization, there may be strong feelings of powerlessness that can lead to depression and hopelessness, disabling one's ability to expect a positive outcome. It is important for patients to have as much control as possible over their space and their legitimate right to be in their space. The culturally responsive health care provider understands and strives to address these needs.

Social Organization

The third cultural phenomenon in the GDTAM, **social organization**, defined as the pattern of relationships among people in a group, is an important manifestation of culture with significant implications for the health care encounter. Social organization is generally associated with ethnicity, with the family serving as the foundation of social organization across cultures. However, the definition of what constitutes family, role assignments in the family, and the effect of gender, age, and relationship on role assignment differ by ethnic group. For some cultures, the traditional nuclear family—father, mother, and children—is considered to be the basic family unit, whereas other cultures are grounded in the extended family system.

In the United States, the definition of family is being reshaped by diversity and changing social norms and the composition of the traditional nuclear family is being redefined. For example, through a second marriage, a woman and man can form a blended family like the Brady Bunch or gay and lesbian life partners can form a family unit through marriage or civil unions in a growing number of states or mutual agreement in other states. A multitude of ways to organize and define the family exist and the health care provider must be prepared to accept and respect the patient's view of what constitutes family and, when appropriate, work in partnership with the family in collaboration with the patient. Family systems of any ilk can be constructive or destructive to the patient.

Irrespective of the particulars of the patient's family structure, the three elements of the systems approach to patient care described in Chapter One facilitate working in partnership with the patient and, when appropriate, his or her family and community: medical homes, interprofessional teams, and patient-centered care. The systems approach, however, has barriers to surmount. Minuchin, Colapinto, and Minuchin (1998) identified the following obstacles to working with the social organization of family and community, as defined by the patient, through a systems approach:

- Bureaucracies tend to give rise to silos of services, such that fiefdoms multiply and care is not integrated.

- Providers are educated to identify individual problems but rarely to deal with the person in context of family and community.

- Social attitudes including moralistic judgments can lead to families being blamed for their problems and viewed as a burden on society or the provider.

These obstacles are best addressed by adopting the systems approach to diversity and cultural competence and Minuchin, Nichols, and Lee's empowerment model (2007), designed to strengthen the informational and supportive capacity of families by including them as appropriate in the patient's care plan.

A case in point is type 2 diabetes prevention and management. The devastation of type 2 diabetes and its frequent companion, obesity, is of epidemic proportions for the American Indian (Palacios, Butterfly, & Strickland, 2006) and also affects African Americans and Latinos at higher rates than European Americans. The keys to diabetes management are monitoring, education, diet, exercise, and medications, as conveyed by the mnemonic MEDEM (Satchen & Pamies, 2006). MEDEM must include consideration of the family to be successful. For example, the patient may not be the cook in his family and may feel obligated to eat what the family member who cooks prepares. As a consequence, the family member who is the cook as well as the grocery shopper may need education regarding diet and family eating patterns. Dietary and other lifestyle choices are made and changed in the context of social systems. The culturally responsive health care provider who works with the system and its members is more likely to experience patient adherence to recommended lifestyle changes.

Religion, which is often closely associated with ethnic identity and reinforced through the family system, is an important aspect of social organization. Religious beliefs and traditions are often salient to the health care encounter. For example, Jehovah's Witnesses are opposed to blood transfusions if the blood is obtained from a blood bank or is a donation, believing that accepting blood from a source other than themselves defies their scriptural teachings. One option developed to meet the needs of the Jehovah's Witness community was bloodless surgery because it was transfusion-free and acceptable to most Jehovah's Witness followers. In the health care encounter, the provider needs to be aware of the impact that a patient's religious beliefs might have on health care in order to respond appropriately to the traditions and beliefs of the patient.

Time

The fourth cultural phenomenon in the GDTAM is time. As with communication, space, and social organization, the ways in which people experience time are socially determined. People from task-focused cultures are more likely to value being "on time," whereas people from relationship-focused cultures are more likely to value being "in time." Giger and Davidhizar refer to these two distinct approaches as clock time and social time. Social time arises out of and emphasizes the value of social interactions. Phillip Bock (1964), an anthropologist, described an American Indian wake in terms of gathering time, prayer time, singing time, and meal time. The nurse who starts and ends her twelve-hour shift on schedule is operating in accordance with clock time norms, which emphasizes the value of "getting the job done." Both approaches to experiencing time are the result of humans structuring and functioning within a system of social organization.

In the United States, clock time is relied on to keep the wheels of commerce turning and to run health care provider organizations efficiently. The commonly heard phrase "time is money" reflects a task-oriented, clock-time emphasis. In a health care encounter, relationship-oriented patients who operate "in time" and are late for their scheduled appointment might anger a task-oriented provider operating within clock-time norms. The "on-time" provider may feel inconvenienced or disrespected, whereas "in-time" patients may feel that the provider is being unreasonable because social-time people consider time to be flexible and expect events to begin when they arrive rather than at a predetermined time.

Now consider the following scenario and address the associated questions for the opportunity to resolve a conflict between on-time and in-time perspectives in a health care encounter. What insights does the GDTAM provide on the conflict between how time is perceived by Mrs. Sanchez and by the health care provider organization and its representatives? How can these insights help to frame a resolution that incorporates a systems perspective?

CULTURAL RESPONSIVENESS SCENARIO THREE

Seventy-two-year-old Mrs. Sanchez had worked hard to organize her ride for her doctor's appointment. Everyone in her family was at work and it had taken her six weeks just to get this appointment. Her nephew Ramon had actually taken time off from work to bring her and, without warning, his tire had blown out and they arrived at the clinic forty-five minutes late. The receptionist at the desk, who Mrs. Sanchez perceived as incredibly rude, suggested that she did not appreciate the opportunity to see her doctor and questioned whether the doctor would be able to see her. After an hour and a half of waiting, Mrs. Sanchez's name was finally called and she began the encounter with her physician wondering if she was being punished for something that was out of her control. She asked herself, should I even bring up the problems that I came to talk about?

Justify Mrs. Sanchez' perspective.

Justify the receptionist's perspective.

Describe the needs they share in common.

Propose a resolution that meets the needs and reflects the value of on-time and in-time perspectives.

Environmental Control

The fifth cultural phenomenon in the GDTAM is environmental control, which refers to whether a person tends to believe that he or she controls or is controlled by external circumstances. The concept that undergirds this cultural phenomenon is known as **locus of control**, which means the extent to which people believe they have mastery over their own experiences and outcomes. Locus of control is defined as either internal or external and, although it can reflect an individual's own personality, locus of control is learned through **enculturation** in the family and the community.

The dominant cultural perspective in the United States generally and in the health care system specifically values an internal locus of control. The belief that we can move obstacles, implement a plan, and thus direct the future outcome is deeply ingrained in the cultures of the health care professions. Cultures that reinforce an internal locus of control can be defined as directive, and cultures that reinforce an external locus of control can be defined as adaptive. And, often, cultural traditions that value social time over clock time also reflect an external locus of control.

Because ethnocentrism, or the belief that your identity group's cultural style is superior to others, is a human tendency, health care providers may prefer working with patients whose locus of control is internal and may even devalue or discount patients who operate from an external local of control. The antidote to ethnocentrism is first to be aware that you have it and then to expand your intercultural experiences so that you can see the truth in alternative perspectives. Cognitive reframing, discussed in Chapter Five, is a helpful technique in the quest to overcome ethnocentrism, a necessary quest because without respect for the patient's style, communication will be ineffective and the process and outcome of care will be adversely affected. As Leininger (1991, 1996) suggests, consider the health care encounter as a negotiation and be open to working with clients to maintain their perspective, to accommodate or negotiate, or to work with clients to change their perspective, when provider and patient both agree that change is necessary.

When it comes to locus of control, internal and external orientations have some truth to them. After all, we cannot control many natural forces in the environment like the weather and, although we can influence our odds of getting certain diseases or our odds of recovery, we simple do not have absolute control. And some of us have more environmental control than others, with that control associated with diversity dimensions such as socioeconomic status, gender role as defined in our family system, or disability status.

For example, communities composed of individuals of color with low socioeconomic status tend to have disproportionate levels of exposure to hazardous wastes and environmental pollutants due to factors such as location of sites for toxic waste disposal and industries that produce pollutants (Satcher & Pamies, 2006). Massey (2004) summarizes findings from myriad research studies, which establish that exposure to pollution and hazardous waste is disproportionately higher in low SES communities and communities of color and documents the associated health risks. When compared with whites, African American, Hispanic, and Asian and Pacific Islander children are exposed to higher mean levels of air pollution. Although asthma mortality and morbidity increased in all US children from 1980 through 1998, African American children were three times as likely to be hospitalized for asthma as whites and more than four times as likely to die from an asthmatic attack (Akinbami & Schoendorf, 2002).

Pregnant women and children living near shorelines may experience higher-than-average levels of exposure to methyl mercury. Consistent consumption of saltwater fish may lead to a concentration of methyl mercury in the developing fetus and in the brains of children, which could affect their neurological development. Freshwater fish in rural areas can also deliver a pollutant, polychlorinated biphenyl (PCB), which is a by-product of manufacturing run-off. This pollutant has been associated with cognitive deficits in infants and behavioral problems and lower academic achievement in children (National Institute of Environmental Health Sciences, 2001).

Lead poisoning is another example of environmental inequity. It is five times more likely to occur in African American children than white children because they are more likely to live in older, deteriorating housing. Lead poisoning even at low blood levels has been associated with neurological defects and low birth weights. Lead poisoning has its effect across the life span and in adulthood has been associated with hypertension and kidney disease (National Institute of Environmental Health Sciences, 2001).

In the health care encounter, it is important for the provider to determine whether environmental exposure may be affecting the health of the care recipient. It is also important to remember that such exposure is not always the "fault" of the patient and, although patients and their families can influence environmental exposure and act to reduce it personally, they do not have absolute control. Culturally competent providers will be able to **decenter**, that is, take into account others' perspectives and, in the health care encounter, will show respect for their own situation and preferred locus of control and that of their patients. In this fashion, common ground and shared purpose can be negotiated in the health care encounter, resulting in a better outcome.

Biological Variations

The sixth and final cultural phenomenon in the GDTAM is biological variations, which refer to factors such as the role of genetics in predispositions to certain diseases, the impact of variations in skin color among ethnic groups on certain clinical assessments (Giger & Davidhizar, 2008), and genetic variations in drug metabolism. **Ethnopharmacology** is an increasingly important field of study that looks at responses to drugs in relationship to genetic variation among ethnic groups. As discussed in Chapter Two, mapping of the human genome has fueled attention to ethnopharmacology and pharmacogenomics, with the goal to maximize therapeutic impact through development of personalized biopharmaceutical interventions that are individually tailored to a person's genetic make-up. Thus, ethnopharmacology and pharmacogenomics are consistent with the systems approach to patient care and have the potential to maximize effectiveness and minimize unwanted side effects. See Chapter Two for more detailed information about our current understanding of the complex relationship among self-reported race and ethnicity, genetics, and health.

Historically, clinical trials for new drugs were performed without sufficient attention to the representation of people of color and women. The same was true in development of standardized assessment instruments, such as those used by speech pathologists in diagnosing a patient. Recently, representation in clinical trials and in samples used to develop standardized test norms has increased because of regulation and developers' recognition of the demographic imperative, discussed in Chapter One of this book.

In 2005 (US Department of Health and Human Services), the FDA provided guidance to drug developers on meeting the demographic rule set forth in the 1998 final rule on investigational new drug (IND) applications and new drug applications (NDAs), which requires IND holders to tabulate in their annual report the number of subjects enrolled in clinical studies of drugs and biologic products by age, race, and gender, and requires sponsors of NDAs to include summaries of effectiveness and safety data for important demographic subgroups, including racial subgroups. This guidance is also intended to assist applicants in preparing biologics license applications and is recommended but not required for developers of medical devices.

Finally, highly pigmented skin color can be difficult, especially for the inexperienced provider, to assess for certain conditions such as pallor or cyanosis. The health care provider should establish a baseline by assessing the least pigmented areas such as the palms of the hands, soles of the feet, the abdomen, and the buttocks. And, regardless of how dark the skin is, there should be an underlying red tone to the skin. Proper lighting is essential in making this assessment. Mongolian spots, which are bluish discolorations often mistaken for bruises, are also more common in African, Asian, Mexican, and Native American newborns than in European Americans (Giger & Davidhizar, 2008).

Knowledge of biological variations, coupled with related clinical experience, will help ensure that the health care provider does not fail to consider biological variations in the health care encounter.

BEING CULTURALLY RESPONSIVE

Learning to be culturally responsive in the health care encounter can be compared to learning to ride a bicycle. The integration and synthesis of the various parts may be difficult at first as the new rider focuses on balance, braking, being observant, pedaling, and steering. Enjoyment of the ride may not be the primary experience during the early learning phase. And, like riding a bicycle, there may be an experience of awkwardness when the provider first uses the GDTAM or another cultural competence framework in the health care encounter.

Although the provider may focus on different aspects of the six cultural competence models discussed in this section at different points during the encounter, communication will be a consistent factor that must be considered in the same way that balance and steering is foremost when riding a bicycle. With practice, there can be satisfaction in the real life health care encounter for patient and provider. This does not eliminate bumps in the road or even crashes as institutional, interpersonal, and intrapersonal "hot button" issues are surfaced through health care encounters in the context of diversity. To become culturally competent in the health care encounter, providers must take advantage of the opportunity to connect with the "other" and experience the privilege of being allowed to touch and participate in the healing of lives through embracing and acknowledging the diversity in oneself and others.

In the Introduction it was noted that the health care encounter represents center stage for cultural responsiveness. The provider must have the desire, do the self-development work, and acquire the knowledge that it takes to be culturally responsive.

As discussed in Chapter Six, mnemonics or memory tools such as LEARN (Berlin & Fowkes, 1983) can help providers ensure that their encounters with patients are culturally responsive. The LEARN mnemonic reminds the health care provider of the five key elements of effective communication in the health care encounter: listen, explain, acknowledge, recommend, and negotiate. The following presents the LEARN mnemonic and a role-playing scenario the reader can use to practice its application.

LEARN APPROACH TO CROSSCULTURAL COMMUNICATION

Listen to the patient's perspective.

Explain and share one's own perspective.

Acknowledge differences and similarities between the two perspectives.

Recommend treatment.

Negotiate a mutually agreed-on plan.

Source: Berlin and Fowkes (1983).

"Hello Ms. Baker. My name is Samantha Jordan and I'm a physician assistant who works here in the clinic. I understand this is your son, Eric. Hi, Eric. Can you tell me what brings the two of you in today?" Ms. Baker describes the difficulty she is having with her son's asthma attacks. Usually she just goes to the emergency room, but it just seems to happen over and over again. Eric is in the fourth grade, but he's twelve years old and because he's out of school so much, he doesn't do well in school. It doesn't look like Eric is going to progress to the next grade and the school system is talking about moving him into special classes in another school for children with problems. Samantha Jordan takes a complete history that includes an exploration of Eric's living environment. She discovers that they live in an old dilapidated house and in some of the rooms the paint is peeling off the walls.

Role-play this scenario in groups of three, rotating among the roles of the patient, his mother, and the physician assistant, who is to apply the LEARN approach to the patient encounter.

What did you learn about crosscultural competence from the role-play?

Did you find the LEARN mnemonic helpful in ensuring culturally responsive care? Why or why not?

SUMMARY

This chapter defined the health care encounter as a planned or unplanned interaction between a provider of health care or related services and a recipient of care or information. The health care encounter was characterized as center stage where the reality of the theories, training, assumptions, and social and cultural barriers are interwoven and enacted by individual providers, resulting in positive or negative health care experiences and outcomes.

Six cultural competence models from the nursing profession were described and their application to self-development and the culturally responsive health care encounter was discussed: Leininger's Sunrise Model, Purnell's Model for Cultural Competence, Campinha-Bacote's Process of Cultural Competence in the Delivery of Health Care Services, Jeffreys' Cultural Competence and Confidence Model (CCC), Andrews and Boyle's Transcultural Concepts in Nursing Practice, and the Giger-Davidhizar Transcultural Assessment Model (GDTAM). Each of the six models emphasizes different but important aspects of the culturally responsive health care encounter.

The six cultural phenomena in the GDTAM—communication, space, social organization, time, environmental control, and biological variations—were described in detail. LEARN, a widely used mnemonic that can improve cultural responsiveness in the health care encounter, was also introduced in this chapter.

Chapter Eight builds on this chapter by discussing language and communication barriers specific to health care encounters with LEP patients, including the provision of interpretation and translation services through a systems approach. Chapter Eight also examines the role of verbal and nonverbal communication in cultural competence, extending the content presented in this chapter on arguably the most important aspect of cultural responsiveness in the health care encounter: communication.

KEY TERMS

consensual validation	power
cultural desire	proxemics
decenter	self-monitor
enculturation	social organization
ethnopharmacology	transcultural nursing
health care encounter	transcultural self-efficacy
locus of control	

REVIEW QUESTIONS AND ACTIVITIES

1. Describe the relationship between cultural competence in the health care encounter and the systems approach to diversity and cultural competence (see Figure 1.2). List five actions a health care organization can take to support culturally competent health care encounters.

2. Referencing Leininger's Sunrise Model, describe a crosscultural health care encounter that would be best resolved by culture care preservation and maintenance. Then, describe a crosscultural health care encounter that should be resolved by culture care repatterning and restructuring. When should a provider strive to maintain a patient's culturally based value, belief, or behavior and when should the provider work with the patient to change it?

3. Referencing Campinha-Bacote's Process of Cultural Competence in the Delivery of Health Care Services, describe five actions a health care organization can take to encourage cultural desire in its clinical staff.

4. Referencing Jeffreys' Cultural Competence and Confidence (CCC) model, describe five actions health care providers can take to build their own transcultural self-efficacy.

5. Compare the Purnell Model for Cultural Competence to Andrews and Boyle's Transcultural Concepts in Nursing Practice Model. What do you see as the main difference in emphasis? Explain your answer.

6. Which of the six cultural phenomena identified in the Giger-Davidhizar Transcultural Assessment Model (GDTAM) do you think is most significant to the health care encounter? Justify your answer.

7. Compare the LEARN mnemonic with another mnemonic you identity through independent research. How are they similar? How are they different? Explain your answer.

REFERENCES

Akinbami, L. J., & Schoendorf, K. C. (2002). Funds in childhood asthma: Pervasive healthcare utilization and mentality. *Pediatric, 110*, 315–332.

Anderson, M. (2003). Trans-cultural perspectives in nursing children. In M. Andrews & J. Boyle (Eds.), *Trans-cultural in nursing*. Philadelphia: Lippincott, Williams, and Wilkins.

Andrews, M., & Boyle, J. (2007). *Transcultural concepts in nursing care* (5th ed.). New York: Wolters Kluwer Health; Lippincott Williams and Wilkins.

Berlin, E., & Fowkes, W. A. (1983). Teaching framework for cross-cultural health care. *Western Journal of Medicine, 139*, 934–938.

Bock, P. (1964). Social structure and language structure. *Southwestern Journal of Anthropology, 20*, 393–403.

Campinha-Bacote, J. (1999). A model and instrument for addressing cultural competence in health care. *Journal of Nursing Education, 38*(5), 203–207.

Campinha-Bacote, J. (2008). Cultural desire: "Caught" or "taught." *Contemporary Nurse, 28*, 141–148.

Carson, V. (2000). *Mental health nursing: The nursing patient journey* (2nd ed.). Philadelphia: W. B. Saunders.

Davidhizar, R., & Giger, J. (1998). *Canadian transcultural nursing: Assessment and intervention*. St. Louis: C. V. Mosby.

Davidhizar, R., & Hart, A. (2005). Pain management. *Healthcare Traveler, 13*(6), 3–41.

Giger, J., & Davidhizar, R. (1990). Transcultural nursing assessment: A method for advanced practice. *International Nursing Review, 37*(1), 199–203.

Giger, J., & Davidhizar, R. (2002). The Giger and Davidhizar transcultural assessment model. *Journal of Transcultural Nursing, 13*(3), 185–188.

Giger, J., & Davidhizar, R. (2008). *Transcultural nursing: Assessment and intervention* (5th ed.). St. Louis, MO: Mosby.

Hall, E. T. (1966). *The silent language.* New York: Anchor Books.

Hayter, J. (1981). Territoriality as a universal need. *Journal of Advanced Nursing, 6,* 79–85.

Jeffreys, R. (2006). *Teaching cultural competence in nursing and health care: Inquiry, action, and innovation.* New York: Springer.

Jeffreys, R. (2010). *Teaching cultural competence in nursing and health care* (2nd ed.). New York: Springer.

Kaegi, L. (2004). What color is your pain? *Minority Nurse,* Summer, 28–35.

Knapp, M., & Hall, I. (Eds.). (1992). *Nonverbal communication in human interaction.* St. Louis, MO: Holt, Rinehart and Winston.

Leininger, M. (1989). Transcultural nursing: Quo vadis (where goeth the field?). *Journal of Transcultural Nursing, 1*(1), 33–45.

Leininger, M. (1991). *Culture care diversity and universality: A theory of nursing.* New York: National League for Nursing Press.

Leininger, M. (1996). Culture care theory, research, and practice. *Nursing Science Quarterly, 9*(2), 71–78.

Leininger, M. (2002). Culture care theory: A major contribution to advance transcultural nursing knowledge and practices. *Journal of Transcultural Nursing, 13*(3), 189–192.

Leininger, M., & McFarland, M. R. (2002). *Transcultural nursing: Concepts, theories, research and practice* (3rd ed.). New York: McGraw-Hill.

Massey, R. (2004). *Environmental justice: Income, race, and health.* Medford, MA: Global Development & Environment Institute Tufts University.

Minuchin, P., Colapinto, J., & Minuchin, S. (1998). *Working with families of the poor.* New York: Guilford Press.

Minuchin, S., Nichols, M. P., & Lee, W.Y.L. (2007). *Assessing families and couples: From symptom to system.* Upper Saddle River, NJ: Pearson.

Montague, A. (1986). *Touching: The human significance of the skin.* New York: Harper and Row.

Murphy, S. (2006). Mapping the literature of transcultural nursing. *Journal of the Medical Library Association, 94*(2) Supplement, E-143–E-151.

Murray, R., & Huelskoetter, M. (1991). *Psychiatric and mental health nursing: Giving emotional care* (3rd ed.). New York: Appleton and Lange.

National Institute of Environmental Health Sciences. International Disparities Reserve. (2001). *Children health disparities fact sheet.* Triangle Park, NC: NIEHS.

National League for Nursing. (2007). *Strategic plan.* New York: National League for Nursing.

Nunez, A., & Robertson, C. (2006). Cultural competency. In D. Satcher & R. Pamies (Eds.), *Multicultural medicine and health disparities*. New York: McGraw-Hill.

Palacio, J., Butterfly, R., & Strikland, C. (2006). American Indians. In J. Hisor, S. Dibble, & P. Minavik (Eds.), *Culture and clinical care*. San Francisco: USCF Nursing Press.

Purnell, L. (2002). The Purnell model for cultural competence. *Journal of Transcultural Nursing, 13*(3), 193–196.

Satcher, D., & Pamies, R. (2006). *Multicultural medicine and health disparities*. New York: McGraw-Hill.

Scott, A. (1988). Human interaction and personal boundaries. *Journal of Psychosocial Nursing, 26*(8), 23–28.

Scott, A., & Dumas, R. (1995). Personal space boundaries and clinical applications in psychiatric mental health nursing. *Perspectives in Psychiatric Care, 3*(13), 14–19.

Thiederman, S. (1986). Ethnocentrism: A barrier to effective health care. *The Nurse Practitioner, 11*(8), 52, 54, 59.

US Department of Health and Human Services. (2005, September). *Guidance for industry— collection of race and ethnicity data in clinical trials*. Rockville, MD: Food and Drug Administration, Center for Drug Evaluation and Research (CDER), & Center for Biologics Evaluation and Research (CBER).

Watson, O. M. (1980). *Proxemic behavior: A cross cultural study*. The Hague, The Netherlands: Mouton Press.

Chapter 8

LANGUAGE ACCESS SERVICES AND CROSSCULTURAL COMMUNICATION

LEARNING OBJECTIVES

- To become familiar with the extent of language differences in the US population
- To appreciate the serious impact that language barriers can have on communication in health care
- To become aware of legislative, regulatory, and accreditation requirements surrounding the provision of language access services (LAS)
- To understand that provision of LAS is a quality of care and safety issue
- To become familiar with the many models and resources available for providing language services in health care

(Continued)

- To become alert to the pitfalls of using untrained interpreters and translators
- To become acquainted with aspects of nonverbal communication and cultural perspectives as they affect communication

This chapter begins with a discussion of language and communication barriers as they relate to interactions between health care providers and the limited-English-proficient patients they serve. It was pointed out in Chapter One that language was one of the dimensions of diversity that was important to consider in the provision of health care. In this chapter we briefly review the extent of linguistic diversity in the United States. There are communication difficulties that are very peculiar to health care and to the relationship between health care providers and patients, and these will next be considered. The threats to equitable care and patient safety that are posed by **language barriers** have received extensive legislative and regulatory attention since about 2000, which will be discussed. Excellent strategies to reduce language barriers will be described along with the highly varied organizational efforts to systematize language access. Resources for information on how to implement **language access services (LAS)** will be given. We will point out that **trained health care** and **medical interpreters** have come to be essential in many health care settings, and clinicians and others have had to acquire skills in managing the interpreted encounter. Some tips on appropriate, effective, and legal use of interpreters will be provided. The professionalization of the medical interpreter and medical translator roles has rapidly evolved since about 2000, and we will review how this has occurred. In the final sections we examine how aspects of language other than just words play important roles in crosscultural health care communication: differences in language style, nonverbal cues, and the complex relationships among language, culture, and meaning.

LANGUAGE USE IN THE UNITED STATES

Often when the subject of language barriers is broached, what immediately comes to mind is the barrier between Spanish speakers and English speakers. However, the linguistic situation in the United States has become much more complicated than the barrier between English and Spanish. Currently, fifty-two million people, 19.4 percent of the US population, speak a language other than English at home; in the western United States, the percentages rises to 34 percent. Of these, 23 million, or 8 percent of the US population, speak English "less than very well," an increase of nearly four million persons with **limited English proficiency (LEP)** from 1998 to 2003 (US Census Bureau, 2003). By the time the Affordable Care Act (ACA) is fully implemented, forty-four million new subscribers will be added to the health insurance rolls; half of these will come from non-English-speaking immigrant communities (Armoruso, 2011). Reflecting the immigration patterns since the 1980s, many languages are involved. In some large urban areas, such as New York, Chicago, and Los Angeles, where more than one hundred languages are spoken, the situation becomes quite complex because some health care catchment areas are populated by many language groups. For example, at Montefiore Medical Center in New York, eighty languages, including Gujarati, an Asian language, and Zapotec, a native Mexican-Indian dialect, are among those spoken by patients. In San Francisco, the LEP population is predominantly Asian, and in Los Angeles, it is overwhelmingly Spanish speaking, though in each of these California cities linguistic pockets of Samoan or Afghani speakers can be found and large groups of Armenian, Vietnamese, and Korean speakers live and receive medical care just five or six miles away. For health care organizations seeking to understand where concentrations of specific foreign-born populations are located, the Migration Policy Institute publishes detailed maps of the percent foreign born in each US county.

An American College of Physicians study (2007) reports that two-thirds of physicians serving adults have LEP caseloads on average about 12 percent of the time and more than half see LEP patients daily or a few times a week. Seventy percent of the doctors interviewed believed that LEP patients couldn't understand health information as well as English-proficient patients. Only 13 percent of pediatricians see no LEP patients (Kuo, O'Connor, Flores, & Minkovitz, 2007). Of course, these physician visits are only a fraction of myriad encounters between LEP patients and nurses, laboratory technicians, case managers, paramedics, health educators, and pharmacists, to name only a few of the vast array of health care personnel involved in face-to-face contact with the public.

The communication challenges within health care even when language barriers are not involved are enormous because the field is made up of a multifaceted array of specialties and subspecialties with their own knowledge bases, terminologies, techniques, and paraphernalia. The structural relationship of hospitals, clinics, doctor's offices, health management organizations, pharmacies, and laboratories to each other is complex and confusing even to the average English speaker. No wonder that research has found that persons who are limited English speakers have enormous difficulty in accessing health services or returning for follow-up services and care (Flores, 2006; Flores et al., 2003).

The health care workforce itself is multicultural and is growing more so rapidly. Shortages in a number of health care fields, such as nursing and pharmacy services, have resulted in recruiting personnel from other countries. Although English is the required language for workers in most health settings, Southeast Asian, Chinese, Korean, Middle Eastern, Spanish, and Caribbean accents are common and a variety of languages can be heard in the lunchrooms and off-duty lounges. "It's the United Nations in our lunchroom and the nurses' lounge," commented one licensed vocational nurse, "and that sometimes makes for difficult teamwork." "Dr. Wong is a wonderful pediatrician, but all but the Chinese nurses have a hard time understanding what he's saying," remarked another (Gilbert, 1996, p. 14).

LANGUAGE DIFFERENCES IN HEALTH CARE ENCOUNTERS

Although language and cultural differences may create some workforce concerns at all levels of staffing, the major language issues in health care are focused on exchanges between patients and health care staff and care providers. Effective and appropriate health care is critically dependent on the ability of patients and providers to communicate clearly with each other. Ease of access to health care services, from understanding eligibility and benefits to appointment making and way finding (the process of organizing spatial and environmental information to help users find their way around a structure), rests on accurate oral and written communication. Even more important, the interactions between clinical professionals and their patients, which include history taking, diagnostic interviews, description of tests, informed consent, and explanation of treatment and prognoses, all require that each party to an exchange fully grasps the meanings and intent of what is being communicated. This is oftentimes difficult when patient and provider speak the same language; it is truly hazardous when they do not (Divi, Ross, Schmaltz, & Loeb, 2007). One family practice physician ruefully remarked that treating patients when a language barrier is present "seems dangerous to me . . . I don't know what they understand and what they don't. It's a little like doing veterinary medicine" (Gilbert, 1999).

Physician Paul Schyve points out (2007):

> The more the care is patient- and family-centered, the more frequent the communication with the patient and the patient's family to understand the patient's perspective and to involve the patient in the treatment team itself. Because much of medical care is really information management, the communication between treatment team members and the patient and patient's family is a core component of health care . . . (p. 360)

Dr. Schyve also notes that the need to communicate effectively is recognized as an element of the quality of care, and that a Joint Commission study (Divi, Ross, Schmaltz, & Loeb, 2007) found that adverse outcomes from medical errors are more serious among LEP patients than English-speaking patients. Clear communication in health care is obviously essential but it is often fraught with special difficulty for the following reasons:

- Health care encounters are often emotionally charged and frequently accompanied by fear, anxiety, pain, denial, and uncertainty on the part of patient and family. These emotions often cause a limited-English speaker to revert to his or her first language or to speak English with difficulty.

- Feelings of confusion and vulnerability on the part of the patient may be intensified through lack of understanding.

- Miscommunication between health care providers and patients can have dangerous consequences, imperiling the safety of the patient and the liability of the provider.

- Health care communication is often focused on subjects of extreme delicacy such as sexuality and sexual behavior, reproductive health, mental health, substance abuse, informed consent, and end-of-life concerns, to name just a few subjects that need to be approached with sensitivity, nuance, and confidentiality.

- Misinterpretation of the other's meaning or intent on the part of provider or patient undermines rapport and trust, and decreases the likelihood of adherence to treatment or follow-up (Karliner, Jacobs, Chen, & Mutha, 2006).

- The language of medicine and health care is often highly technical, reflecting many specialty vocabularies and scientific concepts; some of these terms have no equivalent in other languages (including English!).

When patient and provider don't speak the same languages, the difficulties common to health care exchanges are greatly intensified. Consider the following scenarios:

- A pregnant Hispanic woman with gestational diabetes was accompanied by her mother-in-law to the obstetrician's office. A cousin was enlisted to interpret because neither woman could speak English. When, through the interpreter, the doctor was attempting to discuss the need for the young woman to stick to her diet plan, the mother-in-law interjected that the diabetes was the will of God. On hearing the interpretation of this, the doctor said that even though the diabetes may be the will of God, it was still important for the girl to stick to her diet plan. The mother-in-law was horrified when the cousin interpreted this as "the doctor doesn't care about God. She has to eat what the doctor says."

- A Hmong man presented to his primary care physician with probable symptoms of a venereal disease. When the doctor needed to take a sexual history, the only one available to interpret was the man's seventeen-year-old daughter. The man refused to answer the doctor's questions. The daughter was terribly embarrassed.

- A very angry Spanish-speaking monolingual assaulted his urologist following prostate surgery because he had not understood that possible side effects of the surgery were impotence and urinary incontinence. The urologist was surprised because Mr. Ortiz had assured him that he would read the Spanish-language explanatory literature that he had been given and that covered these possibilities thoroughly. The patient also had signed the required informed consent that contained information on possible risks prior to the surgery. The consent form was written in English but explained by a medical assistant who was thought to be fully bilingual but had no facility with medical terminology.

The first case involves communication errors that could probably have been avoided had a skilled, trained medical interpreter been available to the physician. The indelicate breach of confidentiality that often occurs when family members are asked to interpret is illegal and inappropriate, as in the case of the Hmong father and daughter. The failure to adequately communicate the risks associated with prostate surgery despite having an English language consent form sight interpreted by a bilingual family member resulted in harm to patient and physician.

The use of such **ad hoc** interpreters and translators is dangerous and unfair: dangerous because it invites misinterpretation by a person unfamiliar with medical terminology and unfair because it breaches confidentiality and places the ad hoc interpreter in a situation of extreme role conflict. Non-English-speaking parents have in the past been frequently asked to bring their English-speaking children with them to interpret, a practice that is now considered reprehensible and reflecting a low standard of care (Andrulis, Goodman & Pryor, 2002).

Untrained bilingual medical personnel cannot be expected to accurately translate the complexities of an informed consent document such as occurred in the situation of the prostate patient, Mr. Ortiz. All of these cases, although dramatic, are true and representative of the dilemmas faced daily in clinics, doctors' offices, and hospitals across the United States. More illustrative cases of language barriers can be found in the very readable *In the Absence of Words: A Compilation of Personal Stories Addressing the Language Barriers in Healthcare* (Pacific Asian Language Services/Pals for Health, nd).

Clearly, language barriers cause problematic safety and quality of care issues in sometimes critical and life-threatening circumstances; hence, it is not surprising that failure to provide adequate language access services may result in medical malpractice cases. A study that analyzed medical malpractice claims (Quan & Lynch, 2010) found that in 2.5 percent of a carrier's total claims reviewed, language barriers played a role and the carrier paid almost five million dollars in damages and legal fees associated with the claims. The cases involved many patients' suffering death or irreparable harm. Untrained family interpreters, even sick children, had been asked to interpret in some cases. Failure to translate important documents, such as informed consents, occurred as well. There was failure to document LEP patients' language needs in the medical record. Because the provision of trained medical interpreters and adequately translated documents has now become a widely recognized standard of practice, health care providers and organizations open themselves up to malpractice actions if they fail to provide language access and harm to the patient ensues.

Since 2000 or so, there has been a growing awareness of the lack of health literacy among the population in the United States: for example, much of the general population has little understanding of how and if prescription drugs work, what treatments are available for different health problems, how lifestyle choices affect health, and a plethora of other complexities in the health care field. Health illiteracy is exacerbated by language barriers, particularly when an LEP person is an immigrant or has little education and may not be literate in his own language. However, the strategies for meeting the needs of low literacy are largely distinct from those that address the needs of LEP individuals, although interpreters and translators need to consider the possible effects of low health literacy in patients' target languages (Andrulis & Brach, 2007).

ATTITUDES TOWARD LIMITED-ENGLISH SPEAKERS

In the late 1980s and early 1990s, as the health care industry experienced the effects of increasing language diversity, the situation was often met by annoyance, bewilderment, and resistance. Some health care personnel chose to ignore the issue. "Whatever their language and culture, I treat all patients the same," was the mantra heard from receptionists to surgeons, disregarding the actual impossibility of doing so in the face of language barriers. "I speak urology, not Spanish," was the curt response of a Colorado physician when the subject of language barriers was brought up. "If they want care in the United States, let them learn English" was the remark of a nursing student, continuing, "when in Rome, do as the Romans do." One Fresno nurse, desperate, thought she had found at least a bandage solution, "If they speak Thai, I call a Thai restaurant; if they speak Chinese, I call a Chinese restaurant. At least I might find someone who can interpret a few important words." Others relied on gestures, pictures, and the inevitable raised voice. LEP patients were urged to bring someone with them to interpret for them, ignoring issues of accuracy and confidentiality.

Some of these frustrated responses still occur in today's health care institutions. Prevailing concerns about the legality or illegality of immigrants often color perceptions: "These ladies scream bloody murder when they are having a baby. They aren't even citizens and we have to take them," reported an obstetrical nurse in Los Angeles. Patients and other health care workers mistake the motives of groups whose linguistic styles differ from their own: "Iranians yell at us and make trouble when they have to wait for an appointment," averred a receptionist in the same city. "I feel so sorry for these Somali women," from a San Diego obstetrician, "they don't know what is going on and I feel so helpless in trying my best to assure them with smiles and touches." The language barrier often causes patients to perceive health care personnel as cold and uncaring: "The nurse barely speaks to me when she comes into my room," commented an African American hospital patient about a Filipino nurse. The unfortunate tendency for people to stereotype individuals from specific language or cultural groups is exacerbated by their inability to communicate easily, person-to-person, with individuals from those groups.

"Why don't they learn to speak English?" is a question uttered frequently by health care personnel in some frustration. Many immigrants do try very hard to learn English, and many become reasonably fluent over time. The language schools in most cities are completely and constantly enrolled. Unfortunately, many Americans themselves have limited or no experience with learning a foreign language, and their attitudes often reflect this. Most Americans speak only English or have had just a couple of years of classroom foreign language. Even those who have traveled as tourists to other countries rarely find themselves in situations where English isn't spoken because the language has become the "lingua franca" of the Western world. Persons who have never tried, as adults, to learn a new language often minimize the emotional and cognitive difficulties involved in speaking a second language well enough to function in complex situations. Trying to speak accurately in a non-native tongue is exceedingly fatiguing and the fear of appearing stupid or of embarrassing oneself or others is a constant concern. Relatively few American-born health care providers have had the experience of being immersed in difficult medical or social circumstances in which they couldn't fluently communicate in their native language, so it isn't surprising that their usual empathy is sometimes strained when they are confronted with numerous LEP patients.

Further, settings and circumstances often affect the ability of an immigrant to speak English. A limited-English speaker may readily greet the receptionist, nurse, or doctor in English, but the stress of many health care situations involving emergencies, pain, fear, and uncertainties may strain their capacity to speak the new language. Many non-native English speakers who are reasonably fluent in English will revert to the language they know best and unwittingly "forget" the English they have learned. Gayle Tang, trained as a nurse and one of the nation's foremost experts in medical interpretation and translation, often recounts her experiences in reversion to Cantonese under duress (personal communication). This type of reversion is a normal phenomenon among bilingual persons but one that is not always appreciated by health care personnel.

Finally, it should be pointed out that health care settings are notable for the several pressures that affect them. Health care professionals are expected to demonstrate productivity, a quality that is often defined by the number of patients seen in a given amount of time. Working with an LEP patient expands appointment time five to fifteen minutes. Workforce shortages in a number of critical occupations, such as nurses, mean that workers are often overburdened and that time for training is very limited. Health care organizations are under constant pressure to cut costs while maintaining an acceptable and competitive quality of care. Given these circumstances, it is understandable that the patience and extra effort it takes to deal compassionately with LEP patients might seem to some to be just an added burden in already difficult workplace. Still, it is admirable that many health care organizations have made significant efforts to train their personnel in cultural and linguistic competency and more and more professional educational program are preparing students for meeting persons of varying linguistic and cultural backgrounds (Wynia & Matiasek, 2006; Youdelman & Perkins, 2005).

CHANGING RESPONSES TO LANGUAGE BARRIERS IN HEALTH CARE

In the mid-nineties, when it became clear that "Rome" itself had changed and the polyglot patient population was only likely to increase, considerations of practicality and quality, compassion, and caring began to come to the forefront. It became clear to many that although some immigrants resist learning English, most didn't, though it wasn't always a rapid process. Further, studies had begun to show that language barriers and inadequate interpretation resulted in costly and unnecessary tests, reduced adherence to medical recommendations and treatment, were associated with inadequate preventive care, and a whole laundry list of quality-adverse effects. Advocacy groups began to look at the legal and civil rights issues associated with the persistent inattention to language barriers in health care. Large health management organizations and health plans began to understand cultural and linguistic groups as markets to be wooed.

Two pivotal events occurred. First, the DHHS Office of Civil Rights stated that, under Title VI of the Civil Rights Act of 1964, any health care provider that received federal funds was prohibited from discriminating against persons with limited language proficiency because this would constitute de facto national origin discrimination. Federal courts have also ruled that Title VI prohibits discrimination based on limited English proficiency (DHHS, 2000). This regulation covered Medicaid, SCHIP, Temporary Assistance to Needy Families (TANF), and Medicare services. Under the Affordable Care Act, the Title VI language provisions will apply to health care exchanges under Title I of the ACA, thus to contracts of insurance. These services cover a wide swath of the nation's health services. DHHS provides extensive guidance on what is involved in providing language access services (DHHS, 2000). The next turning point was when the State of California, as a part of its move to have matched state and federal health services covered by health management organizations, stipulated that organizations that contracted to provide these services had to meet language access requirements (MRMIB/HFP, 2007). This requirement was extended in 2009 to apply to private commercial health plans under California Senate Bill 853. The required LAS included a needs assessment, the availability of trained interpreters in the language of the service area at key points of contact, and business and medical documents translated into the appropriate languages. It is notable that this last development probably would not have taken place without the efforts of strong advocacy groups in California mobilizing in this multicultural and multilingual state. The story of this advocacy effort is nicely told by the California Pan-Ethnic Health Network (CPEHN) (2009). CPEHN and numerous ethnic organizations coalesced and brought pressure on state legislators, monitoring the language of the bill and its progress until it was passed by both houses.

Seventeen additional states and the District of Columbia have now enacted legislation covering LAS in health care. The legislation varies from state to state and has been summarized in detail by the National Health Law Program (NHelp, 2003) in *Ensuring Linguistic Access in Health Care Settings: Legal Rights and Responsibilities* and their *Summary of State Law Requirements Addressing Language Needs in Health Care* (NHelp, 2008). Most states, at a minimum, require the availability of interpreters and translated documents.

Other critical milestones in the development of LAS regulation include the DHHS Office of Minority Health publication of standards for culturally and linguistically appropriate services (known widely as the CLAS standards and outlined in Chapter Four of this book) in the *Federal Register* in December 2000 and Clinton's Executive order #13166, "Improving Access to Services for Persons with Limited English Proficiency" (Department of Justice, 2000), which mandated language services in all federal agencies. The Affordable Care Act of 2010 has substantive provisions for LAS, reviewed by Youdelman (2011). An important development occurred when the Joint Commission added new patient-centered communication standards for hospitals: hospitals must collect and enter into the patients' medical records their language and communication needs and provide appropriate language access services (Joint Commission, 2009). The Joint Commission is the nongovernmental agency that evaluates and accredits more than fifteen thousand health care entities in the United States through unannounced inspections of many aspects of a health care organization's services and functions. Because their findings are made public, most health care organizations are most anxious to receive their seal of approval. The Joint Commission has been studying a sample of hospitals to assess their capacity to address the issues of language and culture that affect the quality and safety of patient care. Their findings reported in *Hospitals, Language and Culture*, completed in June 2007 by Wilson-Stronks and Galvez, is available on their website. Judging from this report, there is significant variation in the degree to which hospitals have developed systematic approaches to language access for patients. The report documents a few innovative and appropriate responses to language needs by several hospitals. Additionally, a comprehensive guidance document and checklist for meeting the new standards is contained in *Advancing Effective Communication, Cultural Competence, and Patient- and Family-Centered Care: A Roadmap for Hospitals* (The Joint Commission, 2010). The Joint Commission has on its website a four-part video (downloadable) that explains and discusses the DHSS language-access requirements and the Joint Commission standards.

Another important accreditation organization, the National Committee on Quality Assurance (NCQA, 2010), has set performance measures for interpretation and translation services based on the number of LEP patients served by a managed care organization (MCO) with detailed reporting requirements on language services in MCOs that serve Medicaid, Medicare, and SCHIP populations.

This agency has also set up a best-practices award for outstanding innovations in multicultural health, and many of the awardees from 2006 to 2009 have been health care organizations that have created outstanding strategies to overcome language barriers and provide culturally competent care (NCQA, 2006, 2007, 2008, 2009). Finally, the American Medical Association, as part of its Ethical Force Program, has produced the document, *Improving Communication, Improving Care: An Ethical Force Consensus Report* (2007), detailing how health care organizations can implement language services as part of patient-centered communication.

The plethora of regulations and standards has resulted in some understandable confusion as to what, exactly, a health care provider or organization must do in order to comply with basic LAS requirements. Please consult the resources mentioned in this chapter to learn more. However, the bottom line requirements are summarized in the following.

ESSENTIAL REQUIREMENTS FOR LAS IN HEALTH CARE ORGANIZATIONS

- Have signage and written materials informing patients of their right to have an interpreter at no cost to themselves.

- Have a system for assessing patients' language needs.

- Have a written language policy and disseminate it widely to staff.

- Review the available resources for meeting patients' language needs.

- Create a plan for meeting patients' language needs that includes interpretation and translation needs.

- Avoid using patients' family, friends, and especially minors as interpreters.

- Document patients' language needs in the medical record.

The two major stumbling blocks to the implementation of LAS in health care organizations and among provider clinics and offices has been the (1) cost and time required to provide these services and (2) lack of knowledge about how to plan for, staff, and organize these services. Fortunately, the Federal Center for Medicaid and Medicare Services has worked out a mechanism whereby providers can be reimbursed for these services through federal and state funds, though only for the programs that receive federal funding. The National Health Law Program (2004) has published a how-to manual on the way several states have accessed federal funds for reimbursement of providers for language access services. Ku (2006) has also outlined processes that may be used for reimbursement of language services costs. In California, the Medi-Cal Language Access Task Force (2009), working in conjunction with the California Department of Health Services, has created a planning document focused on generating federal reimbursement of state expenditures on language services. Because the various states accomplish this differently, there are several models for getting reimbursement funds appearing in these several documents. As of 2009, thirteen states had set up processes to access federal funds.

Research has also indicated that the benefits to be derived from providing trained interpreters may far outweigh the costs in terms of patient satisfaction, use of preventive care, and reduced risk of medical errors (Jacobs, Shepard, Suaya, & Stone, 2004; Karliner, Jacobs, Chen, & Mutha, 2006). It is therefore a cost-savings activity for health care organizations that serve patients whose care is not publicly supported.

The second problem, lack of knowledge about how to set up language services, has largely been resolved through detailed how-to guidance materials and model programs that have been developed since 2000, as we will see.

Major Resources for Providing LAS

A combination of carrots and sticks has worked to produce real progress toward effective provision of LAS and improved crosscultural communication in the health care industry since the turn of the new century. Legislation and accreditation requirements constitute the sticks but excellent research, a desire for new markets, and a goal of higher-quality health care for all their patients has motivated many providers to innovate in the area of crosscultural communication. There is no dearth now of strategies, models, and systematic approaches to language access provision for almost every type of health care organization.

Notably, one of the factors that has made it easier for the health care field to adopt new practices in crosscultural communication has been the support of several proactive foundations, particularly The Commonwealth Fund, The California Endowment, the Robert Wood Johnson Foundation, and the National Health Law Program (NHelp). Together and singly they have moved language access services rapidly forward in a short period of time. The California Endowment and The Commonwealth Fund have sponsored research into the effects of language barriers and the use of interpreters. Robert Wood Johnson, through its multi-million dollar Hablamos Juntos funding initiative, has underwritten the testing of a variety of innovative systems for providing language services. Each of these foundations supports websites that provide extensive resources and information on how to plan for, create, and maintain good crosscultural communication in health care.

The National Health Law Program, through support from these foundations, has been especially proactive in providing information and resources, such as the *Language Services Resource Guide for Health Care Providers* (Sampson, 2006), *Language Access in Health Care Statement of Principles: Explanatory Guide* (Martinez, Hitov, & Youdelman, 2010), and *What's in a Word: A Guide to Understanding Interpretation and Translation* (2010). NHelp also provides on its website a listing of all federal and state laws relating to language access in health care. This organization has produced a practical guide for small practitioner groups, *Providing Language Services in Small Health Care Provider Settings* (Youdelman & Perkins, 2005), which gives language access recommendations for the 59 percent of physicians in solo or small group practice. It has also developed a guide for providing language services in pharmacy settings (Wong, 2010). In New York, for example, interpreters must be available for patient-pharmacist consults and prescription labeling is mandatory for the top seven languages spoken. California is working on similar legislation.

The California Primary Care Association (Mataeo, Gallardo, Huang, & Niski, 2009) has published *Providing Health Care to Limited English Proficient Patients: A Manual of Promising Practices*, which gives examples of how language access is provided in a variety of health care settings: rural clinics, migrant health centers, and urban community health centers. Noting that policy making around the provision of language services is a critical first step, a manual, *Straight Talk: Model Hospital Policies and Procedures of Language Access* (Paras, 2005), offers model templates for the design of hospital and health system policies and procedures. For health plans, the American Health Insurance Plans (AHIP) has created *Tools to Address Disparities in Health Communication. Resources to Close the Gap: A Compendium of Resources for Health Insurance Plans, Physicians, and Health Care Organizations* (2006). This document covers a wide variety of topics relevant to setting up language services, from consumer needs assessment to internal and external advisory groups. The *Language Services Resource Guide for Health Care Providers* (Sampson, 2006) prepared for NHelp and the National Council on Interpreting in Healthcare (NCIH) gives information on how to locate interpreters and translators, assessment tools for determining proficiency, and how to locate training for interpreters or staff. The Office of Minority Health has made available the step-by-step and comprehensive *A Patient-Centered Guide to Implementing Language Access Services in Health Care Organizations* on their website. Health care providers no longer can claim ignorance of the laws or an inability to understand how language services can be provided.

A number of useful tools, available to everyone, have been developed to aid crosscultural communication in health care. An "I speak" card and a language identification flashcard are available. The former, developed by Pacific Asian Language Services (PALS) for Health is a pocket card that can be downloaded from their website and presented to the health care provider to identify the language of the speaker. The card also provides information to LEP patients about their rights under the law and instructions to the health care provider. A language identification flashcard has been developed by the US Justice Department and enables LEP persons to identify their languages by checking off a form showing that language.

The Hablamos Juntos project (2010) sponsored by the Robert Wood Johnson Foundation researched, created, and tested a set of downloadable universal symbols in health care. These symbols are a set of graphic representations identifying facilities, departments, and functions that are usable in signage and way-finding directions so that LEP persons can find their way around health care organizations and identify departments and specific facilities. This same organization also produced the More Than Words Toolkit series (2009). Kaiser Permanente's National Linguistic and Cultural Program has developed a set of reference manuals for use in their facilities and available online that translate illustrated anatomical and health care terms into Vietnamese, Korean, Spanish, Russian, Armenian, and Chinese, and The Chinese Community Health Plan in San Francisco has created a resource center where health education materials and other health-related documents in Chinese can be downloaded free from their site.

Model Systemic Approaches to LAS

More approaches to LAS are reported by the National Committee on Quality Assurance in their Innovative Practices in Multicultural Health Awards (2006, 2007, 2008, 2009). Their awards for innovations in multicultural health document how several medium and large nonprofit health plans have implemented model crosscultural communications services. For example, Health Plan Partners of Minnesota has invested five million dollars in creating a language assistance plan for its LEP and deaf members. This included a needs assessment and a review of organizational capabilities and actions to match needs with organizational resources. The plan is operative throughout all clinics and network providers. Networked physicians are provided with training and access to telephonic interpreters (NCQA, 2007).

Kaiser Permanente, Northern California, in collaboration with San Francisco City College, has established a qualified bilingual staff model. Using the organization's own staff, educated through the college, the health plan created a three-level interpreter program. The first level, language liaison, is made up of persons involved in simple, nonmedical interpreted encounters with patients; level-two interpreters, language facilitators, take on more complex clinical or nonclinical interpretations, and level three, designated interpreters, provide simple to complex medical interpretations and translations. The initial program is being implemented in the health plan's mid-Atlantic region as well. The plan has proven to be so successful that, partnering with the Robert Wood Johnson Foundation, more than one hundred college-level instructors throughout the country have been trained and nine hundred interpreters have been certified through the program's partner colleges (NCQA, 2006).

Group Health Cooperative of Puget Sound, Kaiser Permanente, and Aetna Health Plans, among other health plans, identify their members' language preferences and make that information part of the members' permanent record and patient management information systems. This makes it possible to arrange for interpretation when appointments are made, an important means of ensuring that interpreters are available when needed.

Wynia and Matiasek (2006) provided examples of how hospitals are addressing language access needs. These included having dedicated champions advocate for communication programs, collecting information on patient needs, engaging communities, developing a diverse workforce, and tracking performance over time. Small clinics and medical groups have increasingly been able to meet legislated LEP communication standards by a number of strategies. They may hire bilingual staff and offer them the opportunity to take training in health care interpretation. Some communities have set up language banks composed of contract interpreters hired at an hourly rate by clinics and medical offices on an as-needed basis. Telephonic interpreting services are sometimes sufficient for providers who have a small number of LEP patients and they are easily accessed, confidential, and reasonably priced (Youdelman & Perkins, 2005). More recently, some hospitals and clinics have been using remote video-interpreting services wherein the interpreters stay in a fixed location and are accessed remotely as needed. This strategy requires video monitors and equipment to be set up in provider offices or a location convenient to provider offices as well as, when possible, advance scheduling. However, an even more flexible model has recently been innovated. An excellent brief video by the University of California at Irvine (2010) demonstrates just how remote interpreting is conducted at their hospital and clinic. In their remote program, the interpreters stay in one place and are accessed via a portable computer that can be rolled from place to place on a cart. This makes it possible to have quick, on-demand access to interpreters, cutting down on delays in patient care. Although remote interpreting can't always take the place of in person interpreting, more and more health care organizations are using it as an efficient way to augment face-to-face interpreting.

Common to all of the strategies for implementing language services is early assessment of need. Health care organizations must initially determine the major languages spoken by their patients and the approximate proportions of patients who speak each language. This enables the organization to structure its language services systematically, for example, providing face-to-face interpretation by trained on-site or video interpreters for the major target languages, and telephonic interpretation for less-needed languages. A similar triage approach could be used for translations: printed materials in the major languages, perhaps online materials for less-used languages.

Fully bilingual health care professionals, such as doctors, nurses, physician assistants, and health educators, are not interpreters per se because they can speak directly to LEP patients in their languages (language concordance). Some health care organizations are making an effort to match these professionals with LEP patients or are creating fully bilingual clinic modules if the catchment population characteristics make this cost effective. Although use of bilingual clinicians and staff is convenient, cost effective, and more personal for the patient, care must be taken that staff *are* fully bilingual, culturally aware, and are able to convey (or translate) medical terminology and concepts in English and the target language. This usually means that language competency testing rather than self-assessment takes place (Hwang, Ramos, Jones, & Regenstein, 2009). Inadequate knowledge of a target language by well-meaning staff can result in serious medical errors, inadequate and truncated medical encounters, and unwitting steering of conversations through limited vocabulary (Ferguson, 2008).

Kaiser Permanente, with its 6.5 million California multicultural patient population, has found language concordant providers to be an efficient strategy in some locales. In Northern California, the health care organization has developed a new tool to assess the proficiency of physicians' language skills that can be used throughout the national organization (Tang, Lanza, Rodriquez, & Chang, 2011). Additionally, Kaiser's Southern California region has put in place an innovative program that matches patients with physicians who speak their preferred languages fluently and provides incentives for physicians who participate in the program (National Committee on Quality Assurance, 2009). This strategy is particularly useful in areas with high concentrations of patients who speak a specific language. For example, in the Los Angeles area there are dense population clusters of Vietnamese, Armenian, Cantonese, and Spanish speakers. The University of California at Los Angles (UCLA) has begun a pilot program that recruits medical school graduates from Latin America. They are paid a stipend for training in UCLA-affiliated hospitals and preparing for licensure in the United States. They commit to practice for three years in a medically underserved community that can use their bilingual skills (Amoruso, 2011).

Clearly, the provision of language services has become the standard of practice for most health care entities. It is no longer considered an appropriate level of health care quality for providers to struggle through medical encounters with LEP patients solely through gestures, pictures, and ad hoc individuals pressed into service as medical interpreters. The following is a list of LAS resources.

Resources for Information on the Provision of LAS Office of Minority Health Center for Cultural and Linguistic Competence: http://minorityhealth.hhs.gov/templates/browse.aspx?lvl=1&lvlID=3

The California Endowment: http://www.calendow.org/

The National Health Law Program: http://www.healthlaw.org/index.php?option=com_content&id=239&Itemid=196

The Commonwealth Fund: http://www.commonwealthfund.org/

Robert Wood Johnson, Hablamos Juntos: http://www.hablamosjuntos.org/resource_guide_portal/

National Commission for Quality Assurance: http://www.ncqa.org/

Intersect: A Newsletter About Language, Culture, and Interpreting: http://myemail.constantcontact.com/INTERSECT—A-Newsletter-About-Language—Culture-and-Interpreting.html?soid=1103067 601986&aid=WJv_FwQ7rog

AN EXPANDING PROFESSION: THE HEALTH CARE INTERPRETER

What is a health care or medical interpreter? Fifteen years ago practically no one could have answered this question with any certainty. However, because there have been many changes in the way crosscultural communication is now managed by most health care organizations, this new profession is coming into its own. The health care industry has come a long way from the time that people grabbed a janitor or a cook who spoke a patient's language and pressed them into service as interpreters. Whereas the use of untrained persons to make appointments or provide directions may not be as problematic, there are serious issues involved in having such persons interpret for medical encounters or any other health care situation when it is crucial that all parties to an interaction understand completely what is said or what must be done.

Research into the different levels of interpreters used by health care organizations demonstrates that there are costs in terms of patient safety and quality of care when ad hoc and untrained interpreters are used. Untrained interpreters have been found to make serious and clinically significant interpretation errors (Flores, Laws, Mayo, et al., 2003). Ad hoc interpreters are less likely to tell patients about medication side effects and often omit doctor's questions (Flores, 2006). Use of interpreters is associated with better access to clinical services as measured by office visits, prescriptions written and filled, and follow-up services (Jacobs, Shepard, Suaya, & Stone, 2004). A comprehensive review of twenty-eight studies that compared trained interpreters with ad hoc interpreters concluded that professional interpreters raised the quality of clinical care for LEP patients to approach or equal that for patients without language barriers (Karliner, Jacobs, Chen, & Mutha, 2006). The sources of the errors committed by untrained persons are various. Most are unintentional but there have been numerous cases when family members or other untrained persons intentionally withheld difficult or embarrassing information from either doctors or patients.

The more common sources of error are summarized as follows.

COMMON PROBLEMS ASSOCIATED WITH THE USE OF UNTRAINED INTERPRETERS

- Linguistic distortion: inaccurate interpretation of words and concepts

- Lack of familiarity with medical and health care terminology

- Embarrassment over discussions of bodily functions

- Intentional or unintentional editing of clinician's or patient's utterances

- Deletion of information through attempts to paraphrase

- Intimidation and fearfulness, especially on the part of children

- Unwillingness to deal with unpleasant issues or to be the bearer of bad news

- Potential breeches of confidentiality

There are several types of interpreters used by health care providers. The **dual role interpreter** is an employee of the health care organization whose major function is not that of an interpreter but whose usual task is another health care function such as medical assistant, medical records clerk, nurse, or even physician. This person may or may not have been trained in the skills of interpretation but is familiar with some medical terminology in both languages. Relying on a dual role interpreter is probably better than relying on ad hoc persons such as the patient's friends or family, but it is not without problems. First, these persons may have difficulty handling numerous requests for interpretations as well as doing the major tasks to which they are assigned. Workmates and supervisors may resent the time taken away from these tasks to do interpreting. Second, dual role interpreters are likely not to have training in interpretation skills and may not be truly fluent in English and the target language. Several studies have shown that the number of errors made by dual role personnel is almost as great as those made by **ad hoc interpreters.** This is especially the case when the dual role interpreters are entry-level workers such as medical assistants. Although dual role interpreters may appear to be fluent in their language to persons not familiar with the language, the untrained interpreter may speak a regional, slang, or idiomatic version of the target language.

The trained health care interpreter has taken courses in medical terminology and procedures as well as the special skills necessary for effective and accurate interpretation. The trained person most probably will be a face-to-face or telephonic or video interpreter, trained in the consecutive style of interpreting. Using this style, the interpreter alternates between interpreting the speech of the provider and that of the patient in a back-and-forth fashion. Very few health care organizations use UN-style simultaneous interpretation, when the interpreter utters the words of the speaker almost as they come out of the speaker's mouth. Some large health care organizations use face-to-face for those languages encountered very often and telephonic or video interpreters for languages that their needs assessment has indicated occur infrequently. Research is being done to assess the impact that the various types of interpreter services have on the quality of a clinical encounter (Gany et al., 2007). The *Journal of General Internal Medicine* devoted an entire special supplement in 2007 to issues related to language barriers in health care. Researchers have learned that the use of remote, simultaneous interpretation resulted in fewer errors and was faster than other commonly used methods (Gany et al., 2008). A randomized controlled trial revealed that patients felt that remote interpretation protected their privacy well but that patients who experienced any method of interpreting were not as pleased as those who had a language-concordant physician. It was also found that patients with language-discordant providers received less health education and experienced less personal care, though these problems were somewhat mitigated if interpretation was provided (Ngo-Metzger et al., 2007).

As noted, face-to-face interpreters most often interpret consecutively, that is, repeat what the patient or provider has just said. They use the first person, because they are speaking as the person whose utterances are being interpreted. Research has shown that far fewer errors and much better rapport between patient and provider results from the first-person style of interpreting (Gilbert, Roat, Lonner, Perez, & Diaz 2004). The goal of the interpreter is to be a conduit, allowing the provider and patient to control the encounter. In many cases, the interpreter is bicultural as well as bilingual and can help the provider understand culture-specific meanings and attitudes that may potentially cause misunderstandings. Such an interpreter works collaboratively with the provider as part of the health care team.

In response to the growing need for health care interpreters and the legal and accreditation problems that may result in failing to provide them, a large number of telephonic interpreting companies have begun providing communication services across the United States. They make available trained health care interpreters in almost any language in less than a minute to their subscribers. If the provider is equipped with a speaker phone, having a telephonic interpreter on the line is very much like having a face-to-face interpreter in the room and is, in some cases, more comfortable for the patient. A provider-unique telephone code is used to access the interpreter line and the service is charged by the minute. The National Health Law Program provides a listing of telephonic-interpreting companies on their website.

The Bureau of Labor Statistics of the US Department of Labor (2011) reports that interpreters and translators held 50,900 jobs in 2008 and that interpreters and translators can expect much faster-than-average job growth, increasing an expected 22 percent between 2008 and 2018. Training opportunities for health care interpreters are growing rapidly. Many community colleges offer courses in health care or medical interpreting. In addition, there are now several consulting firms that offer week- or two-week-long interpreting courses at the work site. Of particular importance, there are many state interpreters' associations, such as the California Healthcare Interpreters Association, commonly called *CHIA* (2002) and the Massachusetts Medical Interpreters Association as well as the National Council on Interpreting in Health Care (NCIHC), which offer educational meetings and conferences. These organizations have created standards for the health care interpreting profession (California Healthcare Interpreters, 2002; NCIHC, 2005) and they have worked together to create a **medical and healthcare interpreter certification** program (NCIHC, 2005). The NCIHC studied the various training programs used in the United States and in spring 2011 published the national standards for health care interpreter training. These activities suggest that, very soon, the certified health care interpreter will be the benchmark for the health care and medical interpreting field and using such professionalized interpreters will be a best practice standard for health care providers. Bilingual students in the health care fields, especially in the allied health care fields, may wish to look into the growing opportunities in this area.

In addition to training for interpreters, there are now brief trainings for persons who use interpreters. For example, the Office of Minority Health has a one-page handout for working with an interpreter on their training website, Think Cultural Health. The goal of this kind of training is to help providers negotiate an interpreted encounter effectively and efficiently. Three major provider complaints about the use of interpreters in health care are that their use lengthens encounters with LEP patients, the provider feels out of control of the interaction, and the provider feels uncertain about the accuracy of the messages transmitted. These uncertainties are considerably diminished when health care professionals work regularly with trained medical interpreters and acquire skills that make such encounters seem comfortable and natural. However, several specific procedures are taught that, with very little practice, can greatly enhance a person's skill in conducting effective interpreted exchanges. The most important of these are summarized in the following.

TIPS FOR WORKING EFFECTIVELY WITH AN INTERPRETER

- Choose an interpreter whose age, gender, background, and so on makes it easiest to work with the patient.

- Introduce the interpreter to the patient and family and get the patient's permission to use an interpreter. Explain the interpreter's commitment to confidentiality if necessary.

- Position the interpreter behind the patient or behind you, not between you and the patient, so that your attention can be focused on the patient.

- Speak and look directly at the patient, not the interpreter.

- Use the first person and expect the interpreter to do the same: "Mrs. Chan, I want you to think about when the headaches started."

- Don't speak too long without letting the interpreter interpret.

- Learn basic words from the target language that you will use often. Asking interpreters about words or comments that haven't been interpreted prompts attention to detail.

- Come back to an issue if you suspect misunderstanding on the part of yourself or the patient.

- If you come across a cultural belief or behavior that is unfamiliar to you, take some time later to ask the interpreter about it.

- Treat the interpreter as a respected health care professional.

Interpreters are often bicultural as well as bilingual. The target language is their native language and they were often born into the culture that speaks it. They can be especially helpful in assisting health care personnel to understand the aspects of language that go beyond words: style, intonation, volume, pace, and register. Language style has to do with the directness or indirectness with which conversations are carried out. Americans tend to have a very direct, cut-to-the-chase style, often exacerbated in time-sensitive health care surroundings. Some Latin, Asian, and Middle Eastern patients imbue their speech with asides and contextual information that they feel gives the listener the whole picture of, say, why a symptom manifested as it did or came about when it did. English speakers can find this indirection time consuming and vague. Additionally, the intonations of some languages, particularly Asian languages, can be puzzling and abrasive to Western ears, even though the tonal characteristics of these languages carry additional meaning. People from some cultures speak loudly and rapidly when anxious and can give the appearance of being impatient or demanding and those from other cultures can appear subdued and stoic in the same circumstances. The speech of several American Indian cultures seems maddeningly slow in pace to the ears of a non-Indian because it is full of reflective pauses; conversely, the faster delivery of an Anglo provider may seem lacking in considered thought to an Indian. The register of an utterance refers to its formality or idiomatic characteristics. Speakers from many cultures use a more formal register or usage when speaking to authorities or persons of higher stature or even when the subject matter is very serious. They may, for example, resent joking or attempts at lightheartedness as reflected in a health professional's language meant only to put them at ease. Finally, many interpreters are familiar with some of the different dialects that denote the locales from which immigrants come and can interpret the idiomatic usages that characterize these dialects. Familiarity with these many linguistic nuances can prevent misunderstandings between patients and providers. Working frequently with trained, bicultural interpreters has the added advantage of enabling health care providers to become familiar with subtle and important language differences.

Using an interpreter does not mean that the interpreter takes over in the encounter. It is up to the English-speaking health care provider to set the tone of the interaction through greetings, knowing the name of the patient, setting the patient at ease by smiling, and acknowledging responses through nods and an alert gaze. It is good practice, whenever possible, for the provider to learn expressions of greeting, acknowledgment of information, and anatomical terms or other critical words in the target language. Paying close attention to non-verbal expressions, gestures, and body postures is helpful in judging responses and emotions. As people become more skilled in using interpreters, they can manage encounters more efficiently and with greater assurance. They also learn that any extra time that might be involved is a small price to pay for ensuring greater mutual understanding, rapport, and effective and safe patient care.

TRANSLATION IN WRITTEN HEALTH CARE COMMUNICATION

In considering crosscultural communication, it is important to know that there is a difference between language interpreters and language translators because there is a tendency to confuse their functions. An interpreter deals with oral language and a translator with written communication. In many cases, particularly among persons born in the United States, who learned their foreign languages in informal, family settings, individuals who can speak a language cannot function well as translators because they are unfamiliar with the grammar, usage, and spelling of the written target languages. Many are ill-equipped to provide translations of medical or commercial health care documents.

A great deal of communication in health care depends on the written word. To name just a few types of information that are conveyed to clients and patients in written form, there are eligibility and benefits documents, admissions and medical history forms, discharge instructions, laboratory instructions, prescriptions, consent forms, and health education materials. For example, signed consent forms are legally required before invasive, nonemergent procedures are performed on a patient in order to make sure that the patient fully understands the nature of the procedure and its risks and benefits. Frequently, LEP patients are "consented" by an interpreter, trained or untrained, reading the consent document written in English and orally interpreting its content on sight. In one study of the impact of language barriers on documentation of informed consent, it was found that, despite having an interpreted or translated document, fewer LEP patients than English-speaking patients (28 compared to 53 percent) had full documentation of consent, and fewer LEP patients had signed the consent form than did the English-speakers (70 compared to 85 percent) (Schenker, Wang, Selig, Ng, & Fernandez, 2007).

As more laws and accreditation standards mandate that LEP persons be provided with critical documents in their languages, companies that provide translated materials are being widely used by health care organizations to design and translate accurate and culturally appropriate commercial, clinical, and educational documents for their LEP patients. Accurate and effective health care translations are the work of translators who have in-depth knowledge of a language and its dialects and idioms. There are helpful resources available to aid health care organizations to ensure that translated materials are accurate and culturally appropriate, such as the Hablamos Juntos, *More Than Words Toolkit Series* (2009) and *What's in a Word* (2010) produced by the National Health Law Program. The American Translation Association has listings of certified medical translators and companies as well as a guide for how to work effectively with translators. The Hablamos Juntos Program (nd) funded by the Robert Wood Johnson Foundation also has available on its website the Translation Quality Assessment Tool as an aid to health care organizations that require translations of educational or other health care written materials. Fortunately, the health care industry has come a long distance from the time when providers relied on translations by uncertified bilingual employees or "the doctor's wife who knows Spanish"!

Qualified translators are sensitive to cultural issues involved in the design of illustrated documents such as health education or other informational materials that are targeted to specific language and cultural groups. Such materials often picture family groups, interpersonal interactions, even the illustration of diets and foods that need to be appropriate and meaningful to the cultural group to whom the written information is directed. Translators are sensitive to the fact that colors have symbolic connotations that communicate very different meanings across cultural groups. In the United States, white is the color of weddings and purity; in Asian cultures it the color of death and mourning. Black is the color of death, mourning, and evil in Western culture and it is unlucky in Japan. The color green is revered by Muslim populations as a religious color; in the United States, green is associated with plants and ecology. For Chinese, red is the color of happiness, prosperity, and marriage; for the Japanese, something written in red ink means the end of an association or relationship. Numbers have special meanings in different cultures as well. In Europe, thirteen is an unlucky number and many buildings do not have thirteenth floors. In China, four is an unlucky number because it sounds like "to die" in Mandarin and Cantonese. Misuse of colors and numbers can render a message offensive or at the least ineffective or comical. A trained translator will be aware of cultural symbolism.

In both interpretation and translation, documentation is important. Most regulators and accreditation agencies require documentation of how language barriers are handled for each LEP patient. Because health care providers tend to adhere to the concept that if an activity isn't recorded in the medical record, it didn't happen, documentation of language access needs and the provision of language services are important. The primary language of an LEP patient, the names of anyone who provided interpretation, and for whom and what should be recorded in the medical record. Similarly, notes or copies of translated documents given to the patient should also be entered.

COMMUNICATION IS MORE THAN WORDS

If communication were limited to words alone, crosscultural interactions would certainly be much easier to manage through interpretation and translation. But language is embedded in culture in complex ways that are often difficult to perceive and understand. A great deal of any culture's communication is made up of behavior rather than, or in addition to, words. Most communication behaviors are learned out of consciousness. That is, members of a culture pick up these behaviors from their parents and others without actually being aware that they are learning them. Additionally, they almost always perform these behaviors automatically, without being aware that they are doing them. Not surprisingly, cultures vary considerably in terms of these wordless communications, often causing misunderstanding or discomfort in crosscultural exchanges. The information and illustrations in this section expand on the discussion of communication-related issues in the health care encounter in Chapter Seven.

Anthropologists such as Edward Hall have studied these wordless communication differences and the effects they have on crosscultural communication. In *The Hidden Dimension*, Hall (1966) discusses proxemics, or the culturally shaped concepts of how space and spatial distance are used as part of interpersonal communication. He discusses how people of all cultures separate themselves from others inside a personal bubble of space, the dimensions of which differ crossculturally. These spatial bubbles even differ within a culture according to rules that relate to such things as gender and status. In other words, space is used to communicate meaning in that it is used to convey understandings about relationships between people. In crosscultural encounters, these rules are often unknowingly violated. Health care situations frequently call for people's physical proximity, whether it be in a waiting room, exam room, doctor's office, or radiology lab, increasing the probability that some of the rules will be in conflict. Some nurses and medical assistants, for example, have expressed unease over the tendency for Middle Easterners to stand too close to them, infringing on the unspoken American rule of maintaining a professional spatial distance of about four feet. "I feel uncomfortable with people of Arab background because they breathe on me," explained one lab technician. "I know they don't mean to be offensive, but I don't like it. It seems pushy." Arab proximity rules call for much greater closeness between nonintimates of the same sex, and they feel it is impolite not to directly face the person with whom they are speaking. However, a physician may feel rebuffed, when, as taught in medical school, he extends his hand in greeting to new patient, a Middle Eastern woman, and she does not extend hers to meet his. The Muslim rules of who can touch whom guide her behavior and touching or being touched by a man other than a family member is not allowed.

Eye contact during a verbal exchange is another **nonverbal communication** behavior that differs dramatically across cultures. An English person or an American shows attention to what is being said by gazing at the speaker, though the American may shift his gaze more than the English person, causing the English person to wonder if he's really listening. Japanese learn to direct their attention to a speaker's neck while in conversation. Arab men learn that they should gaze intently into the eyes of the speaker and hold the gaze, a practice that can cause unease in some other cultures. If an American directs his eyes away from an American speaker for long, he is seen to be disinterested or shutting the other person out; however, if the one to avert his gaze is a child, this behavior is seen as disrespectful. In other cultures an averted or downward gaze on the part of an adult or child is seen as a sign of respect. It can easily be seen that these differing rules could be upsetting and create uncertainty in a discussion of symptoms, treatment, or prognosis.

Much of the spoken word is accompanied by hand, facial, or body gesturing. People wave good-bye, beckon, give directions, express doubt, approval, success, and disrespect with hands and fingers. Heads nod, shake, and waggle; eyes roll and wink; eyebrows lift; shoulders shrug; mouths smile, pout, and point; noses are held . . . these are imbued with meaning but the meanings often differ culture by culture (Axtell, 1991). Certain gestures such as the thumbs-up gesture or the circled thumb and forefinger gesture have positive meanings in the United States but negative or sexual meanings in other cultures. Beckoning with the palm upward to "come here" or "follow me" is considered rude in some cultures because it is considered the way to call animals! Health care personnel report that one of the most difficult nonverbals to interpret is one of the most common—the smile and the nod. These can mean embarrassment, agreement, disagreement, a cover-up for not understanding, respect for authority, or friendliness. If the situation is serious, aware providers do not take a smile or a nod at face value but will seek other ways to make absolutely sure the patient has understood.

It is unnecessary, not to speak of impossible, for health care providers to learn all of the possible nonverbal or para-language signals prevalent in other cultures. Nonverbal communications also vary within cultures and with the length of time a person has been in the United States. However, when working with persons from cultures other than their own, sensitive providers don't jump to conclusions about what a given nonverbal behavior means. The loud tones and rapid gestures of an Iranian immigrant don't necessarily mean that he is demanding or angry, nor does the quiet attitude and downcast eyes of an Asian mean that she disagrees, is depressed, or isn't paying attention. By the same token, caution should be used in making casual gestures in interactions with persons from other cultures until one is sure how familiar the cultural other is with American nonverbal expression. Many trained health care interpreters are cognizant of nonverbal cues and can be helpful to providers in interpreting what they convey.

Communication of Culture and Meaning

Good interpretation and good translation go a long way toward solving cross-cultural communication problems and language barriers in health care. However, as effective as they are, they can't completely bridge the communication gulfs that are created by cultural perspectives and differences in meaning. This is because language and culture are inextricably intertwined. Through social interaction and socialization processes, values, beliefs, attitudes, gestures, and many culturally specific meanings are encoded in words, forming the basis of knowledge and worldview within a culture. Language is truly the "software" of the mind (Fisher, 1988). A cultural group will draw on this collection of words and knowledge to comprehend others, to share experiences, and to express thoughts, ideas, or wants. Clearly, different languages do not just represent different sounds for the same things. Although many separate words can be interpreted and translated, often-times there remains a residue of meaning in a word or utterance that can't be translated because it is culturally unique. This becomes relevant to health care.

Cultural differences in meaning abound in the understandings of etiology, the causes of disease or disorder. Whereas most clinicians in the United States will look for a direct cause or cluster of symptoms, people in non-Western cultures may see a cause in a seemingly unrelated chain of events. An interesting example of this occurred while one of the authors of this book was making rounds in a pediatric ward with residents and an interpreter. The group clustered around the bed of a six-year-old Mexican boy with gastrointestinal problems. His mother explained through the interpreter what precipitated the problem, describing several events, including a neighborhood car accident witnessed by the child. The residents were puzzled. The medical anthropologist was not. What the mother was describing was a classic case of *susto*, a folk illness brought on by fright or emotional distress. Further questioning confirmed the mother's belief.

Similar cultural chasms often occur when it comes to the meaning of symptoms. Although the patient and clinician may agree that the patient is suffering from headaches, the two may have very different interpretations of frequency, severity, cause, treatment, and prognosis. And, although the physician may form a diagnosis based on neurology, the patient may form his based solely on the location of the headache and find the reason for the headache in a set of negative social relationships in the family.

Whereas it may be true that effective communication occurs when the sender and the receiver understand the words in a message, these cultural differences show that crosscultural communication in health care may remain elusive, at least in part. Bridging a conceptual gap is not easy; however, health care workers can maintain an inquiring, nonjudgmental perspective and pay attention to different patterns of response related to how events or words seem to be understood by different groups of patients. Over time and across patients from the same cultural group, it may be possible to see a patterned response that is culturally mediated. Other strategies for enhancing cultural understanding include forming good working relationships with health care interpreters and expressing a willingness to learn about cultural ideas and explanations. Many health care organizations have also made it possible for staff to receive input from the members of linguistic and cultural communities they serve or have hired outside linguistic and cultural experts to teach continuing education units based on crosscultural health beliefs, behaviors, and explanatory models. Most health care personnel have found these trainings to be useful and enriching.

SUMMARY

If patients and health care providers are not able to communicate well with each other as a result of language and cultural barriers, patient safety and quality of care are compromised. The increased number of limited-English-speaking patients coming to US health care organizations for care has presented these institutions with a number of dilemmas. Since the 1990s, the health care industry has undergone massive changes in the way that crosscultural communication and language barriers are managed. Whereas early on the response was to deny or resist making personnel or organizational change in the face of language differences, concern over quality of care for all patients, advocacy, research, lawsuits, regulation, and accreditation have driven strategies designed to break down language barriers. The health care industry has responded with many innovative procedures and tools created to reduce the communication problems of limited-English speakers and their health care providers. They have been aided in making these changes by funding from large foundations and the state and federal governments as well as willing and compassionate personnel in all branches of health care. Provision of language access services for limited-English speakers has now become a recognized standard of quality health care. New health care professions have been born—health care interpreters and translators—and are growing in stature as organizations and providers recognize what they can contribute to health care quality. They present interesting opportunities for bilingual persons who want to work in the large and growing health care industry. The difficulties of crosscultural communication aren't completely solved by having qualified interpreters and translators. Health care workers need to remain open to learning about cultural beliefs and attitudes that are encoded in the language of cultural groups. Those that do this will be rewarded with enhanced interpersonal rapport with patients and more effective, rewarding work lives.

KEY TERMS

ad hoc interpreters

dual role interpreter

face-to-face interpretation

interpretation

language access services (LAS)

language barriers

language concordance

limited English proficiency (LEP)

medical and healthcare interpreter certification

nonverbal communication

trained health care and medical interpreters

translation

REVIEW QUESTIONS AND ACTIVITIES

1. Think back to your most recent visit to a health care organization. Who was the first person you encountered and what information did you need to give and receive from this person? What difficulties might an LEP person have

had at this point? Now walk yourself through your entire visit, thinking about the same questions with respect to each person you interacted with during your visit. Discuss your responses with the class.

2. Why would the diversity of languages spoken by persons within the health care workforce create teamwork problems among health care staff? What language etiquette could ease interpersonal and professional issues caused by multiple languages spoken by workforce members?

3. Go to the website www.palsforhealth.org cited in your text and download two "I speak" cards in two different languages. Bring them to class and discuss the information on them. What other resources are available on this website?

4. Name several situations in which a family member might be inclined to edit the information the patient gives to a doctor or nurse. By a clinician to a patient? Why would this be a problem?

5. Is your state one of the states that has regulations or legislation around LAS in health care? What are they? Have someone make a copy to bring to class for discussion.

6. Go to the website for the National Council on Interpreting in Healthcare (www.ncihc.org) and download their standards for health care interpreter training and their standards for interpreter practice. Bring to class for discussion.

7. Go to the website of the American Translators Association (www.atanet.org). Download their brochure *Getting It Right* and bring to class for discussion.

REFERENCES

American College of Physicians. (2007). *Language services for patients with limited English proficiency: Results of a national survey of physicians.* Position paper. Retrieved from http://www.acponline.org/advocacy/where_we_stand/policy/lep_paper.pdf

American Health Insurance Plans. (2006). *Tools to address disparities in health: Communication resources to close the gap. A compendium of resources for health insurance plans, physicians, and health organizations.* Washington, DC: Author. Retrieved from http://www.vdh.virginia.gov/ohpp/clasact/documents/CLASact/research/default.pdf

American Medical Association. (2007). *Improving communication, improving care: An ethical force consensus report.* Retrieved from www.ama-assn.org/ama1/pub/upload/mm/369/ef_imp_comm.pdf

Amoruso, C. (2011). Needed: Bilingual health care providers. *Diversity Employers, 19*, 29. Retrieved from http://www.diversityemployers.com/index.php/features2/7-bilingual-healthcare

Andrulis, D., & Brach, C. (2007). Integrating literacy, culture and language to improve health care quality for diverse populations. *American Journal of Health Behavior, 31*(supp. 1), 122–133.

Andrulis, D., Goodman, N., & Pryor, C. (2002). *What a difference an interpreter can make: Health care experiences of uninsured with limited English proficiency.* Boston: Center for Community Health Research and Action, Brandeis University. Retrieved from http://www.hhs.gov/ocr/civilrights/resources/specialtopics/lep/whatadifferenceaninterpretercanmake.pdf

Axtell, R. E. (1991). *Gestures: The dos and taboos of body language around the world.* New York: John Wiley and Sons.

California Healthcare Interpreters Association. (2002). *California standards for healthcare interpreters: Ethical principles, protocols, and guidance on roles & intervention.* Retrieved from http://www.chiaonline.org/resource/resmgr/docs/standards_chia.pdf

California Pan-Ethnic Health Network. (2009). *A blueprint for success: Bringing language access to millions of California.* Retrieved from http://www.cpehn.org/pdfs/Sb853briefScreen.pdf

Chinese Community Health Plan. (nd). Retrieved from http://www.cchphmo.com/chinese/

Department of Health and Human Services. (2000). *Strategic plan to improve access to HHS programs and activities by limited English (LEP) persons.* Retrieved from http://www.hhs.gov/ocr/civilrights/resources/specialtopics/lep/lepstrategicplan2000.pdf

Divi, C., Koss, R. G., Schmaltz, S., & Loeb, J. M. (2007). Language proficiency and adverse events in U.S. hospitals: A pilot study. *International Journal for Quality in Healthcare, 19*(2), 60–67.

Ferguson, W. J. (2008). Un poquito: The benefit and perils of knowing "a little bit" of Spanish when communicating with Spanish-speaking patients. *Health Affairs, 27*(6), 1695–1700.

Fisher, G. (1988). *Mindsets.* Yarmouth, ME: Intercultural Press.

Flores, G. (2006). Language barriers to health care in the United States. *New England Journal of Medicine, 355*(3), 229–231.

Flores, G., Laws, M. B., Mayo, S. J., et al. (2003). Errors in medical interpretation and their potential clinical consequences in pediatric encounters. *Pediatrics, 111*, 6–14.

Gany, F., Kapelusznik, K., Gonzalez, J., Orta, L. Y., Tseng, C. H., & Changrani, J. (2007). The impact of medical interpreter method on time and errors. *Journal of General Internal Medicine, 22*(supp. 2), 319–323.

Gany, F., Ling, J., Shapiro, E., Abramson, D., Motola, I., Shield, D., & Changrani, J. (2008). Patient satisfaction with different interpreting: Methods: A randomized controlled trial. *Journal of General Internal Medicine, 22*(supp. 2), 321–318.

Gilbert, M. J. (1996). *Notes from cultural competence in the clinic training session.* Pasadena: Kaiser Permanente, Southern California.

Gilbert, M. J. (1999). *Notes from culture in clinical settings: What to do.* Training session. Pasadena: Kaiser Permanente, Southern California.

Gilbert, M. J., Roat, C. E., Lonner, T. D., Perez, L., & Diaz, E. (2004). *Dual role interpreters: Costs and benefits.* Unpublished report prepared for The California Endowment, Los Angeles.

Hablamos Juntos. (nd). *Translation quality assessment tool.* Retrieved from.http://www .hablamosjuntos.org/mtw/html_toolkit/pdf/7TQA%20tool-Dec19_GYMR.pdf

Hablamos Juntos. (2009). *More than words toolkit series: Improving the quality of health care translations.* http://www.hablamosjuntos.org/mtw/default.toolkit.asp

Hablamos Juntos. (2010). *Universal symbols in health care.* Retrieved from www.rwjf.org/pioneer/ product.jsp?id=69209

Hall, E. (1966). *The hidden dimension.* Garden City, NY: Doubleday.

Hwang, J., Ramos, J., Jones, K., & Regenstein, M. (2009). *Talking with patients: How hospitals use bilingual clinicians and staff to care for patients' language needs.* Retrieved from http:// www.calendow.org/uploadedFiles/Publications/By_Topic/Culturally_Competent_Health_ Systems/Language_Access/Talking%20with%20Patients.pdf

Interpreters ratify contract with Washington State. (2011, June). *Sky Valley Chronicle.*

Jacobs, E. A., Shepard, D. S., Suaya, J. A., & Stone, E.-L. (2004). Overcoming language barriers in health care: Costs and benefits of interpreter services. *American Journal of Public Health, 94*(5), 866–869.

The Joint Commission. (2009). *The Joint Commission 2009 requirements that support effective communication, cultural competence, and patient-centered care.* Retrieved from http://www .jointcommission.org/assets/1/6/2009_CLASRelatedStandardsHAP.pdf

The Joint Commission. (2010). *Advancing effective communication, cultural competence, and patient- and family-centered care: A roadmap for hospitals.* Oakview Terrace, IL. Retrieved from www.jointcommission.org/Advancing_Effective_Communication/

Kaiser Permanente. (nd.). *Trilingual manuals.* Retrieved from kphci.org/resources/trm.html

Karliner, L. S., Jacobs, E. A., Chen, A. H., & Mutha, S. (2006). Do professional interpreters improve clinical care for patients with limited English proficiency? A systematic review of the literature. *Health Services Research, 42*(2), 727–754.

Ku, L. (2006). *Paying for language services in medicine: Preliminary options and recommendations.* Washington, DC: Center on Budget and Policy.

Kuo, D. Z., O'Connor, K. G., Flores, G., & Minkovitz, C. S. (2006). Pediatrician's use of language services for families with limited English proficiency. *Pediatrics, 119*(4), 920–927.

Martinez, E. L., Hitov, S., & Youdelman, M. (2010). *Language access in health care statement of principles: Explanatory guide.* Washington, DC: National Health Law Program. Retrieved from http://www.healthlaw.org/images/stories/Language_Access_in_Health_Care_Statement_ of_Principles_Explanatory_Guide_2010_Update.pdf

Mataeo, J., Gallardo, E., Huang, V. Y., & Niski, C. (2009). *Providing health care to limited English proficient patients: A manual of promising practices.* Sacramento: California Primary

Care Association. Retrieved from http://www.hhs.gov/ocr/civilrights/resources/specialtopics/lep/providinghealthcaretoleppdf.pdf

Medi-Cal Language Access Services Task Force. (2009). *Providing language services for limited English proficient patients in California: Developing a service system for the state.* Retrieved from http://www.lchc.org/documents/FinalMCLASReport4–09.pdf

MRMIB/HFP. (2007). *Cultural and linguistic services in the health families program.* Retrieved from http://www.mrmib.ca.gov/MRMIB/Agenda_Minutes_102407/7f_CL_summary_10–24–07_FINAL_DRAFT.pdf

National Committee on Quality Assurance. (2006). Innovative practices in multicultural health. Retrieved from http://www.ncqa.org/Portals/0/HEDISQM/CLAS/CLAS_InnovativePrac06.pdf

National Committee on Quality Assurance. (2007). *Innovative practices in multicultural health* Retrieved from http://www.ncqa.org/Portals/0/HEDISQM/CLAS/CLAS_InnovativePrac07.pdf

National Committee on Quality Assurance. (2008). Innovative practices in multicultural health. Retrieved from http://www.ncqa.org/Portals/0/HEDISQM/CLAS/CLASInnovativePrac_08.pdf

National Committee on Quality Assurance. (2009). *Innovative practices in multicultural health care.* Washington, DC: Author. Retrieved from http://www.ncqa.org/Portals/0/HEDISQM/CLAS/CLAS_InnovPrac_09.pdf

National Committee on Quality Assurance. (2010). *Implementing multicultural health care standards: Ideas and examples.* Retrieved from http://www.ncqa.org/Portals/0/Publications/Implementing%20MHC%20Standards%20Ideas%20and%20Examples%2004%2029%2010.pdf

National Council on Interpreting in Health Care. (2005). *National standards of practice for interpreters in health care.* Retrieved from http://www.ncihc.org/assets/documents/NCIHC%20National%20Standards%20of%20Practice.pdf

National Council on Interpreting in Health Care. (2011). *National standards for health care interpreter training.* Retrieved from http://www.ncihc.org/assets/documents/National_Standards_5–09–11.pdf

National Health Law Program. (2003). *Ensuring linguistic access in health care settings: Legal rights and responsibilities.* Retrieved from http://www.healthlaw.org/index.php?option=com_content&view=article&id=120:ensuring-linguistic-access-in-health-care-settings-legal-rights-a-responsibilities&catid=40

National Health Law Program. (2004). *Language services action kit: Interpreter services in health care settings for people with limited English proficiency.* Retrieved from http://www.healthlaw.org/index.php?option=com_content&view=article&id=119:language-services-action-kit-interpreter-services-in-health-care-settings-for-people-with-limited-english-proficiency-revd-feb-04-&catid=40

National Health Law Program. (2008). *Summary of state law requirements addressing language needs in health care.* Retrieved from http://www.lawhelp.org/documents/383231nhelp.lep.state.law.chart.final.pdf

National Health Law Program. (2010). *What's in a word? A guide to understanding interpretation and translation in health care.* Retrieved from http://www.nyhq.org/doc/Page.asp?PageID= DOC000312

Ngo-Metzger, Q., Sorkin, D. H., Phillips, R. S., Greenfield, S., Massagli, B. C., & Kaplen, S. (2007). Providing high quality care for limited English proficient patients: The importance of language concordance and interpreter use. *Journal of General Internal Medicine, 22*(supp. 2), 324–330.

Office of Civil Rights. (2000, August 16). Guidance memorandum: Title VI prohibition against national origin discrimination as it affects persons with limited-English proficiency. *Federal Register, 65,* 50123.

Office of Minority Health. (nd). *A patient-centered guide to implementing language access services in healthcare organizations.* Retrieved from http://thinkculturalhealth.org

Pacific Asian Language Services/PALS for Health. (nd). *In the absence of words: A compilation of personal stories addressing the language barriers in health care.* Retrieved from http://tcenews .calendow.org/pr/tce/document/In_the_Absence_of_Words.pdf

Paras, M. (2005). *Straight talk: Model hospital policies and procedures in language access.* Sacramento: California Health Safety Net Institute. Retrieved from http://www.safetynetinstitute .org/content/upload/AssetMgmt/Site/StraightTalkFinal.pdf

Quan, K., & Lynch, J. (2011). *The high costs of language barriers in medical malpractice.* Washington, DC: National Health Law Program. Retrieved from http://www.pacificinterpreters.com/docs/ resources/high-costs-of-language-barriers-in-malpractice_nhelp.pdf

Robert Wood Johnson. (2008). *Speaking together toolkit.* Retrieved from www.rwjf.org/ qualityequality/product.jsp?id=29653

Sampson, A. (2006). *Language services resource guide for health care providers.* Washington, DC: National Health Law Program.

Schenker, Y., Wang, F., Selig, S. J., Ng, R., & Fernandez, F. (2007). The impact of language barriers on documentation of informed consent at a hospital with on-site interpreter services. *Journal of General Internal Medicine, 22*(supp. 2), 294–299.

Schyve, P. M. (2007). Language differences as a barrier to quality and safety in health care: The Joint Commission perspective. *Journal of General Internal Medicine, 22*(supp. 2), 360–361.

Tang, G., Lanza, O., Rodriguez, F. M., & Chang, A. (2011). The Kaiser Permanente clinician cultural and linguistic assessment imitative: Research and development in patient-provider language concordance. *Journal of Public Health, 101*(2).

University of California at Irvine. (2010). *Video, on demand.* Retrieved from www.uci.edu/ features/2010/06/feature_videointerpreters_100601.php

US Census Bureau. (2003). *DP-2. Profiles of selected social characteristics: 2000.* Retrieved from http://factfinders.census.gov

US Department of Labor, Bureau of Labor Statistics. (2011). Interpreters and translators. *Occupational outlook handbook 2010–11 edition.* Retrieved from www.bls.gov/oco/ocos175.htm

Wilson-Stronks, A., & Galvez, E. (2007). *Hospitals, language, and culture: A snapshot of the nation. Exploring cultural and linguistic services in the nation's hospitals: A report of findings.* The Joint Commission. Retrieved from http://www.jointcommission.org/assets/1/6/hlc_paper.pdf

Wong, D. (2010, October). *Providing language services in pharmacy settings: Law and promising practices.* Paper presented at the Seventh National Conference on Quality Health Care for Diverse Populations, Baltimore, MD. Retrieved from www.healthlaw.org

Wynia, M., & Matiasek, J. (2006). *Promising practices for patient-centered communication with vulnerable populations: Examples from eight hospitals.* Retrieved from http://www.commonwealthfund.org/Publications/Fund-Reports/2006/Aug/Promising-Practices-for-Patient-Centered-Communication-with-Vulnerable-Populations—Examples-from-Ei.aspx

Youdelman, M. (2011). *The ACA and language access.* Short paper #5. Retrieved from http://familiesusa2.org/conference/health-action-2012/toolkit/content/pdfs/ACA-language-access.pdf

Youdelman, M., & Perkins, J. (2005). *Providing language services in small health care settings: Examples from the field.* Washington, DC: National Health Law Program. Retrieved from http://www.commonwealthfund.org/usr_doc/810_Youdelman_providing_language_services.pdf

Chapter 9

GROUP IDENTITY DEVELOPMENT AND HEALTH CARE DELIVERY

LEARNING OBJECTIVES

- To discuss theory and research that undergird the majority and minority group identity development frameworks presented in this chapter

- To distinguish between out-group (minority) and in-group (majority) identities

- To describe the process of group identity development for individuals who are members of a minority or out-group

- To describe the process of group identity development for individuals who are members of a majority or in-group

- To illustrate the impact of group identity status on interactions in diverse health care organizations

- To explain the relationship between group identity status and cultural competence at the individual and organizational levels

A s previous chapters discussed, demographic changes have made diversity leadership and the delivery of culturally and linguistically appropriate care an imperative for health care organizations. But, unlike more-typical business imperatives such as responding to changes in reimbursement policies or technological innovation, health care professionals and the health care delivery organization itself must engage in an unprecedented level of self-exploration to respond effectively to the diversity imperative. The experience of human diversity, after all, is a very personal one, and must begin with understanding ourselves. And, for better or for worse, our self-understanding is expressed through our interactions with colleagues and patients in the process of health care delivery.

In our role as health care providers, we interact with some colleagues and patients who are members of our own identity groups and some who are not. As discussed in Chapter One, identity groups are socially relevant classifications of people such as ethnic, racial, gender, and religious groups. We choose some of our identity groups like membership in a professional association and others, including the immutable dimensions of diversity—ethnicity, race, gender, and sexual orientation—are socially determined to be important and their role in everyday interactions is reinforced through culture. Certain identity groups, generally referred to as majority or in-groups, are assigned higher value and esteem by the larger society. In contrast, minority or out-groups are assigned lesser value and esteem. Majority or in-group members are united by a common identity and shared beliefs, attitudes, or interests, and have the collective social power and influence to exclude outsiders. Minority or out-group members are excluded from belonging to the in-group and, relative to the in-group, are seen as less powerful, socially desirable, or contemptibly different.

In this chapter we discuss the process of group identity development and the role that group identity status plays in health care delivery. Group identity status is defined as the constellation of attitudes and beliefs that shape how we experience and enact our group affiliation. Two models of group identity development undergird our discussion: one focuses on minority identity development and the other on majority identity development. Each model consists of a number of discrete but dynamic statuses and each status reflects a distinctive worldview or constellation of core beliefs about that dimension of diversity. Because core beliefs have a profound influence on our perceptions and our behavior, the group identity status of patients, caregivers, administrators, and the organization itself will influence the extent to which care is perceived as culturally competent and the extent to which delivery of culturally competent care is perceived to be important by organizational stakeholders.

As Cox (1993) explains, "Various group identities play a part in how we define ourselves as well as how others view us" (p. 43). We will use case examples to illustrate the role that group identity development plays in everyday interactions among managers, staff, clinicians, and patients in health care organizations and how these interactions affect the delivery of culturally competent care. The two models of identity development that frame this chapter were developed first in the counseling psychology literature to study racial identity development in the context of black and white and are used in organizational development initiatives and executive coaching by diversity consultants.

RESEARCH HIGHLIGHTS

Cross (1971); Atkinson, Morten, and Sue (1979); and Helms (1984, 1990) have all advanced models of identity development that can be used to illustrate the impact of group identity status on health care encounters and other interactions in health care organizations. Although these models were originally advanced to explain the statuses of majority and minority racial and ethnic identity development in a black-white racial context, they provide a conceptual framework that can be extended to other majority-minority or in-group–out-group identities, such as other racial and ethnic groups, LGBT individuals and heterosexuals, and women and men. In this chapter, majority group and in-group are used as synonyms as are minority group and out-group. Valuing diversity involves understanding how what we believe about our in-group and out-group identities influences the ways in which we interpret, choose, explain, and justify our own behavior and the behavior of others in the workplace.

The examples used in this chapter to illustrate the models are hypothetical or composite examples drawn from experience. Individuals cannot be categorized into an identity status based solely on a few observed behaviors or expressed attitudes. The process of identity development is complex. In fact, Helms (1999) contends that the statuses are dynamic in that they evolve from one another and can appear in different combinations in any given individual. As Helms (1999) explains, our **dominant status** determines our reactions most of the time, whereas our **accessible statuses** are at least strong enough for us to express in some circumstances. It is important not to use your perception of another's identity status to label or stereotype that person.

Research findings point to an association between racial identity statuses, defined by Helms (1995) as the "dynamic cognitive, emotional, and behavioral processes that govern a person's interpretation of racial information in his or her interpersonal environments" (p. 184) and other traits such as self-esteem. For example, status one, conformity, of the Minority Status Group Identity Development Model presented in Table 9.1 and discussed later in this chapter, has been associated with low self-esteem, low feelings of competence, and higher feelings of inferiority, anxiety, and inadequacy. The same researchers found that individuals in statuses one, conformity, and three, resistance and immersion, of the model experienced more personal distress and less-healthy self-actualizing behavior, whereas those in statuses two, dissonance; four, introspection; and five, synergy evidenced attitudes that reflected higher self-esteem, feelings of competence, and low anxiety (Parham & Helms, 1985).

Gushue and Carter (2000) found that status two, dissonance, in the majority status group identity development model presented in Table 9.2 and discussed later in this chapter was associated with heightened anxiety about race and resulted in a better memory for race-related information about people of color, especially when that information contradicted commonly held stereotypes. Status four, liberal, in the same model was found to be associated with "strident non-racism" and a resultant tendency to see other majority group members in a stereotypical way, even when information provided was to the contrary. Thus, research supports the role that identity status plays in beliefs, attitudes, and behaviors that are salient in a diversity context.

It is important to remember that identity status is dynamic, not static or permanent. Human beings are able to adapt and change the way we see ourselves and others and thus can move among the statuses of group identity development. In fact, Thompson and Carter (1997) contend that movement among statuses is indicative of a shift in worldview that occurs in response to experiences, self-reflection, and conscious decisions on the part of the individual.

These same models (Tables 9.1 and 9.2) can be used not only to evaluate and understand interactions among providers and patients but also the overall diversity climate in the health care organization. Chrobot-Mason and Thomas (2002) contend that organizational identity and individual identity development influence one another in the workplace. The researchers explain that a monocultural

TABLE 9.1 Minority Status Group Identity Development

Statuses of Identity Development	Attitudes Toward Self	Attitudes Toward Others of the Same Identity Group	Attitudes Toward Others of Different Minority Groups	Attitudes Toward Culturally Dominant Group
Status one: conformity	Self-depreciating	Group depreciating	Discriminatory	Group appreciating and denial of discriminatory practices
Status two: dissonance	Conflict between self-depreciating and self-appreciating	Conflict between group depreciating and group appreciating	Conflict between acknowledging and identifying mutual experiences and feeling alliance with views held by dominant culture	Conflict between dominant group appreciation and anger and resentment about discriminatory practices
Status three: resistance and immersion	Self-appreciation based on membership in own group	Group appreciating	Conflict between feelings of empathy for other cultural groups' experiences and feelings of cultural centrism	Group depreciating
Status four: introspection	Concern with basis of self-appreciation	Concern with nature of unequivocal appreciation	Concern with cultural-centric basis for judging others	Concern with the basis for group depreciation
Status five: synergy	Self-appreciating	Group appreciating	Group appreciating	Selective appreciation

Source: © Eclipse Consultant Group (2004). Reprinted with permission.

TABLE 9.2 Majority Status Group Identity Development

Statuses of Identity Development	Self-Identity and Awareness of Privilege	Same Identity Group	Attitudes Toward Minority Individuals	Attitudes Toward Minority Groups
Status one: naiveté	Unaware of majority status and privilege	No awareness of group membership	Seeks similarity: "I'm not prejudiced."	Everyone is the same: "People are people."
Status two: dissonance	Beginning to see majority status and privilege	Ambivalence	Approach and avoidance; interpersonal conflict	Emerging awareness of stereotypes; internal conflict emerges
Status three: defensive	Justifies privilege	Justifies superior status	Avoidance and internal or external hostility	Group depreciating
Status four: liberal	Acknowledges privilege	Distances self from majority group	Seeks acceptance	Over-identifies and justifies
Status five: self-exploration	Struggles with personal prejudice	Recognizes positive and negative aspects	Begins to develop authentic relationships	Explores complexity
Status six: transcultural	Realistic self-appreciation	Realistic group appreciation	Has authentic relationships	Reflective appreciation

Source: © Eclipse Consultant Group (2004). Reprinted with permission.

workplace in which differences are either ignored or devalued will encourage individuals at low statuses of identity development to remain there and individuals at higher statuses of identity development to regress. However, a health care organization that has implemented the systems approach to strategic diversity management and cultural competence (see Figure 1.2) will encourage members of the workforce with low-identity development statuses to progress and those at high statuses of identity development to sustain that personal growth. Chrobot-Mason and Thomas (2002) also contend that the dominant racial identity development status of leadership may actually drive the organization's commitment to diversity management and cultural competence: "It is critical to understand the racial identity development of organizational leaders whose influence is manifested in the corporate values that guide diversity practices that shape the organizational climate for diversity" (p. 337). Dansky and her colleagues (2003) drew a similar conclusion based on their study of diversity practices in Pennsylvania hospitals.

MINORITY STATUS GROUP IDENTITY DEVELOPMENT

Table 9.1 shows the model of minority group identity development used by the Eclipse Consultant Group, one of the many independent consulting firms in the country that deliver diversity and cultural competence training and other organizational development interventions to client organizations. The theory that supports Table 9.1 was originally developed by Cross (1971) and subsequently extended by Atkinson, Morten, and Sue (1979). The model has since been extensively studied, refined, and validated (Helms, 1990). Each status in the model is discussed in detail below, and implications for intra- and inter-group relationships in health care organizations are illustrated through hypothetical or composite examples drawn from experience. The examples were developed to show behavior in a health care setting that reflects the theoretical status of group identity development under discussion. Although the Cross (1971) model was originally developed to explain black racial identity development, our illustrations of the model include interactions between majority and minority group members on additional dimensions of diversity, including other racial and ethnic groups, women, and LGBT identity groups.

Conformity

The first status, conformity, occurs when the minority group member attempts to adapt and accommodate to the majority culture. For an individual at this status of identity development, assimilation is the name of the game.

According to the model, minority group members at this status of identity development will reinforce negative stereotypes against their own group if the majority group promotes it. For example, if the majority expresses the perception that blacks are angry and dangerous, the person in a conformity status will appear to agree. If the majority expresses the perception that women are overly emotional and not as well suited to leadership as men, the woman in a conformity status will appear to agree. A black recreational therapist in the conformity status might nod and express agreement when her white colleagues say, "Most blacks are so angry and difficult to get along with. We're glad you're not like them." A female nurse in the conformity status might acknowledge her male colleague's leadership ability while being unable to see the same abilities in her equally qualified female colleagues.

An individual in the conformity status is not fully conscious of the differences as viewed by society or wears a mask to survive in the majority culture. The outcome is that persons in a conformity status tell the majority group member whatever they believe that the majority group member wants to hear. The conformity status reflects a strong identification with the majority group.

How might conformity behavior manifest in a racial and ethnic minority patient? A racial and ethnic minority patient in the conformity status can be seemingly compliant. Patients of color in this status may follow white physicians' orders while in their presence but when left alone, may fail to carry out the orders. For example, a physician tells the patient to take medicine in four-hour intervals; the patient smiles and nods to convey agreement but fails to take the medicine at the prescribed intervals. How might conformity behavior manifest in a female patient? An older female patient in the conformity status may express a preference for a male rather than a female doctor, believing that the male doctor would be better qualified. However, she might refuse care from a male nurse, believing that the nursing role is better suited to a female.

Patients in the conformity identity status may withhold information about their condition and not convey anger or express disagreement with the health care professional. A lesbian patient in a conformity status, for example, may not disclose her sexual identity even when it is salient to the health care encounter.

In order not to appear ungrateful, patients in conformity may attempt to be conciliatory in front of the doctor or nurse. Patients may believe that the doctor knows best and will not question the physician's evaluation. Internally, patients in the conformity identity status may not be consciously aware of any emotional uneasiness about the interaction or may be feeling annoyed and afraid to speak up.

The conformity identity status is framed within the context of deference to majority group authority and is, in part, influenced by sociohistorical experience and culturally transmitted beliefs about the majority group. Soon, however, individuals in a conformity status may discover through experience or the influence of others that there is a price to pay for deference to the majority group's perceived authority.

Dissonance

The second status, dissonance, is characterized by ambivalence and conflict. Individuals in the dissonance status vacillate between rejecting their group and almost simultaneously embracing it. They will make positive and negative comments about their own identity group. They may begin to silently challenge the accepted stereotypes and simultaneously reinforce them.

Dissonance is filled with ambivalence when it relates to attitudes toward one's self. The group identity of an individual in the dissonance status is in a state of flux. For a woman in a dissonance status, thinking may follow along these lines: "Men believe that women are overly emotional and helpless. I'm not overly emotional or helpless and I'm a woman." Alternatively, a gay man in dissonance may vacillate between anger that the health care organization he works for does not offer domestic partner benefits and affirmation of this policy as the status quo and therefore acceptable. New attitudes are in conflict with old ones. Individuals in the dissonance status start to confront the negative messages they've internalized from the majority culture while experiencing emerging feelings of self-acceptance.

Individuals in the dissonance status also begin to surface and question beliefs about majority group behavior. Contradictions are seen in how majority group members treat minority group members relative to majority group members. This questioning of majority group behavior is accompanied by an exploration of negative stereotypes about their own group. Distrust of majority group members surfaces but, initially, is not expressed openly, especially in the presence of majority group members; it is discussed among the minority group in closed settings.

In the health care setting, a Latino service worker in this status may appear to cooperate with white supervisors on the surface but may undercut their authority in front of patients. For example, if a white supervisor criticizes the work, in front of a Latino patient, of a Latino service worker who is in the dissonance status, the worker may be silent and appear compliant in front of the supervisor. However, once the supervisor leaves, the service worker may make ethnically loaded comments about the supervisor to the Latino patient.

Minority individuals in a dissonance status are in conflict about positive acceptance of their own identity group as an important point of reference. One's feelings in this status are ambivalent—a mixture of pride, joy, wonderment, anger, and shame. Minority individuals in a dissonance status recognize that their identity group is like and unlike the stereotypes; some stereotypes fit and some do not.

For example, racial and ethnic minority individuals in the dissonance status become increasingly aware that individual differences within their racial and ethnic group are very broad. Some individuals accept and some reject their racial and ethnic and associated cultural identity. The view of whites as a referent group also changes: in conformity status, whites are seen as the standard of comparison. In a dissonance status, the white standard is questioned and challenged.

A woman patient in a dissonance status might say to another female patient, "I wouldn't go to a female surgeon if you paid me. You know they don't know what they're doing." Moments later the same patient may say, "Did you see how that nurse treated Dr. Johnson (a female surgeon)? She didn't treat Dr. Jones (a male surgeon) that way. Some women sure are prejudiced against our own." On the one hand, female surgeons are denigrated, and on the other, they are most ardently defended. What often propels individuals to resolve their dissonance and confusion in status two is other individuals who share their minority status and intensify the conflict by pressuring them to get off the fence and commit to a favorable minority group identity.

Resistance and Immersion

When the confusion dissipates, status two is more resolved than not. What follows next is the somewhat turbulent period of status three, resistance and immersion. Minority individuals in this status embrace their minority group identity and reject the majority culture. Interactions with majority group members are interpreted in a historical and political context with majority group members being viewed as the oppressor and unilaterally distrusted. However, one's own group is elevated.

Black individuals in resistance immersion revel in ethnic pride and may begin an intense study of black culture prior to, during, and after slavery. They may express their ethnic identity in dress, language, and in some cases through religious affiliation with, for example, the black Muslims, black Jews, black Christians, or black Catholics. People in resistance and immersion may assume ethnic names and disassociate with "slave names." It's a time of deep appreciation for afro-centric behavior, spiritual practices, politics, and professional affiliations.

Similarly, a woman in resistance immersion may revel in her gender's superiority over men. She may reject cultural symbols of women's "oppression" and communicate that through her attire and through expressing disdain for traditional female roles not only for herself, but also for other women. She may bristle at a male colleague who holds the door for her, interpreting his behavior as signifying his underlying belief that she is too weak and helpless to open the door herself. Male behavior is suspect and interpreted in a social and political context of presumed male domination.

Recall that minority patients in a conformity status may not cooperate with minority health care professionals, even dismissing them as not having authority. In the resistance and immersion status, minority patients may demand to see a health care professional from their own identity group and, likewise, refuse to cooperate with majority health care professionals. A woman patient in a resistance immersion status, for example, may refuse treatment from male health care professionals. Such behavior may be confusing to majority *and* minority health care providers, who lack understanding of the role that identity status development plays in majority-minority interactions in health care delivery.

One key change that characterizes status three, resistance and immersion, from status two, dissonance, is the minority person's blatant rejection of the majority group as a reference point for self-identification. The confusion and conflict in status two dissipates in status three, and individuals emerge to fully embrace their own identity group. The person also rejects, unilaterally, any comments from a majority group member about the minority group. An example is that of a female billing clerk in the resistance immersion status with a reputation for viewing every disagreement with her male colleagues as motivated by gender bias and freely expressing the internal disgust and anger she experiences to her colleagues. The person in resistance and immersion is immersed in self-acceptance and self-justification.

There may be a total rejection of the majority culture, and this rejection may be angrily expressed. Without exception, majority group members may be perceived as the enemy. One lesbian nurse reflected status three when she made the following comment during a diversity training session: "There's no way I'd trust a straight doctor. They're so bigoted that they could never accept me for who I am and provide the same quality of care as they do for their straight patients. I see this happening all the time in this hospital!"

Unlike their response to individuals in the conformity or dissonance status, majority group members are more likely to openly express fear or anger toward or to avoid interactions with individuals who are in resistance and immersion. Subordinates of supervisors who are in the resistance and immersion status may perceive the supervisor as always siding with members of his or her identity group when conflicts arise and feel that, as majority group members, they are the victims of "reverse discrimination."

Some minority group members remain in resistance and immersion for long periods of time, whereas others move through the status rather quickly. Several interpersonal factors may influence individuals to move forward, such as relationship pressure from a close friend who has moved through status three, pressure from a majority group member who has sustained contact with the person in resistance and immersion status through this turbulent time, ongoing work relationships in which the minority individual has to rely on or assist a majority person through crisis, or a peak experience of a profound nature that upsets the status three person's worldview, such as having one's life saved by someone who is a majority group member. Experiences such as these are referred to as trigger events, defined as situations that lead a person to question and potentially change his or her belief system.

Introspection

Once individuals begin to actively question whether unilateral acceptance of their own minority group and rejection of the corresponding majority group really reflects their interpersonal experience with both groups, they enter status four, introspection. In this status, they fully accept their own minority group as the point of reference for their identity and concurrently question the need for polarization or rejection of the corresponding majority group. They begin to realize that identity groups are neither all good nor all bad. Questions such as the following are reviewed and are beginning to be resolved in status four:

Is it possible to accept my minority identity group and still relate to some members of the dominant culture?

Can I trust any member of the majority identity group?

Is my group's perspective right all of the time?

Are some aspects of my identity group's beliefs, values, or behaviors counter-productive or destructive to our group?

Is it possible to be positively identified with my identity group and still reject some of the members of my own group?

People in an introspection status will begin to trust individual majority group members who are able to listen to and validate their concerns about bias and social inequity. Once they discover that some majority group members can be trusted, the belief that all majority group members are biased is shattered. The introspection status generally builds the minority individual's ability to differentiate between majority group members who can be trusted and those who cannot. In addition, they can articulate the effects of institutional bias or discrimination on their group. For example, a Latino vice president illustrated the introspection status when she shared the following perception with a white male counterpart with whom she is developing a close working relationship: "I think our hospital has a poor track record for hiring community people who are black and Latino. The problem seems systemic. We need to confront our employment practices and look at both recruitment and retention. I'm not ready to discuss this issue with the rest of the leadership team, but I would like to know what you think." She now trusts her white counterpart enough to raise a racially and ethnically sensitive issue. Similarly, a gay human resource manager in the introspection status might raise the issue of domestic partner benefits with a trusted colleague in the human resource department or a female hospitalist might raise issues of gender and salary equity with a trusted medical director. When the self-reflection that is characteristic of introspection status is no longer foremost in the minority individual's life and trusting relationships with individual majority group members are firmly established, the door opens to the dominant identity status referred to as synergy in the Eclipse model.

Synergy

Status five, synergy, is characterized by self-acceptance, appreciation of other minority identity groups, and open communication with majority identity group members. Status five individuals see value in other identity groups but their own personal group identity is clearly established and cherished. Those in the synergy status speak freely about their identity group as advocates who are not defensive but who do see group identity issues in a sociopolitical context.

Imagine this scenario: A white male radiology technician says to his white female supervisor, "Only blacks and women get promoted to supervisory positions in this place. I don't have a chance even though I'm qualified." The white female supervisor responds in a nondefensive tone by asking, "How many people of color or women do you know in supervisory positions? I am only aware of three out of the forty-five on the non-nursing staff. I can see you really think you are at a disadvantage as a white man. Help me to understand your point of view." Or this: A heterosexual male nurse says to his gay male nurse colleague, "I just don't understand why those gays have to be so obvious about their sexual orientation. Can't they just keep their sexual orientation private? Why do they have to kiss and hold hands right in front of me?" The gay male nurse colleague calmly responds, "I'd like to hear more about how you feel. Do you feel the same when a heterosexual patient kisses his spouse?"

Health care professionals in the synergy status can serve as leaders and as role models in health care organizations that are committed to diversity and cultural competence. Consider the following examples of the kinds of contributions that minority group individuals who experience their minority identity status from the perspective of synergy can make in the workplace:

- A black health system CEO in the synergy status successfully mentors emerging leaders of all races. She has recruited many talented young managers to the health care network. They, in turn, have made impressive contributions to diversity leadership and to the overall success of the organization.

- A Chinese American director of community relations has developed a strategy that dramatically increases racial and ethnic minority participation in the hospital's patient education initiatives. Patient education programming previously drew interest only from white residents of the racially and ethnically mixed service area. The director has helped a diverse group of health educators to develop crosscultural communication strategies that meet the needs of the increasingly diverse and multicultural audience. The hospital's market penetration has increased significantly.

- A gay patient transport worker in the synergy status is a popular peer trainer in the health care organization's cultural diversity initiative. He received an organizationwide award for his role in promoting intergroup understanding and improving employee morale.

How we experience our own minority status group identities has a profound impact on interpersonal relationships in health care organizations. Understanding the minority status identity development process can provide insight into the challenges and complexities of intra- and inter-group dynamics in health care organizations. And these dynamics are critical to the delivery of culturally competent care.

MAJORITY STATUS GROUP IDENTITY DEVELOPMENT

Majority group members also engage in a developmental process that, if it progresses, can result in a positive majority group identity (Helms, 1990). This developmental process occurs because majority status group members, like their minority group counterparts, encounter and are shaped by individual, institutional, and cultural bias (Helms, 1990). These three manifestations of bias can be described as follows:

- **Individual bias** consists of attitudes, beliefs, and behaviors that reinforce the presumed superiority of the majority and inferiority of the minority. Review Chapter Five for some commonly held individual biases that have been uncovered by the Implicit Attitude Test (IAT), a widely used implicit bias assessment tool.

- **Institutional bias** refers to policies, laws, and regulations that have the effect of systematically giving the advantage to the majority and disadvantaging the minority.

- **Cultural bias** refers to societal beliefs and customs that reinforce the assumption that majority culture—for example, dialect, traditions, and appearance—is superior and minority culture is inferior.

Helms (1990) explains how these three sources of bias influence white racial identity development as follows:

Because each of these three types of racism is so much a part of the cultural milieu, each can become a part of the White person's racial identity or consciousness ipso facto. In order to develop a healthy White identity, defined in part as a non-racist identity, virtually every White person in the

United States must overcome one or more of these aspects of racism. Additionally, he or she must accept his or her own Whiteness, the cultural implication of being White, and define a view of Self as a racial being that does not depend on the perceived superiority of one racial group over another. (p. 50)

The same can be said for men regarding their majority gender identity status development or for heterosexuals regarding their majority sexual identity status development.

Helms (1984, 1990) formulated a model specifically to describe the process of white racial identity development. Unlike the bigotry explanation of white racial identity, which divides whites into two categories, overtly racist or not overtly racist, the Helms (1984, 1990) model explains the richness and complexity of white racial identity development and describes the process whereby whites can come to terms with their whiteness as individual members of a racial group. As with the minority model discussed previously, this model can be extended to other majority identities such as male gender or heterosexuality.

Helms's pioneering work can assist health care professionals in understanding the interpersonal dynamics of whites and other majority group members in organizations. Helms (1984, 1990) explains that whites must move through two phases of racial consciousness in order to develop a positive white nonracist identity. The first phase is called "the abandonment of racism" and the second, "establishing a positive white identity" (Helms 1984, 1990). Each phase is characterized by three statuses.

The model of majority status group identity development shown in Table 9.2 builds on Helms's earlier work. Each status in the model is discussed in detail in the following sections and implications for intra- and inter-group relationships in health care organizations are illustrated. As with the minority identity development model discussed previously, the majority model is illustrated with hypothetical or composite examples drawn from experience. The examples are intended to reflect the theoretical status of identity development under discussion and to illustrate the impact that majority identity status can have on intra- and inter-group dynamics in the health care organization.

The Acknowledgement of Privilege

The first phase of majority identity development, referred to by Helms (1984, 1990) as abandonment of racism and renamed here as acknowledgment of privilege, is characterized by three statuses: naiveté, dissonance, and defensiveness. This phase reflects the process of moving from not being conscious of the social and personal significance of one's own majority group identity to the conscious acknowledgment of one's own majority group identity and its broader social and personal significance.

Naiveté

In status one, naiveté, majority group persons are unaware of the implications of the corresponding minority group identity. And, more important, they do not perceive their own majority group as having an identity per se. White persons in the naiveté status may minimize racial identity and instead focus on national identity—that is, on being an American—and may make statements like the following: "Why can't we all just be Americans? I don't understand why these minority groups are making a fuss about racial pride." A man in the naiveté status may not recognize, for example, that his female colleagues experience work-life balance challenges that are often more pronounced and personally challenging than his due to the impact of commonly held gender expectations on roles and responsibilities in the family. Or a heterosexual woman in the naiveté status may not recognize that her lesbian colleague's relationship with her life partner's mother is akin to hers with her husband's mother and, thus, not understand or support calls for more flexible bereavement leave policies in the health care organization that employs them both.

White people in naiveté status believe that they are color blind, yet at the same time insist that minority groups should assimilate into the dominant culture. One white nurse reflected the naiveté status when she was overheard expressing the opinion that Latino patients had far too many visitors at once, crowding whites out of the visiting area. She asked her colleagues, "Why can't they follow the rules and have just one or two visitors like the rest of us?"

Majority group individuals in the naiveté status do express individual bias but in an unsophisticated fashion. They are unaware that comments they make can be perceived as biased at all. For example, a white diabetic patient characterized the naiveté status when he expressed surprise and wonderment that the nutritionist who came into his room to deliver predischarge education on diet was African American. The white patient said innocently, "Wow, you're black! I can't wait to tell my wife that I saw a black nutritionist!"

If a white person in this status of majority identity development engages in sustained contact with one or more individuals from the corresponding minority group, he or she is likely to be made aware of majority group entitlements. This awareness will confront the naiveté of the person who professes to be unbiased and believes that equal opportunity is open to all. The individual in naiveté status may trigger anger or resentment in colleagues or patients who are members of the corresponding minority identity group. A female colleague of a male physician who is in the naiveté status may express anger or hostility at the type of comments she might hear from the male physician, such as, "I don't see that women physicians experience any more challenges than we do" or "We treat all physicians alike regardless of their gender."

Suppose a newly formed Asian Pacific employee resource group in a health care organization requested that displayed artwork depict racial and ethnic minority groups as well as whites. Now suppose that a white manager in the naiveté status is unable to understand why this is important and says, "People are people." Then suppose a Vietnamese American colleague confronts the naiveté by asking, "How would you feel if we had only pictures of Asians in our building?" If confronted often enough, the white person in the naiveté status will begin to experience discomfort and question his or her own naiveté.

Institutional entitlements are then more apparent to the majority group person. For example, a white social worker emerging from the naiveté status may be appalled to learn that his white patients had been given extensive information on what to expect after a heart bypass, whereas Latino and African American patients were rarely given any information on what to expect after surgery. He may have been shocked when he questioned the nurses and physicians about the difference in protocol and was told that "they [the nonwhites] rarely follow instructions anyway."

Once the majority group person in the naiveté status begins to acknowledge that members of his group receive different treatment than the corresponding minority group, they start to notice how deeply negative beliefs from the past shape present intergroup relations. A male accounts payable clerk illustrated emergence from the naiveté status when part of a small group of male employees were laughing at a joke about women. The clerk became aware that a woman employee had overheard and was offended. The male clerk felt ashamed. Jokes about gender and other behavior that he once had perceived as funny now come under self-scrutiny.

Feelings of discomfort, anxiety, and shame toward one's own group's behavior are awakened in majority group people who are emerging from the naiveté status. When discussing issues with majority or minority group individuals, they are caught in a dilemma: "If my group is responsible for these problems, what can I as an individual do to correct them? And what responsibility does the minority group have for creating and maintaining its own problems?" Sustained contact between the majority group individual in the naiveté status leads to further exploration of group identity in an increasingly complex context.

Dissonance

Anxiety and discomfort mark the beginning of status two, dissonance. White people in dissonance status may realize, perhaps for the first time, that they do see color, and that other whites see it, too. Majority group individuals in dissonance begin to suspect that there might be an element of truth in their minority friends' and colleagues' perceptions of bias and unequal opportunity. If, through personal choice or through circumstance, they maintain contact with members of the corresponding minority group, and if that contact is consistent at work or in social situations, then they start to notice that others are reacting to their intergroup relationships.

For example, a white nurse manager shared in a diversity training session that her neighbors scurried over to ask if she was planning to sell her house to a black colleague who had just departed with her husband and children after an enjoyable afternoon visit. She was shocked by her neighbors' questions. When she invited white colleagues and their families to her home, the neighbors had never inquired about plans to sell her house.

Once majority group individuals in dissonance become aware that other members of their majority identity group are assigning meaning to their intergroup relationships, they must make a choice between continuing the intergroup relationship and facing rejection by some of their fellow majority group members or succumbing to pressure and limiting the relationship. If the former is chosen, they can continue to struggle with what it means to be a majority group member in the context of diversity. If the latter course of action is chosen, they may attempt to retreat into a world in which interactions with the members of the corresponding minority group are avoided. A heterosexual in dissonance may avoid interactions with gay colleagues or a male physician may choose to mentor only male colleagues.

However, retreating to a homogenous world as a coping mechanism has become an increasingly difficult option for individuals in the dissonance status to exercise due to the changing demographics discussed throughout this book.

Sustained contact with members of the corresponding minority group will cause majority group individuals in dissonance to experience more anxiety, especially as they continue to learn about the human experiences of LGBT, racial and ethnic minorities, and female colleagues. On the surface, majority group individuals in dissonance status want to identify with their minority associates and be accepted as individuals who are not considered to be biased. Under the surface, they gradually become aware that some minority people have strong negative feelings toward the majority group and, perhaps, toward them by association.

Acceptance by some minority individuals and rejection by others, in addition to the majority person's growing self-awareness of his or her majority identity, can cause feelings to intensify: "Did I make the right choice to continue my close association with this minority group person? Should I admit I made a mistake and drop the association?"

White persons in status two experience cognitive dissonance or internal conflict (Festinger, 1957) wherein their treasured belief that "all people are created equal" clashes with their growing awareness that women, racial and ethnic, and LGBT group members are not regarded as equals in our society, so either they are inferior or the way they have been treated is wrong. One way for those in dissonance to reduce conflict is to limit contact with minority group members to the greatest extent possible. Dissonance may lead a straight service worker who used to take coffee breaks with her lesbian coworkers to begin to cluster only with her straight coworkers. Dissonance may explain why a white speech pathologist who carpooled to an in-service training with her black colleague then avoided sitting with her at the training where all other participants were white.

Another way to reduce cognitive dissonance is by attempting to identify with the corresponding minority group through imitation or taking up the cause of social justice as a way to show acceptance of the minority group. Around other majority group members, the individual experiencing dissonance may espouse liberal views and acknowledge past inequities. Another action of individuals in the dissonance status can be to engage in patronizing discussions with individuals from the corresponding minority group in an attempt to demonstrate how much they understand challenges and tensions. These discussions can be accompanied by offers of unsolicited advice on how the minority individuals can improve some aspect of their personal style in order to be accepted by the majority group. A white social worker in dissonance, for instance, may suggest that her Latino colleague consider accent reduction therapy to be better accepted by white patients. Then during a department meeting, she may express the opinion that more services and more sensitive care is offered to white patients than to Latino patients.

Attempts to "help the underdog" are sometimes really strategies designed to reduce the anxiety that majority group people in dissonance feel about their own group's unearned privileges. These strategies may eventually result in the person being rejected by both identity groups: minority group members may accuse them of being paternalistic and phony and majority group members may accuse them of overidentification with minority causes. Rejection by both groups often results in a strong defensive response by the person operating from dissonance status, which brings dissonance status to a close and initiates status three, defensive.

Defensive

A key characteristic of status three, defensive, is that the majority person's anger about being rejected by minority and majority group members is mixed with a growing awareness of his or her own personal majority group identity. Anger may be openly expressed and targeted at the corresponding minority group or the individual in the defensive status may be angry and resentful but not openly expressive of feelings. In the health care field, white patients in this defensive status may refuse care from black nurses or question the credentials of racial and ethnic minority physicians or allied health professionals.

In one health care organization, male managers were encouraged to hire or promote more women into supervisory positions to achieve greater diversity in management ranks. Almost all of the current supervisors were men and a majority of support staff were women. Shortly after a strongly qualified female billing clerk won promotion to supervisor over a well-liked male colleague, a male employee reflected the defensive status by expressing the opinion that the female billing clerk was promoted based on gender. Here the employee was assuming that gender was not a factor in hiring any of the previously promoted male supervisors and that promoting a woman automatically meant that management was filling a quota. Majority group members in the defensive status often do not recognize double standards for minority identity groups and consequently they tend to feel cheated.

Therefore, status three is characterized by Helms (1984, 1990) as a "return to racism," or for purposes of this more general discussion, a return to entitlement. Charges of reverse discrimination will often be advanced as a rationale to maintain the status quo. For majority group individuals in the defensive status, *different* comes to be equated with *deficient* and they may start to rationalize that minority employees have lower standards and that majority privileges exist because majority group members have earned the privileges by working harder and smarter.

If the dissonance experienced previously was resolved by retreating back into a homogeneous context, the individual is likely to maintain a defensive posture and may develop overtly biased attitudes and behaviors. However, progression to a more advanced status is possible if the person in the defensive status maintains contact with other majority group members who are at more advanced statuses of majority identity development or if they maintain contact with members of the corresponding minority group who have worked through their own group identity. In one health care training session, a white male nurse reported a decrease in the number of racially loaded comments made by other nurses once he revealed that his fiancée was Filipino. Prior to that, staff, operating from the defensive status, regularly talked about racial and ethnic minorities in a derogatory way.

Establishment of a Positive Majority Group Identity

The second phase of majority identity development, referred to by Helms (1984, 1990) as establishment of a positive white identity and referred to here as establishment of a positive majority group identity, is also composed of three statuses: liberal, self-exploration, and transcultural.

Liberal

Two distinct areas of fundamental change characterize the liberal status. The first is the relationship the majority group person has to other majority group members and the second is the majority group person's relationship with people from the corresponding minority group.

Majority group individuals in the liberal status recognize institutional bias and other forms of exclusion that are ingrained in the health care organization's system. For instance, a white supervisor in the liberal status in an accounting department may notice that the music piped into the department by the health care organization appears to be enjoyed by most of the white staff but many of the black staff bring headsets.

A white person in the liberal status is able to see how double standards operate at the institutional level. For example, a white nurse in the liberal status may conclude that the hospital's visitation policy disadvantages Latino patients who, she has observed, tend to exhibit closer relationships with their extended family than white patients generally do.

Initially, the majority group person in the liberal status confronts other majority group members who deny the existence of institutional bias, and it is common for the individual to actively work to bring about major shifts in the system to achieve balance. Here's an example: one health care organization that had only men at the director level was attempting to hire another director quickly, before an anticipated hiring freeze went into effect. No women were included in the quickly assembled applicant pool. As a result, a male vice president, whose dominant gender identity status was liberal, approached the executive council and pressured the group to extend the application deadline so that a gender-diverse pool of qualified applicants could be developed.

On a personal level with LGBT individuals, for example, the heterosexual person in the liberal status may attempt to create an intellectual bond by acknowledging homophobia and heterosexual collusion in creating and sustaining institutionalized discrimination. There is also a curiosity about the LGBT experience. Heterosexual people in the liberal status try to deepen their knowledge about the LGBT experience and their understanding of LGBT issues by asking LGBT individuals to teach them about sexual identity. In addition, heterosexuals in the liberal status may assume that every LGBT individual is an expert on homophobia. The heterosexual person in a liberal identity status may join political causes to end homophobia and may also glorify what they perceive to be LGBT culture as a way of showing support.

Sustained contact and honest interactions with minority group members are very important in this status. The white person in the liberal status, for example, has to confront the desire to "save the world" while simultaneously struggling with understanding white racial privilege at an institutional and personal level. A white lab technician in the liberal status might therefore reveal to a black friend that he only goes to Latino or African American doctors, because whites usually avoid them and he wants to show others in his family how stupid they are for avoiding them. However, the individual in this status may be surprised to learn that the black friend is not impressed, saying that white people need to stop working so hard trying to prove that black people are equal. The individual may be asked, "If you believe they are equal, then why do you have to keep proving it?"

If contact with people from the corresponding minority group is maintained, majority group individuals in the liberal status may begin to notice that their friends and colleagues from the corresponding minority group may become annoyed when asked to validate their need to help correct past injustices. Women friends or colleagues, for example, may tell the male operating from liberal identity status to talk to other men if they want to know about sexism or to look inside themselves at their own unconscious attitudes toward women.

If majority individuals in the liberal status do turn inward, awareness of their own majority identity can be awakened through self-reflection and through relationships with other majority group members who have struggled with internalized bias and come to terms with unearned privilege because of their membership in the majority group. It is at this point that majority group people start to explore their majority identity with others who share that identity and are involved in a similar process.

Self-Exploration

At this juncture, the majority group individual has now entered status five, self-exploration, and the internal struggle is formed by the question, "What does it mean to be white and nonracist?" or "What does it mean to be male and nonsexist?" or "What does it mean to be heterosexual but not homophobic?" The majority group person in the self-exploration status may begin to seek out other majority group members who are trying to answer the same question. For example, a white physician in this status may regularly meet with other white physicians to discuss sources of racial and ethnic bias in their approaches to medical care delivery. Or a straight nurse may meet with other straight nurses to discuss attitudes, policies, and practices that interfere with the delivery of culturally competent care to LGBT patients.

The relationships that majority group individuals in the self-exploration status develop with individuals in the corresponding minority group also take on a different dimension. For example, instead of asking racial and ethnic minority group members to describe their experiences with racism, white people in this status start to disclose their own experiences within a racial and ethnic context and acknowledge passive forms of internalized bias and awareness of the consequences of being different. For instance, a white building engineer in the self-exploration status may reveal to a black coworker that he had stood by silently while white coworkers at a previous place of employment wrote racist graffiti on black building engineers' lockers. Or a white phlebotomist in the self-exploration status of white racial identity development might reveal in a diversity training seminar that she has seen other white phlebotomists treat black patients roughly but white patients gently, acknowledging that she had never brought up her observations in meetings or mentioned them to any coworkers. The white building engineer and phlebotomist may be able to engage together in dialogue and self-disclosure about their own experiences as in-group members on the diversity dimension of race and, perhaps as, out-group members on other diversity dimensions. In this fashion, individuals in self-exploration strive to unravel and understand the complexity of group identity, both their own and others'.

In this status, whites address the question, "What does it mean that I am white?" Men address the question, "What does it mean that I am a man?" Heterosexuals address the question, "What does it mean that I am a heterosexual?" Although majority individuals in the liberal status operate from the head and view issues from the outside in, majority individuals in the self-exploration status operate from the heart and view issues from the inside out.

Transcultural

In status six, transcultural, the often-intense self-exploration that occurs in the previous status has subsided, and the individual has successfully developed a positive majority identity. Transcultural white people are able to recognize internalized forms of racism within themselves and acknowledge the impact personally and professionally in the context of the health care organization and the community as well as US and global culture. Racial and cultural issues are now understood at a deep level; transcultural whites do not need to defend, glorify, or rescue themselves or other whites. Similarly, transcultural men do not need to justify or deny the privilege that is so often afforded to the male gender as it is to the white majority culture. And transcultural heterosexuals have come to terms with the institutionalized privilege that they experience daily due to their majority sexual identity. Institutional exclusion of others is observed and challenged in constructive ways and the integrity of others who are different is no longer denied or questioned.

Majority individuals who have arrived at the transcultural status are now able to discuss issues of privilege and entitlement comfortably and help to develop a workplace that is flexible enough to include people with different life experiences and who are at different statuses of identity development. Differences associated with race and ethnicity, gender, and sexual orientation as well as other diversity dimensions can be observed in others and valued as different, without being evaluated as inferior. There is an appreciation for the complexity of identity groups. For example, being male (majority group) and black (minority group) or female (minority group) and white (majority group).

As with minority group members in the synergy identity status, transcultural majority group members can serve as leaders and role models in health care organizations that are engaged in diversity leadership. Consider the following examples of the kinds of contributions that transcultural majority group members can make in the health care organization.

- A heterosexual physical therapist in the transcultural status becomes equally comfortable delivering care to her homebound LGBT or straight patients. She is aware of and successfully monitors her own stereotypes and assumptions and, consequently, treats each person as an individual, respecting the uniqueness of each. Her exemplary performance produces accolades for the home health care agency by the local LGBT community and area media outlets.

- A white director of nursing in the transcultural status forms a close friendship and working relationship with the black director of patient services. The two colleagues freely discuss the similarities and differences between their racial and ethnic identity groups. Their collaboration results in a nationally recognized model for culturally sensitive patient care.

- A male human resource director in the transcultural status encourages a group of female nurses who want to form a support group to share concerns about their status relative to the predominately male physicians. At their request, he carries their concerns to a higher level, resulting in fundamental changes in policy, improved morale, and establishment of the first affinity group in the organization.

- A Latino security officer in the transcultural status successfully mediates a dispute between Latino and white officers. His efforts avert potentially costly, time-consuming, and publicly embarrassing litigation.

USING THE MODELS

Coming to terms as individuals with our majority and minority group memberships is a complex and personal process. Health care professionals who actively engage in the process will be more astute observers of their own and others' interpersonal dynamics in today's increasingly diverse health care organizations. Culturally competent health care delivery requires that we understand how identity status affects patient and provider perceptions and interactions in the process and outcome of care.

The theories and illustrations presented in this chapter have aimed to simplify the developmental statuses from which we each experience our group identities. Every individual will not exhibit all of the characteristics of the statuses presented here; neither does everyone begin at the first status and progress through the last. In the real world, the same person may exhibit behaviors that reflect two or more statuses of identity development. For example, a white person whose expressed beliefs, attitudes, and behaviors generally fit the description of the liberal phase may occasionally respond to a given situation with behaviors indicative of earlier or of later statuses. People can regress to earlier statuses as a result of life stresses or situational demands.

The racial identity development of biracial individuals does not occur in accordance with either the majority or the minority model (Poston, 1990). Although the minority identity development model (Atkinson, Morten, & Sue, 1979) expanded Cross's (1971) original framework to include other racial and ethnic minorities, research has not supported its application to all ethnic and racial minority groups (Gibbs, 1987; Morten & Atkinson, 1983). Even greater challenges are presented by attempts to apply the models to other majority-minority identity groups, such as between men and women or between heterosexuals and LGBT individuals. Certain details of the identity development experience described by the models will not fit the reality of individuals from these groups.

The models, however, do provide some valuable insights. The models are clearly most useful in explaining how members of an out-group, that is, a minority identity group that has been the target of prejudice, stereotypes, or discrimination, and members of the corresponding majority or in-group that was not similarly disadvantaged respond to their group identities and how their resultant identity status affects interpersonal dynamics in health care delivery.

Reality further complicates application of the model in the workplace because multiple and overlapping group and personal identities are operating at once in interpersonal interactions. For example, a black woman manager may have all of the following group identities: black, woman, professional, Catholic, heterosexual, and American. She will also have aspects of her personal identity such as personality or temperament that, like group identities, will affect her interpersonal relationships in the workplace. Group affiliation and identification is clearly an important aspect of each person's identity and diversity leaders and caregivers alike can clearly benefit from greater awareness of the process of minority and majority identity development.

Self-awareness of how we experience our in-group and out-group identities plays a pivotal role in cultural competence by enabling each of us as an individual to successfully manage ourselves and interact effectively with others in the context of diversity. And the pathway to self-awareness of our own dominant and accessible group identity statuses is through self-reflection:

- First, identify your major group affiliations, including race and ethnicity, gender, and sexual orientation.

- Second, for each group affiliation determine whether it is an out-group minority identity such as black or Latino, female, or LGBT or an in-group majority identity such as white, male, or heterosexual.

- Third, reflect on your attitudes, beliefs, and behaviors toward yourself as a member of the identity group as well as toward people who share your group affiliation and people who do not. Be frank and honest with yourself. Consider what you *really* feel, think, and do, not what you believe you "should" feel, think, and do.

Review the status descriptions in Table 9.1 for your out-group minority identities and in Table 9.2 for your in-group majority identities.

- Which status best describes your dominant group identity status?

- Which statuses best describe your accessible group identity statuses?

- How do you know? What evidence do you have to support your self-characterization?

Your dominant and accessible statuses most likely will be different for each of your group identities. An LGBT African American, for example, may be in dissonance for sexual identity and synergy for racial identity as his or her dominant identity status. As you self-reflect to determine your current dominant and accessible identity statuses for each of your group affiliations, it is important to remember that the identity statuses are a developmental process. For example, if you have characterized your dominant white majority racial identity status as transcultural but cannot describe how you arrived at that status, reconsider your self-characterization. You can be more assured that your self-characterization is valid if you can describe the times in your life when your dominant status was naiveté, dissonance, defensive, or liberal *and* identify the trigger events and experiences in your life that moved you into transcultural status. Be sure to also focus on your accessible statuses. Even if, for example, you have accurately characterized your dominant minority racial identity status as synergy, chances are you still express attitudes, beliefs, and behaviors that are characteristic of conformity, dissonance, resistance and immersion, or introspection under certain circumstances.

We begin developing our group identity statuses in our families, communities, and other social networks. So, another way to test the veracity of your self-characterized status is to characterize the dominant and accessible statuses of your family members and others in your inner circle. It is likely that you share dominant and accessible statuses. If your self-characterization differs significantly from your characterization of your inner circle's group identity status, it can be an impetus to reconsider your self-characterization. You can also test the accuracy of your self-characterization by sharing it with trusted others: those who share and who do not share your group affiliation. It is also important to observe your own thoughts, feelings, and actions in contexts in which your group affiliation is salient. This also will give you clues about your dominant and accessible identity statuses.

No dominant or accessible identity status is right or wrong; each is simply a different constellation of attitudes and beliefs that shape how we experience and enact our group affiliation. However, health care professionals who actively engage in a process of personal development that results in a dominant status of synergy for their out-group minority identities and transcultural for their in-group majority identities are best equipped to understand, respect, and validate others, irrespective of identity status or group affiliation, and thus to deliver culturally competent health care.

SUMMARY

This chapter defined group identity status as the constellation of attitudes and beliefs that shape how we experience and enact our group affiliation. Research that undergirds the process of group identity status development was reviewed and the effect of the group identity status of health care professionals and patients on interactions in the health care delivery organization were described.

Two models of identity status development were discussed: the minority status group identity development model (Table 9.1) and the majority status group identity development model (Table 9.2). Although these models were originally advanced to explain the statuses of minority and majority racial identity development for black and white people, they provide a conceptual framework that can be extended to other majority-minority or in-group–out-group identities, such as other racial and ethnic minority groups, heterosexual and LGBT individuals, and women and men. For both models, each identity status was described and illustrations in a health care organization context were provided, using examples of racial and ethnic minorities, women, and LGBT individuals to illustrate the minority model statuses and examples of white, male, and heterosexual individuals to illustrate the majority model statuses.

Certain cautionary notes were emphasized. People cannot be categorized into an identity status based solely on a few observed behaviors or expressed attitudes because the process of identity development is dynamic and complex. It is important not to use your perception of another's identity status to label or stereotype that person. Multiple and overlapping group and personal identities are operating at once in interpersonal interactions, adding complexity to every interaction. Application of the models to diversity dimensions other than black-white race have not yet been validated through research but do have practical utility.

The need for health care professionals to become aware of and develop their dominant and accessible identity statuses for each of their major group affiliations was emphasized and related to cultural competence in health care delivery.

Culturally competent health care delivery requires that we understand how identity status affects patient and provider perceptions and interactions in the process and outcome of care.

Most important, group identity status is not immutable; it can be changed through experiences, self-reflection, and conscious decisions on the part of the individual.

KEY TERMS

accessible statuses

cultural bias

dominant status

group identity status

individual bias

in-groups

institutional bias

out-groups

REVIEW QUESTIONS AND ACTIVITIES

1. Dr. Taylor Cox observes that "most individuals have relatively high awareness of the identity that most distinguishes them from the majority group in a particular setting and considerably less awareness of other identities." Explain how Dr. Cox's observation relates to differences in the process of majority and minority group identity development (Cox 1993, p. 50).

2. Review Table 9.1 and the scenarios in the text. For each identity development status in the model, provide one illustration of behavior for a racial and ethnic minority, female, or LGBT patient operating from that identity status. For each illustration, suggest how a provider could respond in a culturally competent manner.

3. Review Table 9.2 and the scenarios in the text. For each identity development status in the model, provide one illustration of behavior for a white, male, or heterosexual health care professional operating from that identity status. For each illustration, suggest how a manager or supervisor or the health care organization itself through policies and procedures could respond in a culturally competent manner.

4. Review the three manifestations of majority group bias identified by Helms: individual, institutional, and cultural. Give one example of each type of bias

in a health care organization. Then, explain the impact of each of your examples on human resource management or culturally and linguistically appropriate care. Finally, describe the action that leadership can take to address the bias.

5. Janet Helms, pioneering researcher in white racial identity development, says that almost every white person in the United States must overcome individual, institutional, and cultural racism in order to emerge with a healthy white racial identity status. Do you agree or disagree with Dr. Helms? Explain your answer.

6. Using the models, characterize your own majority and minority group identity statuses separately for each of the following diversity dimensions: race and ethnicity, gender, and sexual orientation. What is your dominant identity status? What are your other accessible statuses? Remember that your dominant and accessible statuses are not likely to be the same for all three diversity dimensions. Explain your self-characterizations and describe how you evolved from one stage to another throughout your lifetime. Are you comfortable with your current group identity statuses as you perceive them? Why or why not? What could you do to further develop your group identity statuses if you wanted to?

REFERENCES

Atkinson, D. R., Morten, G., & Sue, D. W. (1979). *Counseling American minorities: A cross-cultural perspective.* Dubuque, IA: William C. Brown.

Chrobot-Mason, D., & Thomas, K. M. (2002). Minority employees in majority organizations: The intersection of individual and organizational racial identity in the workplace. *Human Resource Development Review, 1*(3), 323–344.

Cox, T. (1993). *Cultural diversity in organizations: Theory, research, and practice.* San Francisco: Berrett-Koehler.

Cross, W. E., Jr. (1971). The negro-to-black conversion experience: Toward a psychology of black liberation. *Black World, 20*(9), 13–27.

Dansky, K., Maldonado, R. W., DeSouza, G., & Dreachslin, J. L. (2003). Organizational strategy and diversity management: Diversity-sensitive orientation as a moderating influence. *Health Care Management Review, 28*(3), 243–253.

Festinger, L. (1957). *A theory of cognitive dissonance.* Palo Alto, CA: Stanford University Press.

Gibbs, J. T. (1987). Identity and marginality: Issues in the treatment of biracial adolescents. *American Journal of Orthopsychiatry, 57*(2), 265–278.

Gushue, G. V., & Carter, R. T. (2000). Remembering race: White racial identity attitudes and two aspects of social memory. *Journal of Counseling Psychology, 47*(2), 199–210.

Helms, J. E. (1984). Toward a theoretical explanation of the effects of race on counseling: A black and white model. *The Counseling Psychologist, 12*(4), 153–165.

Helms, J. E. (1990). Toward a model of white racial identity development. In J. E. Helms (Ed.), *Black and white racial identity theory, research and practice* (pp. 33–48). New York: Greenwood Press.

Helms, J. E. (1995). An update of Helms' white and people of color racial identity models. In J. G. Ponterotto, J. M. Casas, L. A. Suzuki, & C. M. Alexander (Eds.), *Handbook of multicultural counseling* (pp. 181–198). Thousand Oaks, CA: Sage Publications.

Helms, J. E. (1999). Another meta-analysis of the white racial identity attitude scale's Cronbach's alphas: Implications for validity. *Measurement & Evaluation in Counseling and Development, 32*, 122–137.

Morten, G., & Atkinson, D. (1983). Minority identity development and preference for counselor race. *Journal of Negro Education, 52*(2), 156–161.

Parham, T. A., & Helms, J. E. (1985). Relation of racial identity attitudes to self-actualization and affective states in black students. *Journal of Counseling Psychology, 32*, 431–440.

Poston, C. (1990). The biracial identity development model: A needed addition. *Journal of Counseling and Development, 69*(2), 152–155.

Thompson, C. E., & Carter, R. T. (1997). Race, socialization, and contemporary racism manifestations. In C. E. Thompson & R. T. Carter (Eds.), *Racial identity theory: Applications to individual, group, and organizational interventions* (pp. 1–14). Mahwah, NJ: Lawrence Erlbaum.

PART FOUR

CULTURAL COMPETENCE AND THE HEALTH CARE ORGANIZATION

Culturally competent health care professionals depend on the health care organization and its leadership to provide a context that supports, develops, and values their work. That is why Chapter Ten, "The Centrality of Organizational Behavior," focuses on organizational behavior (OB), defined as study of the impact that leaders, teams, culture, climate, and infrastructure have on organizational performance. Even with culturally competent clinicians and a strong regulatory infrastructure, health care organizations will differ in their performance with respect to diversity management and cultural competence due to variations in OB. OB research supports the contention that health care organizations with a culture of inclusion that is reinforced and continually improved through the systems approach to diversity management and cultural competence will result in higher-performing organizations and, ultimately, be more successful in ameliorating disparities.

Chapter Eleven, "The Business Case and Best Demonstrated Practices," follows with an overview of the business case for the systems approach to diversity and cultural competence, as conceptualized in this book's Figure 1.2. Buttressed by the experience of not only health care organizations but also organizations in other sectors of the US economy, the connection among strategic diversity management, cultural competence, and improved organizational performance is being made. Improvements in productivity, patient or customer satisfaction, competitive advantage, team performance, and employee recruitment and retention are among the key advantages touted by organizations that are committed to the systems approach. The National Business Group on Health, the Office of Minority Health, and the Agency for Health Care Research and Quality identify three criteria that support the business case for cultural competence: an expanded market share of minority patients, reductions in the cost of health services and increases in the efficiency of service delivery, and reduction of health disparities and improved health outcomes for minority populations.

Pioneering organization within and outside of health care have developed best demonstrated practices and access to information about these practices is straightforward. Case studies of high-performing organizations are presented in Chapter Eleven along with a discussion of the importance of assessment, benchmarking, and the continuous quality improvement practice, Six Sigma. The ultimate goal here is to apply standard quality improvement methods to diversity and cultural competence initiatives because, unless we set goals and measure performance, we cannot be sure that we are achieving our targets.

The final chapter in Part Four, Chapter Twelve, "The Future of Diversity and Cultural Competence in Health Care," looks ahead. It is clear that the diversity-associated disparities in health and health care and in career accomplishment and satisfaction discussed throughout this book will continue unless systematic action to ameliorate these disparities is taken by each and every health care organization. A number of trends support the expectation that the systems approach to diversity and cultural competence in health care will become the norm rather than the exception in the future. The demographic imperative is well established: diversity is increasingly nuanced, complex, and multifaceted; support for inclusion is broad based and growing, especially among the young; mandates continue to grow in breadth and depth; the business case for diversity and cultural competence continues to build; and global interest in diversity and cultural competence in health care is growing. Tools such as force field analysis are invaluable to health care organizations that want to strengthen forces in their organization that support an emphasis on diversity and cultural competence and work against factors that would derail or weaken such an emphasis. When all is said and done, health care professionals, like the readers of this book, will shape the future of the systems approach to diversity and cultural competence in health care and hold the keys to ameliorating disparities.

Chapter 10

THE CENTRALITY
OF ORGANIZATIONAL
BEHAVIOR

LEARNING OBJECTIVES

- To explain why a focus on organizational behavior (OB) is central to the systems approach to diversity and cultural competence

- To define organizational behavior and describe its theoretical underpinnings

- To summarize the research that connects organizational behavior with outcomes for the workforce, patients, and the organization itself

(Continued)

- To define organizational development (OD) and its relationship to OB

- To describe a three-step framework—enable, cultivate, and reinforce—to provide an optimal organizational context for culturally and linguistically competent health care delivery

n Chapter One we introduced the systems approach to diversity and cultural competence and illustrated that approach at the health care organization level with Figure 1.2. We defined a *system* as a structure of interconnected people, policies, and practices designed to work in concert to achieve a common goal and the *systems approach* as the process of considering how different parts of a whole influence and integrate with each other, viewing problems in a system as affecting the system overall. We explained that, despite the fragmentation of the US health care system in general, health care organizations are self-empowered to implement the systems approach to diversity management and culturally and linguistically appropriate health care delivery. The systems approach in a health care organization does the following:

- Originates with leadership's **diversity sensitive orientation (DSO)**, which is expressed in a strategic plan that is data driven, evidence based, and revised through feedback on performance.

- Requires diversity management practices that focus on the workforce, policies, and practices. These are the building blocks of strategic diversity management.

- Results in a culture of inclusion in which a diverse workforce can perform to its highest potential, collaborate, and successfully resolve conflict.

- Ensures that the organization provides a context in which culturally and linguistically appropriate care is the norm and patient satisfaction is paramount, resulting in improved health outcomes for diverse individuals.

The **theory** and **research** that supports Figure 1.2 derive from the academic discipline, **organizational behavior (OB)**, which is defined as study of the impact that individuals, teams, culture, climate, and infrastructure have on organizational performance. OB can enable or impede a culture of inclusion. Even with culturally competent clinicians and a strong regulatory infrastructure, health care organizations will differ in their performance with reference to diversity management and cultural competence due to variations in organizational behavior. The OB research summarized in this chapter supports the contention that health care organizations with a culture of inclusion that is reinforced and continually improved through the systems approach to diversity management and cultural competence will be higher-performing organizations.

Unfortunately, evidence from research also indicates that health care organizations have generally approached diversity and cultural competence as a series of separate and uncoordinated programs rather than a strategic and integrated process that permeates every aspect of the organization. Language lines to provide interpreter services, for example, will be less effective in improving patient care when implemented as a separate program than if implemented as one component of a multifaceted systems approach. The systems approach, not isolated programs, is more likely to produce lasting and measurable improvement in organizational performance because all parts of the organization are working in unison to achieve a common goal.

This chapter summarizes what we know from research about the linkages among the systems approach, organizational behavior and inclusion, and organizational performance. Systematic attention to organizational behavior is essential in health care organizations that strive to ameliorate disparities in the process and outcome of care for patients, families, and communities *and* in the career accomplishments and satisfaction of diverse managers, clinicians, and staff.

The need for health care organizations, managers, and professionals to take a systems approach and focus not only on culturally competent care but also on its precursor and partner, strategic diversity management, is evidenced not only by research but also by best demonstrated practices and the experience of seasoned executives and diversity management professionals, as discussed in Chapter Eleven. An American Management Association article based on the book *Building on the Promise of Diversity* written by R. Roosevelt Thomas (2006), whose research propelled the corporate diversity management movement in the 1990s, puts it this way: "Diversity is a reality in America today. Whether you let diversity be a drain on your organization or a dynamic contributor to your mission, vision and strategy is both a choice and a challenge. To build on the promise of diversity demands that you practice strategic diversity management (SDM), which is, at its core, the craft of making quality decisions in the midst of the differences, similarities and tensions that make up diversity."

As Figure 1.2 illustrated, it is in fact strategic diversity management that will ensure that care is culturally and linguistically appropriate. And it is OB that drives the culture of inclusion that results in culturally competent care and better outcomes for diverse patients.

THE SCIENCE OF ORGANIZATIONAL BEHAVIOR

OB is a research discipline that is grounded in theory from the behavioral sciences, including psychology, sociology, social psychology, anthropology, and political science. It is one of the disciplines within the broader category of management research. Management researchers study all types of organizations, including health care delivery organizations ranging from community-based clinics to hospitals, nursing homes, and others. **Organizational development (OD)** is the practical application of OB theory and research. Diversity vice presidents, directors, managers, and consultants in health care and other organizations are OD practitioners whose role is to help C-suite leadership create a culture of inclusion through diversity management.

OB relies on scientific evidence derived from research to test theories, which are essentially models of how things work in the real world. Research uses rigorous methods to test theories, methods that control for factors that could serve as alternative explanations for an observed relationship. Research also relies on replication of findings through multiple studies to build a strong evidence base to support theory.

Outcomes the OB researcher wants to predict are referred to as **dependent variables**, and **independent variables** are the factors the researcher investigates to see whether they cause the outcome. OB researchers who focus on diversity management in health care delivery organizations want to predict whether outcomes are improved by systematic implementation of diversity management practices and the provision of culturally and linguistically appropriate services. This is often referred to as the **business case**, which will be discussed in greater detail in Chapter Eleven.

OB researchers deal in likelihoods or tendencies rather than in absolutes. Due to the complexity of human motivation and behavior, **contingency variables** invariably moderate the connection between dependent variables and independent variables. When OB is applied to diversity management and cultural competence, consideration of contingency variables is especially important. For example, Richard (2000) found that racial diversity—the independent variable—was positively associated with improved financial performance—the dependent variable—in the banking industry but only for firms that were pursuing a growth strategy, that is, the contingency variable. In fact, the opposite effect of demographic diversity was observed for firms that were downsizing. In the next section, we will review OB research and emphasize the critical role that contingency variables play in explaining the impact that OB has on the performance of health care organizations as it relates to diversity management and cultural competence.

ORGANIZATIONS AS CONTEXTS FOR BEHAVIOR

In previous chapters we summarized how disparities in the process and outcome of patient care and in career accomplishments and satisfaction are associated with significant dimensions of diversity such as race and ethnicity, gender, sexual orientation, socioeconomic status, and language. We will now explore a critical question: Can organizational behavior ameliorate these disparities? OB research answers with a resounding "yes!" However, the "yes" is qualified with "but" because of the need to consider contingency variables, including an organization's strategic orientation, culture, and leadership commitment to the systems approach.

In short, because organizations provide the context in which human behavior at the workplace occurs, differences between organizations not only moderate the effect of demographic diversity itself on performance but can also even change the impact of specific diversity initiatives—for example, cultural competence training for primary care physicians—on key dependent variables such as patient satisfaction. The need to translate research into evidence-based practice that improves the performance of health care organizations is a recurring theme in this chapter as we highlight and summarize the business and health care management research and explore linkages among demographic diversity, organizational behavior, and performance. Chapter Eleven builds on this base by discussing the business case for the systems approach to strategic diversity management and presenting best demonstrated practices from health care and other organizations.

Figure 10.1 provides a conceptual framework for the impact that organizational behavior has on disparities. The framework was developed from a comprehensive review of the OB literature as it relates to diversity management in health care delivery organizations (Dreachslin, Weech-Maldonado, & Dansky, 2004). Demographic diversity and diversity management practices affect individual-, group-, and organization-level outcomes. Individual outcomes, including career experiences, workplace perceptions, and employee satisfaction, affect and are affected by group outcomes, including the quality of group task performance and group communication. These outcomes, in turn, affect and are affected by organization-level outcomes including financial performance and access and quality of care for diverse patients, families, and communities.

In fact, without strategic diversity management, OB research indicates that demographic diversity will do more harm than good. The bottom-line impact of demographic diversity on organizational performance is clearly stated by Williams and O'Reilly (1998) based on their review of forty years of research. Subsequent research continues to lend support to their conclusion: "the preponderance of empirical evidence suggests that diversity is most likely to impede group functioning. Unless steps are taken to actively counter these effects, the

FIGURE 10.1 Conceptual Framework for the Impact of Organizational Behavior on Disparities

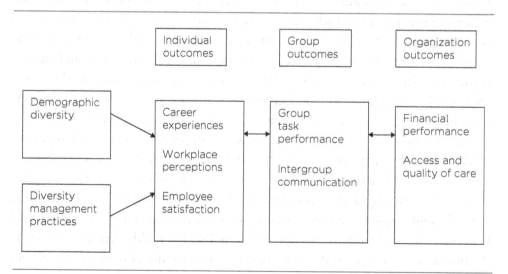

Source: Dreachslin, Weech–Maldonado, and Dansky (2004). Reprinted with permission.

evidence suggests that, by itself, diversity is more likely to have negative than positive effects on group performance" (p. 120).

If demographic diversity does more harm than good, why not just avoid it? The short answer is because we cannot. Workforce and population demographic shifts don't allow health care organizations to avoid demographic diversity and managing diversity effectively is a business imperative. What negative effects does demographic diversity have on performance? What organizational behaviors counter the negative effects of demographic diversity on performance? How can organizations apply OB research to capitalize on the hidden potential of diversity to improve performance and ameliorate disparities? The rest of this chapter focuses on answering these questions.

OB RESEARCH HIGHLIGHTS

Highlights from OB diversity research are presented in this section. First, we focus on the role of leadership in influencing the extent to which strategic diversity management is emphasized in an organization. Then, we explore when diversity improves and when it hinders team performance. Finally, we describe the need for additional research into the relationships among OB, strategic diversity management, and organizational performance.

Leadership and Diversity Management Strategies

OB research lends support to the contention that leadership commitment is the cornerstone of a successful diversity management strategy and drives the systems approach. A case in point: according to a recent Commonwealth Fund–sponsored study, diversity leadership predicts hospital adherence to the US Department of Health and Human Service's Office of Minority Heath's national standards for culturally and linguistically appropriate services in health care (CLAS) (Weech-Maldonado et al., 2007a). This study and its implications will be discussed in greater detail in the section titled, "Can Culturally Competent Health Care Professionals 'Go It Alone'?"

Perhaps leadership is so important because leaders set strategic orientation, which in turn determines how and where an organization will invest its human and financial resources. The strategic orientation known as diversity leadership is defined as "a differentiation strategy that is responsive to demographic shifts and

FIGURE 10.2 Diversity-Sensitive Orientation and Organizational Performance

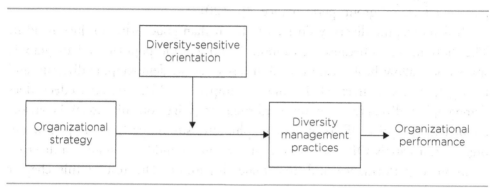

Source: Dansky, Weech-Maldonado, DeSouza, and Dreachslin (2003). Reprinted with permission.

changing social attitudes among both the patients and the workforce . . ." (Dreachslin, 1999, p. 428). This responsiveness is reflected in organizational practices and priorities.

Dansky and her colleagues (2003) concluded that a diversity-sensitive orientation (DSO) on the part of leadership "is a significant predictor of the extent to which hospitals engage in diversity management practices" (p. 250). DSO is a measure of the degree to which meeting the needs of a diverse population and recruiting and retaining a diverse workforce drive an organization's strategy. Figure 10.2 is a visual representation of this study's findings. Similar to what Richard (2000) found in the banking industry, Dansky and her collaborators found that a hospital's strategic orientation is an important predictor of diversity leadership, with hospitals that have a high external strategic orientation engaging in more diversity management practices than those whose strategic orientations are internally focused. However, as Figure 10.2 illustrates, Dansky and her collaborators (2003) also found that DSO moderates the impact of organizational strategy. Consequently, organizations with an external strategy *and* leadership with high DSO engaged in more of the diversity management practices that are associated with high performance in the context of diversity.

The researchers interpret their findings as follows (Dansky, Weech-Maldonado, DeSouza, & Dreachslin, 2003):

Diversity-sensitive orientation can be likened to a corporate-level attitude. DSO shapes diversity management the way attitudes shape behavior. Organizations must be actively interested in, and receptive to, the idea of workforce diversity if they are attempting to shape the management of their diversity efforts. There needs to be shared consensus within the organization regarding DSO if diversity management efforts are to be successful. In other words, there should be a large measure of agreement or overlap among the members of organizations in the degree of their sensitivity toward diversity. The stimulus for such shared consensus needs to arise from top management because it is responsible for planning and directing organizational strategy. If organizations truly desire to increase their DSO, they can identify and hire executives who value diversity, begin initiatives aimed at educating its entire workforce, and reward managers whose behaviors reflect and embrace diversity management. (p. 251)

The studies of Dansky, Weech-Maldonado, DeSouza, and Dreachslin (2003) and Weech-Maldonado et al. (2007a, 2007b) support the recommendation that health care organizations adopt a business strategy to systematically manage workforce diversity and provide culturally and linguistically appropriate services to patients in order to improve overall performance. However, very few health care organizations are actively engaged in a strategic approach to diversity management and cultural competence that is leadership driven. In a survey of diversity management practices in Pennsylvania hospitals, Maldonado, Dreachslin, Dansky, DeSouza, and Gatto (2002) concluded not only that hospitals were relatively inactive but also that hospitals in racially and demographically diverse service areas were not significantly more active than those that were in less diverse areas. Weech-Maldonado and colleagues' more recent (2007a, 2007b) studies also found low levels of diversity management activity in California hospitals. But, the California study did find that hospitals with higher levels of racial and ethnic diversity among inpatients were more likely to engage in diversity management practices. In the Pennsylvania study, hospital's senior managers were asked to identify the extent to which they engage in the diversity management practices that Dreachslin (1999) identified as best practices in health care and business organizations. In the California study, diversity management activity was assessed by the cultural competency assessment tool for hospitals (CCATH) developed with funding from the Office of Minority Health to assess adherence with the national CLAS standards.

Previous research (Motwani, Hodge, & Crampton, 1995; Muller & Haase, 1994) into diversity management in health care organizations found similar levels of inactivity. Similar to the Pennsylvania hospital study cited previously, Muller and Haase (1994) concluded that the activity that did occur appeared to be driven by regulatory compliance rather than by leadership and strategy. Motwani, Hodge, and Crampton (1995) found that, although 70 percent of the employees surveyed believed that diversity and associated cultural issues were important, less than 40 percent believed that their managers were aware of the impact these issues had on the organization.

What explains this lack of widespread engagement in the systems approach to diversity management and cultural competence? A number of different factors are likely at work, including the following:

- The evidence base from OB research that supports performance improvement through diversity management is not straightforward because of the moderating effects of contingency variables, which may discourage some health care leaders from adopting a strategic approach. For example, unmanaged diversity does more harm than good and factors such as whether an organization is growing or downsizing and the nature of the organization's culture influence the ways in which diversity affects organizational performance.

- DSO appears to be a key determinant of engagement in diversity management practices (Dansky, Weech-Maldonado, DeSouza, & Dreachslin, 2003). Consequently, the DSO of leaders must increase for strategic diversity management to become widespread in health care. However, DSO is an attitude and attitudes are difficult to change.

- OB research must be conducted in organizations themselves to better assess and identify critical success factors for diversity initiatives in a fashion that is more relevant to organizations and their leaders (Foster Curtis & Dreachslin, 2008).

Teams and the Performance of Groups

Well-functioning teams are critical to optimal performance in today's health care organizations. Management decision making, patient care, and other key functions all require teamwork. Teams are essential to the success of the promising new approaches to health care delivery discussed earlier in this book, including patient-centered care, medical homes, and interdisciplinary health care teams. But demographic diversity presents some unique challenges to organizations and the teams that drive their behavior. This section summarizes the extensive body of OB research that explores the impact of demographic diversity on team, and consequently, organizational performance. Diversity management practices to improve performance through more effective management of team diversity are also discussed.

With the exception of functional area diversity (for example, marketing, sales, operations, and information technology), Williams and O'Reilly's (1998) comprehensive literature review concluded that diverse teams experience higher levels of conflict than homogeneous teams. This conflict interferes with performance, and leaders of diverse teams rate their own competence as leaders lower than do leaders of more homogenous teams.

Advocates of strategic diversity management reference the **information value of diversity theory**, which contends that diversity will result in more ideas and, consequently, more creative solutions. Others reference **social categorization** and **similarity-attraction theories**, contending that diversity is likely to impede group functioning and result in poorer outcomes because people have a natural tendency to form in-groups and out-groups and are attracted to other people they perceive as similar to themselves. Williams and O'Reilly's literature review (1998) lends support to social categorization and similarity-attraction theories. However, the impact that diversity will have on group performance is contingent on how that diversity is managed, supporting the contention that diversity can improve group performance only if appropriately leveraged (Maznevski, 1994; Williams & O'Reilly, 1998).

Maznevski (1994) analyzed eleven studies of high-performing diverse groups and concluded, "The common element in high performing groups with high member diversity is integration of that diversity. In all of these studies, diversity led to higher performance only when members were able to understand each other, combine, and build on each other's ideas" (p. 532). How can a leader achieve integration in a diverse group and thus capitalize on the information value of diversity? Maznevski (1994) recommends using effective communication as an integrating mechanism, contending that, for homogeneous groups, their homogeneity itself is an integrating mechanism. She offers the following preconditions for effective communication in diverse groups:

- *Common ground and shared purpose:* Group members must share a common goal and their perspectives on the situation or work task at hand cannot be so unlike that they see things totally differently. However, if group members see things exactly the same way, there is no information value in group communication. The more divergent group members' viewpoints, the more difficult it is to communicate effectively.

- *Ability to decenter:* Group members must each be able to acknowledge and validate the perspective of every other group member, even when it is distinctly different from their own. Empathy is a natural outcome of the ability to decenter. A group member who is able to decenter can communicate in terms that a colleague with a very different perspective can understand and can also accurately interpret and accept communication from that same colleague.

- *Motivation to communicate:* At a minimum, group members must each want to communicate to one another. Motivation to communicate is not synonymous with motivation to achieve consensus. It refers only to the motivation to voice and share perspectives in the group.

- *Agreement on behavioral norms:* Diverse groups will likely need to devote more time at the onset establishing rules for appropriate communication than homogenous groups. How conflict is to be resolved, how the leader is to be chosen, how feelings and ideas are to be expressed, and other norms such as attendance at group meetings, timeliness, tone of voice, and physical proximity are among the norms that must be negotiated. Culturally homogenous groups, however, are more likely to already share norms on communication rules such as these and thus take less time at the onset forming them.

- *Ability to attribute difficulties appropriately:* When communication fails, group members must learn to attribute the failure in a way that leads to a solution. By seeing a communication failure as due to a changeable element of the situation rather than the nature or temperament of another group member, effective communication can be facilitated. Of course, sometimes a group member's personal attributes are the source of communication breakdown. However, effective communication in diverse groups requires that group members first explore and change situational aspects such as when and where the group meets and how and when information is shared, and knowledge is built through training and professional development before concluding that ineffective communication is due to a group member personally.

- *Confidence:* Important, members of a diverse group must believe that they have the skills, knowledge, and abilities they need to engage in effective communication with one another.

Group leaders, through training and professional development, can develop and hone these preconditions for effective communication within themselves and team members. In this fashion, the OB research finding that integration is key to high-performing diverse groups can be applied to enhance teamwork in health care organizations. Other OB research studies of diversity and team performance reinforce the importance of integration and communication skills, such as those identified by Maznevski (1994). For example, Oetzel (1998, 2001) concluded that to mediate potential negative effects of team diversity and to realize the information value of diversity, leaders should focus on building group interdependence and team process skills. Pelled, Eisenhardt, and Xin (1999) found that racially diverse groups that worked longer together experienced less emotional conflict over time. In a similar vein, Harrison, Price, and Bell (1998) found that surface-level demographic diversity was overcome by deep-level shared values in diverse teams that have worked together over a long time. An innovative study of team identity and race supported the contention that race can effectively be "erased." Kurzban, Tooby, and Cosmides (2001) found that their research subjects could overcome their initial tendency to categorize by race when a team membership identity was established as an alternative shared identity for the people they observed in the experiment. OB research studies such as these indicate that diverse interprofessional and multidisciplinary health care teams can work effectively together to delivery culturally competent care, given the appropriate communication skills, knowledge, and abilities, and provided Maznevski's (1994) preconditions for teamwork are developed, used, and reinforced.

Dreachslin, Hunt, and Sprainer (2000) used focus groups to study how team diversity influenced nurse, patient-care technician, and patient-care assistant perceptions of communication effectiveness within bedside-care teams. As Figure 10.3 illustrates, the researchers found that leadership style was the driving factor. In teams whose leaders worked to ensure effective communication through integrative mechanisms like those discussed previously and directly and openly acknowledged and valued team diversity, member perceptions of team communication effectiveness were higher and team members expressed less social isolation, less selective perception, and fewer stereotypes.

In summary, although OB research clearly supports the contention that diverse groups are more challenging to lead, it also indicates that diverse groups can perform as well as or better than homogenous groups, contingent on effective leadership. As Figure 10.3 illustrates, human diversity naturally results in a broader

FIGURE 10.3 Relationship Among Diversity, Leadership, and Effective Communication

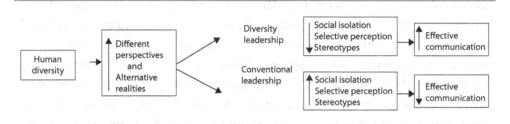

Source: Dreachslin, Hunt, and Sprainer (2000). Reprinted with permission.

array of perspectives and worldviews or realities, which can be personally challenging for diverse group members to bridge—so challenging, in fact, that research has firmly established that, in the absence of external motivation to the contrary, individuals will chose to associate with similar others (see, for example, Baugher, Varanelli, & Weisbord, 2000; Byrne, 1971). Leaders and organizations, therefore, need to not only intervene to ensure that diverse groups are well integrated but also must make a conscious effort to motivate, require, and encourage team diversity. Growing diversity in the workforce and patient base are driving this action as a business imperative. OB research can provide guidance to leaders who want to capitalize on the power of diversity while minimizing its potential drawbacks.

Need for Additional Research

The body of OB research available to support evidence-based practice in strategic diversity management for health care organizations continues to grow. However, a gap remains. Kochan and his colleagues (2003) made another important recommendation based on their research into the impact of demographic diversity on business performance in four Fortune 500 companies: a call for more field-based research in real organizational settings. Kochan and his colleagues (2003) suggest not only that executives work with independent external researchers, but also recommend a more analytical approach to strategic diversity management within organizations themselves. Kochan and his fellow researchers (2003), who studied the effect of diversity and its management on performance ex post facto, were unable to document links unambiguously among demographic diversity, diversity management practices, and improvement in organizational performance:

Despite the widespread availability and use of human resource information systems, we found that basic HR data about individuals or groups could not be readily linked to business-level performance data. Unable to link HR practices to business performance, HR practitioners will be limited in what they can learn about how to manage diversity effectively, and their claims for diversity as a strategic imperative warranting financial investments weakened accordingly . . . Currently organizations typically assess their diversity efforts by simply comparing attitudes, performance, advancement, pay, and so on, among different groups of employees. These comparisons can be useful, but they are only a first step. Equally important but very different questions are: Under what conditions do work units that are diverse with respect to gender or race outperform or underperform work units that are more homogenous? What conditions mitigate or exacerbate diversity's potential negative or positive effects? (p. 18)

Foster Curtis and Dreachslin (2008) reviewed the managing diversity literature published between 2000 and 2005 and found only thirty-eight published articles that examined the effectiveness of specific diversity interventions implemented in organizations. Similar to Kochan and his colleagues, they also called for more field-based research:

The impact of diversity interventions on organizational performance must be more consistently tracked and objectively measured. Because of the evidentiary limitations of the current literature, specific characteristics of effective diversity interventions remain largely untested. The opportunities continue for human resource and organizational development professionals and their organizations, in collaboration with academic researchers, to build a more rigorous and extensive body of published research that directly addresses the impacts of diversity interventions. Academic settings may provide the context for more rigorous experimental designs, and increased collaboration between academicians and practitioners can test the results in the real world by providing access to more diverse field research. The addition of an independent evaluation component in the design of diversity interventions, with advocacy by human resource and organizational development professionals within their organizations to facilitate publication of the findings, would substantially improve the body of knowledge. (p. 25)

A number of obstacles to heeding calls such as these for more field-based research exist. Organizations may be unwilling to put their diversity initiatives to the test, fearing litigation potential or other adverse outcomes. Kochan and his collaborators (2003), for example, spent two years attempting to recruit twenty Fortune 500 companies to participate in their research, ending up with only four. Because the organizations did not agree to a common data set, the researchers had to conduct four separate case studies and use existing data from each organization to assess the impact of diversity and diversity interventions on organizational performance. The result was a less rigorous design and fewer generalizable results, both of which hinder publication in highly regarded journals. Foster Curtis and Dreachslin (2008) point to the need for "sufficiently long lead times prior to initiatives' implementation to allow for research design, organizational approvals, and where necessary, funding . . ." (p. 25). These requirements, which are part and parcel of the process of academic research, may also serve as barriers to collaboration.

Despite the limitations of the current body of OB research into diversity management and organizational performance, health care organizations can use existing research to improve their performance. The next section describes a practical three-step process—enable, cultivate, and reinforce—by which leaders can bridge the gap between OB research and practice through the systems approach.

CAN CULTURALLY COMPETENT HEALTH CARE PROFESSIONALS "GO IT ALONE"?

The obvious answer to this question is absolutely not! How *could* a health care professional consistently deliver culturally competent bedside care without organizational support? Image trying to deliver LAS without language lines or interpreters or exhibiting cultural competence in health care encounters without training and alongside other clinicians who do not share your personal commitment to cultural competence.

The goal of ameliorating disparities in health is an important driver of the growing focus on culturally and linguistically competent care. But culturally competent clinicians, even when supported by regulation and public policy, cannot "go it alone." Health care organizations also have to engage in a leadership-driven systems

Note: Content in the section "Can Cultural Competent Health Care Professionals 'Go It Alone'?" originally appeared as Dreachslin, J. L., & Hobby, F. (2007). Racial and ethnic disparities: Why diversity leadership matters. *Journal of Healthcare Management, 53*(1), 8–13 and is reprinted and adapted with permission.

approach to strategic diversity management for the efforts of clinicians, regulators, and public policy makers to pay dividends for patients, community, staff, and other stakeholders. In an article in the summer issue of *Bridges*, a newsletter by the Institute for Diversity in Health Management (IFD), the essential linkages and critical differences between diversity and disparities were discussed. The article concluded:

> Diversity issues such as language differences, religious differences, cultural differences, gender, race and ethnic differences are not disparities in and of themselves. They are just differences. When they are not understood, valued and appreciated for their impact on the delivery of patient care, the healing process and communication/trust, they become contributors to disparities and unequal medical outcomes. (Hobby & Dreachslin, 2007, p. 6)

In this section, we explore this conclusion and offer a framework for OD to put lessons learned from OB research into practice in the health care organization. We contend that ameliorating disparities requires not only culturally competent clinicians but also leaders who create an organizational context in which cultural competence is enabled, cultivated, and reinforced. In short, health care organizations in the United States need leaders who excel in the context of diversity. As the research in this and previous chapters supports, without effective diversity leadership and a systems approach, even the most culturally competent clinicians will not be able to perform to their full potential.

But first, a caveat: disparities in health outcomes associated with diversity are driven not only by organizational behavior but also by social factors that are beyond the control of any single health care organization. Therefore, although *eliminating* disparities is a worthy and necessary goal, it may not be immediately realistic given the historical legacy and current sociopolitical climate in the United States. However, organizations, through their behavior, can work toward greatly *ameliorating*, that is, reducing, disparities in health outcomes.

The Institute for Health Policy (IHP) identified four drivers of disparities in health outcomes (Meyers, 2007):

1. *Individual socioeconomic circumstances*, including education, income, wealth, and occupation

2. *Physical and cultural community environment*, including community assets, health-related norms, residential segregation by race or income, healthy foods, exercise/play areas, public safety, and pollution/toxins

3. *Personal management of health*, including health behaviors, health resources, and health beliefs

4. *Health care financing and delivery*, including health policy and health care professionals and organizations (p. 9)

As the IHP report explains, "within the four policy arenas, a great many factors influence disparities in health and health care. Although this complexity presents challenges in that no one actor can control or impact all of these factors, it also creates opportunities for many different actors to contribute to solutions and necessitates collaborative approaches" (Meyers, 2007, p. 23).

In this chapter, our focus is on how C-suite leadership can apply OB research through OD, with the goal of ameliorating disparities in the process and outcome of care as well as in career satisfaction and accomplishment within a health care organization. Leaders can do this through a three-step process of OD: enabling, cultivating, and reinforcing the positive actions of culturally and linguistically competent health care professionals. Figure 10.4 is a graphic representation of the model discussed in the following sections.

Enable

Given the right infrastructure, clinicians who are motivated to deliver culturally and linguistically competent care are empowered and enabled to do so. The key areas for executive action through OD are policies and procedures, physical plant and technology, and people.

FIGURE 10.4 Organizational Behavior to Build Inclusion and Ameliorate Disparities

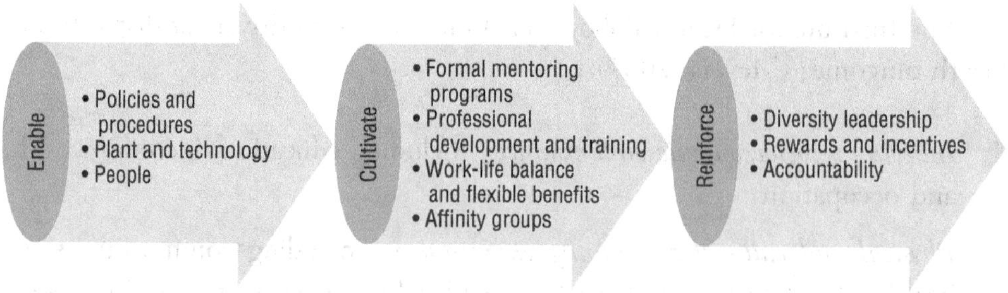

Enable
- Policies and procedures
- Plant and technology
- People

Cultivate
- Formal mentoring programs
- Professional development and training
- Work-life balance and flexible benefits
- Affinity groups

Reinforce
- Diversity leadership
- Rewards and incentives
- Accountability

Policies and Procedures

Policies express an organization's intentions and provide a blueprint for action. They are, in effect, a written version of the organization's "diversity talk." Procedures, however, are the organization's "diversity walk." Diversity leaders aim for concordance between policy and procedure and strive to implement policies and procedures that conform to best practices. On the patient care side, for example, every organization needs a basic, formal written policy on the use of interpreter services at its facilities. This policy must conform to CLAS standards developed by the Office of Minority Health of the US Department of Health and Human Services (HHS, 2001). In fact, Title VI of the Civil Rights Act of 1964 has consistently been interpreted by the courts as prohibiting discrimination against patients who have limited English proficiency (HHS, 2004). Health care organizations that receive federal financial aid must comply with this provision (see http://www.hhs.gov/ocr/civilrights/resources/specialtopics/lep/).

An organization's standard operating procedures must reflect the written policy. This means that the patient's family and friends are not relied on to provide interpreter services and that frontline staff, irrespective of shift or department, have access to appropriate support from face-to-face professional interpreters, trained bilingual staff, or language lines, that is, telephone-based interpreter services provided by a vendor. Essential policy and procedure requirements for language-access services were discussed extensively in Chapter Eight of this book.

Other policies and practices must also be evaluated against the CLAS standards as well as for their impact on other diverse patients served. Visitation policies may need to be revisited and revised to address any unintended negative impact on, for example, gay and lesbian families or extended families. Food services are another area in which policies and procedures can enhance or inhibit cultural competence. The timing of the evening meal during Ramadan, for instance, can potentially make or break a Muslim patient's perception of his in-patient health care experience.

Physical Plant and Technology

The physical environment in the health care organization is also key to realizing the intentions of clinicians to deliver culturally and linguistically appropriate care. For example, if waiting rooms are too small to accommodate extended families, even the most flexible visitation policy will not provide an optimal experience. A similar negative perception is created when displayed artwork does not reflect the community served or when race, ethnicity, and primary language data are collected but the information system does not support their use in care planning or delivery.

People

People complete the picture. HHS researchers (2006) concluded that *concordance*—matching the demographics of employees to the community served—may improve public health by "increasing access to care for underserved populations, and by increasing opportunities for minority patients to see practitioners with whom they share a common race, ethnicity, or language. Race, ethnicity, and language concordance, which is associated with better patient-practitioner relationships and communication, may increase patients' likelihood of receiving and accepting appropriate medical care" (p. 3).

But, as discussed in detail in Chapter Three, concordance is not the norm in health care organizations and the lack of concordance is caused by myriad drivers that can only be addressed through a systems approach at the policy and organizational levels. However, to aim toward concordance alone is not sufficient because cultural and linguistic competence is an attitude and a skill set that can be developed in each of us. Just because a caregiver shares an identity group with his or her patient does not mean that the caregiver is culturally competent. And, people, regardless of their personal diversity, can best build and use their cultural and linguistic competence in organizations that nurture it.

Cultivate

Human resource policies and procedures are important to the diversity leadership infrastructure. Ultimately, they affect those who deliver patient care and, thus, the patient experience itself. Dreachslin and Foster Curtis (2004) identified the following human resource policies and procedures as essential to the recruitment and retention of a high-performing, diverse workforce:

- *Formal mentoring programs.* Such programs ensure that the human tendency toward similarity-attraction does not adversely affect the quality and diversity of the pipeline.

- *Professional development and training.* This builds human capital through enhanced technical and interpersonal skills, including cultural competence and diversity management at all levels of the organization.

- *Work-life balance and flexible benefits.* Intangible advantages like these aid in the recruitment and retention of diverse staff.

- *Affinity groups.* Such groups address the social and emotional needs of diverse staff and capitalize on the power of diversity.

Reinforce

According to The Commonwealth Fund study referenced earlier in this chapter, diversity leadership is the most important predictor of hospital adherence to CLAS standards (Weech-Maldonado et al., 2007a). In the study, four corner-stones defined diversity leadership:

- Strategic plan
  - Goals for diversity in two areas:
    - Recruitment and retention of a culturally diverse workforce
    - Provision of culturally and linguistically appropriate patient care
- Performance metrics
  - Routine assessment of diversity goal achievement as part of strategic planning
- Accountability
  - Dedicated person, office, or committee assigned responsibility to promote diversity goal accomplishments
- Community involvement
  - Annually report to the community about the hospital's performance in meeting the cultural and language needs of the service area

Most important, the study found that adherence to CLAS standards resulted in significant increases in satisfaction for all patients, irrespective of race, ethnicity, or primary language (Weech-Maldonado et al., 2007b). This finding supports the argument that the systems approach to diversity and cultural competence can heighten patient perceptions of high-quality health care.

Rewards for management participation and CEO commitment are two more motivators according to existing literature and the experiences of organizations recognized for their high performance as diversity leaders. First, people engage in behavior that is positively reinforced. As Cole (2006) explains in an article in *DiversityInc Magazine*, "A CEO's vision for diversity is a critical first step, but there will be no substantial progress unless management has specific, quantifiable goals tied directly to awards and penalties" (p. 14). Second, and most important, CEO commitment is the alpha and the omega of organizational efforts to ameliorate disparities through diversity leadership. As Kim (2006) explains, "The greatest emphasis in the four areas measured on The DiversityInc Top 50 Companies for Diversity list is on CEO commitment because a CEO's support of diversity initiatives, in terms of public pronouncements and personally holding managers accountable for progress, is the deciding factor in the success of those diversity strategies" (p. 23).

Disparities can be reduced through the focused and dedicated evidence-based action of leaders and organizations that excel in the context of diversity. By engaging in organizational behaviors that enable, cultivate, and reinforce cultural and linguistic competence, diversity leaders can do their part to reduce disparities in the process and outcome of care.

SUMMARY

Health care organizations, through their behavior, create a context that can facilitate or hinder the optimal performance of a diverse workforce in delivering high-quality care to diverse patients. In OB research the influence of contingency variables is important to consider because situational factors such as whether an organization's strategy is internal or external can moderate the impact of OB on outcomes such as these.

OB research is generally more supportive of social categorization and similarity-attraction theory than of the information value of diversity theory. Diverse groups experience more conflict that interferes with group functioning than do homogeneous groups and, in the absence of organizational motivations to counter the tendency, people will gravitate toward similar others. However, OB research also indicates that diverse groups can perform as well as or better than homogeneous groups, given a supportive organizational content and effective leadership, which is the bedrock of the systems approach to diversity and cultural competence.

The practical utility of the growing body of OB research that pertains to diversity management would be enhanced by more field-based research in real organizational settings. The nuanced business case for diversity can be more clearly articulated when researchers and practitioners collaborate to document links among demographic diversity, diversity management practices, and changes in organizational performance through field-based research.

When implemented within a systems approach, strategic diversity management practices can help ensure that organizations provide a context in which clinicians' efforts to ameliorate racial and ethnic and other group disparities in the process and outcome of care can be optimized. Through a three-step process—enable, cultivate, and reinforce—leaders can demonstrate a strong DSO and ensure that the health care organizations they lead adhere to best practices in strategic diversity management, thus providing an optimal context for culturally and linguistically competent care to be delivered.

KEY TERMS

business case

contingency variables

dependent variable

diversity sensitive orientation (DSO)

independent variables

information value of diversity theory

organizational behavior (OB)

organizational development (OD)

research

similarity-attraction theory

social categorization theory

theory

REVIEW QUESTIONS AND ACTIVITIES

1. Research indicates that organizations with an external strategic orientation are more likely to engage in diversity management practices than those with an internal strategic orientation. Explain this finding.

2. Explain why contingency variables are so important in translating OB research into evidence-based practice.

3. Research strongly supports the conclusion that demographic diversity is more likely to interfere with than to facilitate group functioning. Explain this finding.

Identify three actions that a leader of a diverse group could take to overcome obstacles to high performance.

4. Research indicates that hospitals' diversity management activities are more driven by regulatory compliance than by leadership and strategy. What are the implications of this finding?

5. For each of the following key areas—policies and procedures, plant and technology, and people—identify one action that a health care delivery organization can take to improve performance in the context of diversity. For each action, explain why you believe it would be effective and how it would contribute to culturally competent patient care.

6. A study of adherence to the CLAS standards found that CLAS adherence was associated with increased satisfaction for all patients, irrespective of race, ethnicity, or primary language. Explain this finding.

7. Do you agree with this chapter's conclusion that "disparities can be reduced through the focused and dedicated evidence-based action of leaders and organizations that excel in the context of diversity"? Justify your answer.

REFERENCES

American Management Association (AMA). (2006). *How to practice strategic diversity management*. New York: AMA. Retrieved from http://www.amanet.org/training/articles/How-to-Practice-Strategic-Diversity-Management-SDM.aspx

Baugher, D., Varanelli Jr., A., & Weisbord, E. (2000). Gender and culture diversity occurring in self-formed work groups. *Journal of Managerial Issues, 12*(4), 391–407.

Byrne, D. (1971). *The attraction paradigm*. New York: Academic Press.

Cole, Y. (2006). Holding managers accountable for diversity success. *DiversityInc Magazine*, Special Issue, Fall, 14–19.

Dansky, K., Weech-Maldonado, R., DeSouza, G., & Dreachslin, J. (2003). Linkages between organizational strategy and diversity management practices: Diversity-sensitive orientation as a moderating influence. *Health Care Management Review, 25*(3), 351–368.

Dreachslin, J. L. (1999). Diversity and organizational transformation: Performance indicators for health services organizations. *Journal of Healthcare Management, 44*(6), 427–439.

Dreachslin, J. L., & Foster Curtis, E. (2004). Factors affecting the career advancement of women and racially/ethnically diverse individuals in healthcare management. *Journal of Health Administration Education, 21*(4), 441–484.

Dreachslin, J., Hunt, P., & Sprainer, E. (2000). Workforce diversity: Implications for the effectiveness of health care delivery teams. *Social Science and Medicine, 50*, 1403–1414.

Dreachslin, J. L., Weech-Maldonado, R., & Dansky, K. (2004). Racial and ethnic diversity and organizational behavior: A focused research agenda for health services management. *Social Science and Medicine, 59*, 961–971.

Foster Curtis, E., & Dreachslin, J. L. (2008, March). Diversity management interventions and organizational performance: A synthesis of current literature. *Human Resource Development Review, 7*(1), 107–134.

Harrison, D. A., Price, K. H., & Bell, M. P. (1998). Beyond relational demography: Time and the effects of surface and deep level diversity on work group cohesion. *Academy of Management Journal, 41*(1), 96–107.

Hobby, F., & Dreachslin, J. L. (2007). Diversity and disparities: Parallel challenges for 21st century health care. *Bridges, 13*(3), 5–6.

Kim, W. (2006). Candid advice from CEOs on diversity. *DiversityInc Magazine*, Special Issue, Fall, 23–28.

Kochan, T., Bezrukova, K., Ely, R., Jackson, S., Joshi, A., & Jehn, K., et al. (2003). The effects of diversity on business performance: Report of the Diversity Research Network. *Human Resource Management, 42*(1), 3–21.

Kurzban, R., Tooby, J., & Cosmides, L. (2001). Can race be erased? Coalitional computation and social categorization. *PNAS, 90*(26), 15387–15392.

Maldonado, R. W., Dreachslin, J. L., Dansky, K., DeSouza, G., & Gatto, M. (2002). Racial/ethnic diversity management and cultural competency: The case of Pennsylvania hospitals. *Journal of Healthcare Management, 47*(2), 111–126.

Maznevski, M. L. (1994). Understanding our differences: Performance in decision-making groups with diverse members. *Human Relations, 47*(5), 531–549.

Meyers, K. (2007). *Racial and ethnic health disparities: Influences, actors, and policy opportunities.* Oakland, CA: Kaiser Permanente Institute for Health Policy.

Motwani, J., Hodge, J., & Crampton, S. (1995). Managing diversity in the health care industry. *The Health Care Supervisor, 13*(3), 16–24.

Muller, H. J., & Haase, B. E. (1994). Managing diversity in health services organizations. *Hospitals and Health Services Administration, 39*(4), 415–434.

Oetzel, J. G. (1998). Explaining individual communication processes in homogeneous and heterogeneous groups through individualism-collectivism and self-construal. *Human Communication Research, 25*(2), 202–224.

Oetzel, J. G. (2001). Self-construals, communication processes, and group outcomes in homogeneous and heterogeneous groups. *Small Group Research, 32*(1), 19–54.

Pelled, L. H., Eisenhardt, K. M., & Xin, K. R. (1999). Exploring the black box: An analysis of work group diversity, conflict and performance. *Administrative Science Quarterly, 44*(1), 1–28.

Richard, O. C. (2000). Racial diversity, business strategy, and firm performance: A resource-based view. *Academy of Management Journal, 43*(2), 164–177.

US Department of Health and Human Services (HHS). (2001). *National standards for culturally and linguistically appropriate services in health care.* Washington, DC: US Government Printing Office.

US Department of Health and Human Services (HHS). (2006). *Guidance to federal financial assistance recipients regarding Title VI prohibition against national origin discrimination affecting limited English proficient persons.* Retrieved from http://www.hhs.gov/ocr/civilrights/resources/specialtopics/lep/

US Department of Health and Human Services (HHS). (2006). *The rationale for diversity in the health professions: A review of the evidence.* Washington, DC: US Government Printing Office.

Weech-Maldonado, R. W., Dreachslin, J. L., Dansky, K., DeSouza, G., & Gatto, M. (2002). Racial/ethnic diversity management and cultural competency: The case of Pennsylvania hospitals. *Journal of Healthcare Management, 47*(2), 111–126.

Weech-Maldonado, R., Elliott, M. N., Schiller, C., Hall, A., Dreachslin, J. L., & Hays, R. D. (2007a, November 5). *Organizational and market characteristics associated with hospital's adherence to the CLAS standards.* Presentation at the American Public Health Association Annual Meeting, Washington, DC.

Weech-Maldonado, R., Elliott, M. N., Schiller, C., Hall, A., & Hays, R. D. (2007b, November 5). *Does hospital's adherence to the CLAS standards predict diverse patients' experiences with inpatient care?* Presentation at the American Public Health Association Annual Meeting, Washington, DC.

Williams, K. Y., & O'Reilly III, C. A. (1998). Demography and diversity in organizations: A review of 40 years of research. *Research in Organizational Behavior, 20*, 77–140.

Chapter 11

THE BUSINESS CASE AND

BEST DEMONSTRATED

PRACTICES

LEARNING OBJECTIVES

- To present the business case for diversity management and cultural competence from the health care provider organization's point of view

- To describe the similarities and differences in the business case for health care organizations and the business case for organizations in other sectors of the US economy

- To trace the origins of the business case for strategic diversity management

(Continued)

- To present case examples of organizations that have received national recognition for excellence in diversity management and cultural competence

- To describe the role of pre- and post-intervention assessment and benchmarking performance against best demonstrated practices in the systems approach to diversity management and cultural competence

- To illustrate how a focus on metrics coupled with quality improvement approaches such as Six Sigma and its five step DMAIC process—define, measure, analyze, improve, and control—can be used by health care organizations to enhance organizational performance and ameliorate disparities in the process and outcome of care.

n Chapter Ten we reviewed the theory that undergirds the systems approach to strategic diversity management and cultural competence. We also summarized the research that supports that theory, which connects organizational behavior, inclusion, and strategic diversity management through a leadership-driven systems approach with improved organizational performance. Chapter Eleven builds on this foundation by describing how a growing number of organizations have arrived at the same conclusion: that the leadership-driven systems approach to managing patient and workforce diversity, first introduced in Chapter One, is a business imperative. Improvements in productivity, reductions in disparities, improved patient and customer satisfaction, competitive advantage, team performance, and employee recruitment and retention are among the key advantages touted by organizations that are committed to the systems approach. In health care, the business case for diversity and cultural competence is conceptualized somewhat differently than in other sectors of the US economy and the differences and similarities will also be discussed.

In this chapter, we summarize the business case for the systems approach to strategic diversity management and cultural competence, describe the practices of high-performing organizations that have received national recognition for their commitment to the systems approach, and explain the role of assessment and **benchmarking** in evaluating and improving the impact of strategic diversity management and associated cultural competence initiatives. The chapter ends with an explanation of how health care organizations can, through a focus on **metrics**, defined as a set of measures that quantify results, tie strategic diversity management to quality improvement by using approaches such as **Six Sigma**, which is "a data-driven, methodical program of continuous and breakthrough improvement focused on customers and their critical requirements" (Billington & Billington, 2003), and its five-step **DMAIC** process—define, measure, analyze, improve, and control—to enhance organizational performance and ameliorate disparities in the process and outcome of care.

EVOLUTION OF THE BUSINESS CASE

The business case for diversity and cultural competence was first taken up by for-profit businesses in the corporate sector. These pioneering for-profit organizations represent many different types of businesses from food services and facilities management to banking, manufacturing, and biopharmaceutical companies and more. What they have in common is diversity sensitive orientation (DSO), driven by C-suite leaders who believe managing a diverse workforce and meeting the needs of a diverse customer base is a strategic imperative that should be addressed systematically and can serve as a **distinctive competence**, thus building the organization's reputation and improving performance.

Although the products and services delivered by health care provider organizations differ from those in the corporate sector, health care organizations can adopt **best demonstrated practices** in strategic diversity management and cultural competence that are in place in any organization to benefit their workforce, patients, and community. An important objective of this chapter is to identify high-performing organizations from health care as well as other sectors of the US economy and describe those best demonstrated practices that are worthy of widespread adoption by health care provider organizations. We begin with an overview of the current evidence base that undergirds the business case for the systems approach to cultural competence and diversity management in health care organizations.

THE BUSINESS CASE FOR CULTURAL COMPETENCE IN HEALTH CARE

Health care is one of the major industry sectors in the United States, consuming 17 percent of the nation's gross national product. And although the business case for cultural competence in health care viewed from the providers' and consumers' perspectives shares much in common with the business case for diversity management, there are important differences. According to the National Business Group on Health (2003), the Office of Minority Health (Alliance of Community Health Plans Foundation, 2007), and the Agency for Health Care Research and Quality (2006), arguments supporting the business case for cultural competence rest on three criteria:

- An expanded market share of minority patients

- Reductions in the cost of health services and increases in the efficiency of service delivery

- Reduction of health disparities and improved health outcomes for minority populations

We will briefly explore each of these.

Cultural Competence and Expanded Health Plan Market Share

As was made clear earlier in this book, the population of the United States is diversifying rapidly and heretofore minority populations increasingly are becoming a larger proportion of the population. Health care plans and organizations have not until recently tapped this growing market because they regarded minority groups as "niche" markets, they viewed minorities as difficult or expensive to serve, or pressures to serve minority patients were not coming from health care consumers or employer purchasers. However, the National Business Group on Health (2009b) points out that the working-age population is projected to become more than 50 percent minority in 2039, increasing from 34 percent minority in 2008.

Employers cannot ignore the needs of their minority employees when they purchase health insurance because minorities make up a growing proportion of their workforces. The National Business Group on Health has considered the implications of this for more than ten years. Beginning with *Why Companies Are Making Health Disparities Their Business: The Business Case and Practical Strategies* (2003), this group of business leaders has studied health care disparities among the employed population and has recommended ways for employers to address this issue. In their publication *Eliminating Racial and Ethnic Health Disparities: A Business Case Update for Employers* (2009b), they note that health benefits packages for employees and dependents have grown ever more costly, and if the health plans they offer to their employees do not recognize or consider the needs of specific populations, they may be wasting their health care benefits dollars. The authors point out as an example Verizon, who, as part of their annual health plan contract renewal negotiations, requires potential contractors to demonstrate their methods of assessing and closing gaps in care for racial and ethnic groups. They list PepsiCo, Prudential Financial, and Marriott as corporations that make attention to the health of their diverse workforce an aspect of their human resources efforts. In 2011 the National Business Group on Health, in association with the Urban Institute, conducted new research that showed how a significant percentage of total health care costs are attributable to health disparities: 3.7 percent for managers and professionals and 5.2 percent for nonmanagerial employees. Their most recent publication (2011), *An Employer's Guide on Reducing Racial and Ethnic Health Disparities in the Workplace*, contains a detailed checklist for employers to use in reducing health care disparities among their employees, including asking potential health plans to provide them with data on how they track the services to minority consumers, demonstrate with metrics the efficacy of their services to minority members, provide patient satisfaction data by race and ethnicity, and give information regarding their certification status (National Commission on Quality Assurance [NCQA], Joint Commission) for implementing disparities-directed initiatives.

The NCQA (2011) has created a multicultural health care distinction award to be given to health plans that meet their standards on race and ethnicity data collection, language access services, and use of HEDIS measures to reduce health disparities. Plans receiving the distinction awards are allowed to advertise this commendation with a special seal. Educating benefits-selection committees in human resources about the need to include diversity-related services in contract negotiations with health plans is made much simpler by referencing NCQA's standards and multicultural health care distinction program.

With the implementation of the Patient Protection and Affordable Care Act of 2010, many millions more minorities will purchase health insurance for the first time. The health insurance exchanges outlined in the ACA will bring even more minorities into health plans. In order to be competitive in attracting this huge influx, health plans will have to target minority consumers and be able to advertise the quality of services to potential purchasers. This legislation also stipulates that health care organizations are required to collect data on the race and ethnicity of patients as well as the languages spoken, to use those data to assess disparities in health access and outcomes, and to devise strategies to reduce disparities when they are found. Potentially, those health care organizations that can document high-quality care to minorities will have an advantage in the greatly expanded market.

Proof of business expansion in minority markets due to adoption of cultural competence strategies has not been widely documented. However, several case studies of minority market penetration have surfaced. Kaiser Permanente was able to expand its Chinese membership in San Francisco through creating an all-Cantonese-speaking adult primary care unit (NCQA, 2006) and is expanding its Latino membership as a result of a physician-patient language concordance program throughout Southern California (NCQA, 2009). Holy Cross Hospital in Silver Springs, Maryland, was able to expand its maternity program to meet the needs of Latinas resulting in an increase of two thousand births annually (Alliance of Community Health Plans Foundation, 2007).

Stability of enrollees in employer-based and publicly funded health plans (Medicaid, Medicare) is low: enrollees tend to switch from one health plan to another. Maintaining a stable membership base is cost effective. For example, disenrollment from Medicaid and Medicare programs creates a financial problem for some health plans because the Centers for Medicare and Medicaid Services (CMS) offer additional revenue for Medicaid and Medicare Savings Program enrollees. Faced with disenrollment rates among Chinese seniors of 12 percent, the United Health Care Plan of New York mounted an outreach and education program for Chinese seniors. In three years' time they were able to cut disenrollment rates in this population to 6 percent (NCQA, 2008). Improving the patient-satisfaction levels of diverse health plan enrollees by targeted services may thus be one way of stabilizing health plan membership.

Although these few documented cases of bottom line benefit from cultural competence initiatives are not dramatic, it is anticipated that as more employers make addressing diversity health needs a criterion for selecting health plans, plans with cultural competence programs will be increasingly sought out. And health care organizations that provide health care services under contract or as fully owned subsidiaries of these health plans will be pressured to implement the systems approach to diversity management and cultural competence to remain in the provider network.

Reductions in the Cost of Health Services and Increases in the Efficiency of Service Delivery

Thomas LaViest and colleagues at Johns Hopkins School of Public Health (2009), using data from the federal *Medical Expenditure Panel Survey*, estimated that if health care disparities had been eliminated, the direct medical cost savings between 2003 and 2006 would have been $229.4 billion. Realizing such savings through diversity and cultural competence and other initiatives at the organizational and local level going forward is a major challenge.

Guadalupe Pacheco, senior health advisor to the director of the Office of Minority Health, remarked in the preface of *Making the Business Case for Culturally and Linguistically Appropriate Services in Health Care* (Alliance of Community Health Plans, 2007), "One of the most frequently cited impediments to progress is the reluctance to implement projects that often come with developmental and operational costs while also having an uncertain business benefit for the implementing organization" (p. 4). Brach and Fraser (2002), in their analysis of the business case for culturally competent care, make a similar point: "The emphasis on solvency can stymie efforts to implement cultural competence techniques unless they are proven to pay for themselves" (p. 23). In an era of rapidly escalating health care costs, diversity and cultural competence programs must compete with many other priorities and may lose out if they cannot be shown to be at least revenue neutral or cost effective in the short and long terms.

What are some of the service-related costs that diversity and cultural competence strategies might be expected to affect? Reduction of communication-related medical errors, need for fewer tests, decreased use of emergency services for nonemergent conditions, reduced length of hospital stays, reduced hospital readmissions, and more efficient patient flow during clinic hours might be some areas to pursue. Long-term cost savings could also result from greater use of prevention tests and procedures by minority populations. Unfortunately, with the exception of studies on the costs and benefits of different types of language access services, rigorous cost-benefit analyses of cultural competence innovations in service delivery have not been forthcoming. A group at the Hopkins Center for Health Disparities is hoping to remedy this problem through the Cultural Quality Collaborative (CQC), which is a collaborative of hospitals around the country that are working on formal assessments of cultural competence programs.

Cost-benefit studies of language access services have been those aspects of culturally competent care that have been most frequently studied. For example, Contra Costa County in California was able to reduce its per-minute interpretation costs from $1.69 per minute for contracted services to $.75 by using remote video interpretation and at the same time increase the number of patients per day that they could serve (Alliance of Community Health Plans, 2007). Jacobs, Sadowski, and Rathouz (2007) studied the impact of an enhanced interpreter service intervention on patient satisfaction, hospital length of stay, adherence to follow-up, use of emergency services, and hospitalizations following discharge. They learned that the intervention, costing $234 per patient, did not significantly increase or decrease hospital costs. However, attending physician–patient language concordance reduced return emergency visits and costs. An earlier study (Jacobs et al., 2001) conducted in an ambulatory HMO setting revealed that patients who used the interpreter services had a significantly greater increase in office visits, prescription filling, flu immunizations, and rectal exams compared to a control group. Another study in a pediatric emergency department found that the presence of a language barrier between doctors and patients created a $38 increase in charges for testing and a twenty-minute longer visit than when no language barriers existed (Hampers, Cha, Gutglass, Binns, & Krug, 1999). It seems that the cost effectiveness of language access services may be contingent on place and measures used. It may be some time before we have a good grasp of where and what kind of language-access services represent the best cost-benefit situation.

Overall, though the little available research is positive, it appears that much more research still needs to be done to have a firm grasp of how much or how little cost benefit is associated with the provision of culturally competent service delivery.

Reduction of Health Care Disparities and Improved Health Outcome for Minority Populations

Of all the business case criteria, reduction of health disparities and improved health outcomes across diverse populations is the most important and is the goal that distinguishes health care from other businesses. In health care organizations, public and private, through old and new strategies, the end goal of diversity management and cultural competence must be visible and demonstrate improvements in the health of all population groups. In an era when almost every health care intervention and practice must be evidence based, finding the metrics for demonstrating the efficacy of diversity and cultural competence programs on health outcomes has so far not been easy.

What exactly is meant by evidence based? The term means that a medication, treatment, process, or procedure has been proven scientifically by agreed-on measures to effect positive change in a health outcome. Moreover, in these days of comparative effectiveness research, the strategy under consideration must often prove to be more effective than competing positive measures. The so-called gold standard of providing proof of the efficacy of a strategy has generally been the double-blinded, randomized clinical trial. Though this method has become the usual test for assessing the efficacy of pharmaceuticals and many procedures, it is nearly impossible to require this level of proof for many health care interventions due to an inability to control for intervening variables that might distort results. A clinic or a hospital is not a laboratory where every aspect of an intervention can be controlled. Still, "it seems like it should work," based on theory, intuition, or good intentions, is far from evidence based. When good health, life or death, and medical costs are concerned, a reasonable proof of effectiveness is critical.

An initial examination of the evidence base for cultural and linguistic competency (Goode, Dunne, & Bronheim, 2006) concluded that "the current evidence provides information about intermediate outcomes of short-term interventions, but none directly address the ultimate outcome of decreased incidence of a disease for a population or a decreased morbidity or mortality" (p. vii). Early detection and prevention interventions were the health issues that were most frequently the focus of cultural competence interventions. Culturally sensitive patient education programs demonstrated increased behavior changes compared with programs that were not designed with a target audience in mind. However, the authors point out a notable lack of scientific rigor in the studies they reviewed.

It is certainly true that some of the best evidence for the effectiveness of cultural competence interventions has come from organizations that introduce targeted patient outreach programs directed to specific populations and that subsequently measured changes over time using HEDIS data. The Health Disparities Improvement Project undertaken by L.A. Care is a case in point. This community outreach program improved African American and Latino member participation in health education programs and positive changes in HEDIS data in breast cancer screening, cervical cancer screening, and prenatal and postpartum care (NCQA, 2009). The Midwest Health Plan Caring for Culture, Caring for

Women Initiative (NCQA, 2009) produced consistent improvement over four years' time in prevention testing among Spanish- and Arabic-speaking women. Along similar lines, Aetna (NCQA, 2008) mounted a pilot program designed to increase the rate of clinically acceptable blood pressure measurements among their African American health plan members with hypertension by providing culturally competent disease management support as well as culturally sensitive information and tools. An intervention and control group comparison was part of the study design. At completion, results showed that 31 percent of the intervention group had blood pressure less than 120/80, compared with 22 percent of the control group; other benefits showed an increase in blood pressure monitoring and medication use in the intervention group (NCQA, 2008).

It has been widely assumed that training health care professionals in the attitudes, knowledge, and skills of cultural competence is one mechanism for reduction of disparities and better care for all groups of patients. We presented considerable information on training practices and models in previous chapters of this book. However, the linkage between cultural competence training of providers and patient outcomes is very difficult to measure. Reviews of educational projects that hoped to show linkages between cultural competence training with better patient outcomes (Beach et al., 2005; Lie, Lee-Rey, Gomez, Bereknyei, & Braddock, 2011; Price et al., 2005) report that the studies ranged from low to moderate in scientific rigor, and most did not control for intervening variables, though some showed a positive result. The issue of controlling for intervening variables is the major one facing an attempt to establish a linkage between cultural competence training of health care professionals and patient outcomes. Physician characteristics that have nothing to do with cultural competence training may be at play as would any number of outside variables affecting patient outcomes. To overcome these difficulties, huge sample sizes or more rigorous study designs, including control groups, would need to be involved to demonstrate that specific interventions or organizational practices produce changes in health care outcomes. That said, it is clear that this problem is true for many educational and process interventions in health care and not just cultural competence training.

Betancourt and Green (2010) have offered an approach that has considerable merit and includes focusing on a specific clinical condition in a delimited population; teaching measurable, well-supported competencies; controlling for intervening variables; assessing patient and provider satisfaction; and evaluating specific measurable outcomes. Thus, it would appear that relatively small, carefully focused studies could establish the training and patient outcomes that either support or do not support cultural competence training. Currently, the National Quality Forum (2011) is engaged in creating disparities sensitive measures that will serve to detect not only differences in quality of care across institutions, but also differences in quality of care among populations and social groupings. Over time, as standardized measures of quality of care for diverse populations evolve, linking these to cultural competence training and other organizational practices may become more feasible and routine.

On a somewhat brighter note, the same reviewers who found little evidence yet of cultural competence training's positive impact on the health status of diverse patients did find clear evidence that cultural competence training improves the knowledge, skills, and attitudes of health care professionals as well as positively affect levels of patient satisfaction. What is still lacking is evidence that these attitudinal and behavioral changes affect health outcomes, though it is not too much of a stretch to expect that they do.

It appears that the business case for cultural competence, as providers and consumers of health care understand it, is in the making but not yet made. Employers and consumers are only now beginning to see the cultural competence of health plans and health organizations as a criterion for choosing health care providers, cultural competence strategies are yet to be proven robustly cost effective, and linkages between cultural competence interventions and disparities reduction are promising but not solidly drawn. Six Sigma and DMAIC, discussed in the following sections, and other rigorous techniques for assessing quality and effectiveness in health care organizations themselves will help build the evidence base by testing the impact of cultural competence interventions as they are actually practiced. It is hoped that the readers of this book will carry much of this work forward.

How Different *Is* the Health Care Business Case?

In health care, diversity management commonly refers to human resource management (HRM) and other practices related to recruitment and retention of a diverse workforce, whereas cultural competence refers to practices related to meeting the needs of diverse patients, families, and communities. In other industries, diversity management refers not only to HRM and other practices related to recruitment and retention of a diverse workforce but also to practices related to meeting the needs of a diverse customer base.

The business case is built on much the same rationale for health care provider organizations, which are often not-for-profit, and for organizations in other sectors of the economy that are for-profit businesses. The rationale is this: diversity management and cultural competence improve organizational performance. For nonprofit health care organizations and for-profit businesses, irrespective of the product or service they deliver, the goal is expanded market share and reduction in cost along with increases in efficiency. And, for health care organizations and for-profit businesses, an excess of revenue over expenses is essential to survival. In business, this is called *profit* and is used to pay dividends to shareholders, to reinvest in the company, or to pay bonuses to executives and employees. Making a profit *is* the ultimate goal of a for-profit business. However, for nonprofit health care organizations, profit is *not* the ultimate goal but a necessary means to achieve the ultimate goal of improving the health status of patients and communities.

Due in part to this difference in ultimate goals, some health care administrators and professionals believe they have nothing to learn from the best practices in diversity management that are engaged in by for-profit businesses in other sectors of the US economy. After all, they are in business to make money and health care provider organizations are in business to improve the health of patients and communities. Although understandable in light of this fundamental difference in ultimate goals, this perspective is short sighted because it can result in health care organizations being closed off to learning about innovative diversity management and cultural competence practices that could, if implemented, contribute to improving the health of patients and communities. As the organizing framework—the systems approach to diversity and cultural competence—of this book indicates (see Figure 1.2), diversity management practices and cultural competence lead to improved performance. So, whether the ultimate goal is profit or improved health, attention must be paid to implementing the systems approach to diversity management and cultural competence.

From diversity and cultural competence training to recruitment and retention strategies, diversity metrics, initiatives to improve customer service, and rewards for management and staff participation in diversity and cultural competence initiatives, the fundamental building blocks of successful diversity management are transferable among industries and organizations. In this spirit, the best practices described in this chapter are derived not only from high-performing health care provider organizations but also from organizations in other sectors of the US economy. Although our ultimate goals may differ, the road to achieving them in the context of human diversity is the same.

WORKFORCE, HRM, AND THE BUSINESS CASE

The business case as conceptualized by US corporations began with a focus on HRM and recruitment and retention of a diverse workforce. This focus was grounded in the assumption that a well-managed and diverse workforce would be more productive than a homogeneous one and would, therefore, build market share and improve customer satisfaction in the context of growing population diversity.

Landmark Publications

Two landmark publications are widely credited with fueling the diversity management movement in US corporations in the early 1990s: the Hudson Institute's report, *Workforce 2000: Work and Workers for the 21st Century* (Johnston & Packer, 1987) and Roosevelt Thomas's *Harvard Business Review* article, "From Affirmative Action to Affirming Diversity" (1990). Both publications focus primarily on the workforce and HRM.

The Hudson Institute report drew attention to changing workforce demographics with respect to gender, race, ethnicity, and age. Five demographic trends in the workforce were noted from their analysis of census data:

- Slow growth

- Rising average age

- Increasing participation of women

- Growing proportion of workers of color

- Growing proportion of immigrants

Additionally, Johnston and Packer (1987) discussed the skills gap between the preparation of the available workforce and the requirements of available jobs. Especially noteworthy was their observation that the skills gap was particularly wide for African Americans and Latinos. Chapter Three described the continuing impact of these demographic trends and the skills gap on health care and other industries.

Roosevelt Thomas is founder and senior research fellow of the American Institute for Managing Diversity, a nonprofit organization established in 1984 to build expertise in diversity management through research, education, and community outreach. Thomas is widely considered to be the originator of the strategic diversity management movement and his groundbreaking article, "From Affirmative Action to Affirming Diversity" (1990), was instrumental in transforming business discourse from its earlier focus on compliance with government regulations pertaining to equal opportunity and affirmative action in recruitment to an emphasis on the value that diversity can bring to business. Thomas (1990) explains that the value of diversity can be realized only if organizations focus on building an organizational culture and management practices that are conducive to the high performance of a diverse workforce.

Thomas (1990) contended that an affirmative action pipeline perspective can generate "a self-perpetuating, self-defeating, recruitment-oriented cycle" (p. 8). The recruitment-oriented cycle Thomas described begins with recognition of the need for more diversity in the pipeline, resulting in generally successful recruitment-oriented interventions coupled with "great expectations" for a high-performing diverse workforce. However, he explained, these well-intended efforts instead most often progress to disenchantment when the company's diverse recruits express frustration with their career advancement and with the company's culture and management practices. This, Thomas explains, results in a dormancy stage in which smoldering disaffection is privately rather than publicly acknowledged by management, who question whether there is any action that can be taken to address gaps in career advancement and satisfaction. This stage, he explains, "can continue indefinitely, but is usually broken by a crisis of competitive pressure, governmental intervention, external pressure from a special interest group, or internal unrest" (p. 10). If, in response to crisis, the company concludes that the problem is recruitment, the affirmative action cycle just repeats itself. Instead, Roosevelt advocated learning to manage diversity by replacing the melting pot metaphor with a new approach that emphasizes the value of diversity. He offered the following rationale:

First, if it ever was possible to melt down Scotsmen and Dutchmen and Frenchmen into an indistinguishable broth, you can't do the same with blacks, Asians, and women. Their differences don't melt so easily. Second, most people are no longer willing to be melted down, not even for eight hours a day—and it's a seller's market for skills. Third, the thrust of today's nonhierarchical, flexible, collaborative management requires a ten- or twenty-fold increase in our tolerance for individuality. (p. 12)

Thomas set forth ten guidelines to optimize performance of a diverse workforce beginning with changing motivation for corporate action from legal compliance to an emphasis on the business case for a diverse workforce. From there, he explained, organizations should clarify their own vision of a diverse workforce and expand their definition of diversity beyond race and gender to include other diversity dimensions such as age, education, personality, and functional area, thus making it clear that every individual is complex, multifaceted, and by nature different from one another. He explains that the objective is "not to assimilate minorities and women into dominant white male culture but to create a dominant heterogeneous culture" (pp. 15–16). The remaining guidelines outlined the steps Thomas recommended to create, sustain, and ensure the high performance of the new dominant heterogeneous culture. Thomas (1990) concluded that "the reason you then want to move beyond affirmative action to managing diversity is because affirmative action fails to deal with the root causes of prejudice and inequality and does little to develop the full potential of every man and woman in the company" (p. 23).

Five companies' experiences were summarized to illustrate the real-world process required to put his theory of movement from affirmative action to affirming diversity into action. Roosevelt Thomas (1990) drew attention to the actions of early pioneers in diversity management, described the limitations of affirmative action, offered companies a blueprint for action, and thus fueled the valuing diversity movement. His work laid the foundation for the leadership-driven systems approach that undergirds this book and is followed by organizations that have received national recognition for their performance. Health care provider organizations can learn from the experience of these early pioneers, including Digital Equipment Corporation (DEC) and Hewlett-Packard (HP), described briefly in the following section.

Early Pioneers

DEC, a computing company that merged with Hewlett-Packard in 2002, was among the first organizations to move from an affirmative action paradigm to a valuing diversity paradigm. In the context of growing white male backlash against DEC's affirmative action and equal employment opportunity initiatives, the company hired Barbara Walker, diversity consultant and lawyer, to address the growing tensions in the workforce. She facilitated small group discussions among senior management on racial and cultural stereotypes and over time expanded these conversations to include other diversity dimensions. Walker's discussion groups created a positive buzz in DEC's manufacturing division, prompting Walker to involve even more managers in the discussions. These informal discussion groups grew into a widespread and formal program that was central to DEC's commitment to diversity. By nurturing the diversity sensitivity of these managers, who later assumed executive leadership positions in the company, the foundation for a systems approach to strategic diversity management was laid (Piturro & Mahoney, 1991; Solomon, 1989).

Hewlett-Packard (HP) is also recognized as a diversity pioneer. Solomon (1989) identified HP as being among a small number of corporations whose commitment to diversity preceded the Hudson Institute report discussed in the previous section. Others cited by Solomon included Honeywell, McDonald's, Proctor & Gamble, Avon, and Xerox, each of which has received national recognition for diversity management.

BEST DEMONSTRATED PRACTICES

Organizations that endorse the business case for diversity management and cultural competence often seek recognition for their success in differentiating themselves through their distinctive competence in strategic diversity management and cultural competence. A search of trade journal publications inside and outside of health care will uncover an array of best practices and case studies of nationally recognized strategic diversity management and cultural competence in action. One well-known and easily accessible source for this information is the DiversityInc top fifty companies for diversity list and the thirteen associated specialty lists including the DiversityInc top five hospital systems list, which was added to the portfolio in 2010. Interestingly, the same five hospital systems appeared on the list for two years running (2010 and 2011), with the Mayo Clinic replacing Brigham and Women's Hospital on the list in 2012. Similarly, five of the ten highest ranking companies on the top fifty companies for diversity

TABLE 11.1 DiversityInc Top Five Hospital Systems, 2010–2012

	2012 Rank	2011 Rank	2010 Rank
Henry Ford Health System	1	1	1
University Hospitals	2	5	4
Cleveland Clinic	3	4	5
Mayo Clinic	4	-	-
Massachusetts General Hospital	5	3	3
Brigham and Women's Hospital	-	2	2

list maintained this rank for all four years from 2009 until 2012: AT&T, Ernst & Young, Kaiser Permanente, PricewaterhouseCoopers, and Sodexo. This consistency is indicative of the leadership-driven systems approach each of these nationally recognized organizations undertakes. The top five hospital systems, along with their 2012, 2011, and 2010 rankings, are displayed in Table 11.1.

DiversityInc Selection Criteria

Although DiversityInc does not disclose the details of its proprietary approach to selection, their website provides an overview of the methodology. Unless otherwise cited, information in this section was gleaned from the website www.diversityinc .com or the online version of *DiversityInc Magazine*, accessed through the website.

Participation in the competition for top fifty recognition is building, with 535 companies vying for inclusion in 2011 as compared to 317 companies in 2007. The 2011 applicants each completed a three-hundred-plus-question survey, sent without charge to any company that requests it, provided the company has more than one thousand employees. The same survey is used to select companies for the thirteen specialty lists, including the top five hospital systems (Table 11.1).

With strong emphasis placed on CEO commitment, the survey assesses performance in four areas: CEO commitment, human capital, corporate and organizational communications, and supplier diversity. Each question on the survey has a predetermined weight and survey questions are empirical, designed as objective performance metrics, not subjective opinions or perceptions. For example, the survey doesn't just ask companies if they are committed to unbiased promotion; rather, it compares the demographics of the workforce to that of managers promoted to their first management position. Above-average scores in all four areas of assessment is a must for top ranking.

In 2007, a new criterion was instituted: only companies that offer domestic partner benefits to same-sex couples are eligible for inclusion on the top fifty or any of the specialty lists, including the top five hospital systems list. As Frankel reports, DiversityInc considers such benefits to be "inexpensive and painless to implement and yet are crucially important to the recruitment and retention of LGBT employees" (p. 22). In addition to health care for domestic partners, DiversityInc advocates bereavement leave, adoption assistance, family leave, disability and life insurance, pension plans, education and tuition assistance, credit-union memberships, and relocation expenses for LGBT domestic partners. The same article cites this statistic: 53 percent of Fortune 500 companies offered domestic partner health care benefits in 2007, compared to 40 percent in 2003, at a cost varying from 0.5 percent to 2 percent of total benefits costs. Two percent or less of total employees enroll in these plans (Frankel, 2007).

In an article that reports case examples from the top fifty, Millman (2007) offers some specifics in each of the four performance areas evaluated. CEO commitment is evidenced by practices such as tying management compensation to diversity, CEO meeting regularly with employee-resource groups, and having the CEO chair the diversity council. Human capital is evidenced by factors such as representation and unbiased promotion rates for people of color in management; work-life benefits such as floating religious holidays, job sharing, and alternative career tracks for family care; active recruitment of LGBTs and people with disabilities; and formal mentoring programs that include training for mentors. Corporate and organizational communications is assessed by practices such as mandatory diversity training for the workforce and management and employee-resource groups that are used for recruitment and marketing. Supplier diversity is measured as a percentage of procurement spent with businesses owned by women and people of color and other factors such as the presence of initiatives to train or mentor suppliers.

DiversityInc contends that "bottom-line results support the commitment for diversity," pointing out that the 2007 DiversityInc top fifty companies for diversity list outperformed the NASDAQ, Dow Jones Industrial Average, and the Standard and Poor's 500 over a ten-year period. And, as discussed throughout this book, a growing body of academic research supports the business case that links diversity management with improved customer satisfaction, market share, efficiency, and profits. In addition to the evidence base summarized in the overview of the health care–specific business case previously described, other research that supports the business case within and outside of health care is also presented in Chapter Ten.

Top Three on the 2012 DiversityInc Top Fifty Companies for Diversity List

Information in this section and the top five health systems section that follows was obtained by accessing http://www.diversityinc.com and following the top fifty companies and top five health systems links and by accessing information publicly available on each organization's website, unless otherwise noted.

One: PricewaterhouseCooper (PwC)

DiversityInc's company profile cites PwC's work-life balance policies, employee service to nonprofit organizations, and mentoring programs among the accomplishments that help PwC maintain its longstanding prominence as an exemplar of diversity leadership. DiversityInc states that "what sets PwC apart from most other organizations is its concise and consistent ability to communicate, internally and externally, the importance of diversity to the organization. From its thought-provoking 'Who Am I?' series to its annual Diversity in Business Leadership Conference for high-potential PwC employees, the company's message on diversity is always business-related, relevant, and crystal clear." As with Sodexo, Kaiser Permanente, and other top fifty companies, executive commitment is key. Bob Moritz, chairman and senior partner, is quoted as follows on PwC's DiversityInc top fifty company profile: "We believe that our commitment to diversity, inclusion, and flexibility will create significant value for our clients, our stakeholders, our firm and our people."

Two: Sodexo

Sodexo, a leading provider of food and facilities management services headquartered in Gaithersburg, Maryland, boasts an extensive list of awards and recognition for its long-term commitment to the systems approach to diversity management. In addition to its number one ranking on the 2010 top fifty list and number two ranking in 2011 and 2012, Sodexo was honored with the 2012 Catalyst Award for its efforts to recruit, advance, and develop diverse women in the workplace and also ranks on the following DiversityInc top ten lists:

recruitment and retention, supplier diversity, blacks, Latinos, executive women, LGBT employees, people with disabilities, and global diversity. DiversityInc's profile of Sodexo cites Sodexo's continuing strong commitment to diversity, explaining that diversity and inclusion is one of Sodexo's six strategic imperatives, with 25 percent of executive bonuses tied to diversity objectives. More remarkably, these diversity bonuses are awarded irrespective of Sodexo's overall financial performance. As Sodexo's DiversityInc profile states, "This company continues to set the bar on diversity management through its highly developed metrics, insistence on holding executives accountable for diversity results, and extremely strong diversity leadership."

Sodexo's 2011 *Diversity & Inclusion Annual Report* cites the company's progress, including continuing growth in the already impressive representation of women and racial and ethnic minorities in management from 2007 to 2011. In 2011, 25 percent of managers were racial or ethnic minorities and 45 percent were women. CEO commitment is also central at Sodexo, as DiversityInc states, "For George Chavel, president and CEO of Sodexo North America, diversity is extremely personal and the essential key to his company's business success." Sodexo's Spirit of Mentoring program "gets two dollars back in enhanced employee retention and productivity" for every dollar invested. Sodexo "pays it forward" through its work as diversity "teacher and advocate" to its food and facilities management services clients, many of which are hospitals and health systems.

Sodexo has identified ten key elements that are fundamental to its approach to diversity and inclusion. These elements are visually represented in Figure 11.1. By emphasizing and continually improving performance in each of these areas, Sodexo reinforces diversity and inclusion as integral to its core business. Sodexo's diversity and inclusion journey is chronicled in a Harvard Business School case study entitled "Shifting the Diversity Climate: The Sodexo Solution." For an in-depth look at Sodexo's evolution as a leading proponent of the systems approach, refer to the case study (Thomas & Creary, 2011).

Three: Kaiser Permanente

Headquartered in Oakland, California, Kaiser Permanente is a nonprofit health care delivery system composed of insurance plans and a network of 35 hospitals and 454 medical offices. With facilities in nine states and Washington, DC,

FIGURE 11.1 Sodexo's Ten Key Elements for Inclusion and Systemic Cultural Change

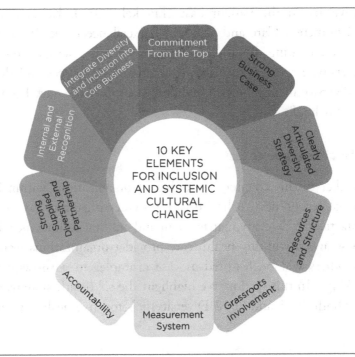

Source: Sodexo. Reprinted with permission.

Kaiser serves 8.8 million members. Kaiser Permanente has earned a place on the top fifty list every year since 2006 and evidences strong performance in all four areas assessed: CEO commitment, human capital, corporate communications, and supplier diversity. Kaiser Permanente has a history of breaking barriers, as attested to in the company profile on DiversityInc: "Kaiser has always stood up for equal opportunity. The company's founder, Henry J. Kaiser, recruited more than 20,000 blacks from the South for his shipbuilding effort during World War II, making sure they had health care in a racially integrated setting, which was unique at the time. Kaiser hired its first woman physician, Chinese immigrant Beatrice Lei, in 1946, and its first black physician intern, Wendell Lipscomb, in 1951, breaking barriers."

DiversityInc states that Kaiser "has the most diverse management—at all levels—of any company we've seen. Its top level of management is 38 percent black, Latino and Asian and 25 percent women. Kaiser has exceptionally strong diversity leadership from its chairman and CEO, George Halvorson, who leads the National Diversity Council and aims to align the diversity in the work force with the diversity in the patient base (Frankel, 2011). Kaiser's Institute for Culturally Competent Care and Centers of Excellence reflect its ongoing commitment to ameliorating disparities in health outcomes across multiple dimensions of diversity. Examples of Kaiser Permanente's practices and their positive impact on diversity management and cultural competence have been referenced throughout this book.

Top Five Health Systems List

As stated earlier in this chapter, a number of organizations within health care award national recognition to health care provider organizations for best demonstrated practices in diversity management and cultural competence. Practices in some of these award-winning health care provider organizations were described earlier and others will be featured as case examples in a subsequent section, "Benchmarking." In this section, we highlight the six health systems that appear on either or both 2011 and 2012 DiversityInc's top five health systems lists.

Henry Ford Health Systems

Headquartered in Detroit, Michigan, Henry Ford Health Systems ranked at the top of DiversityInc's health systems list for 2010 to 2012, and also ranked at number twenty-six on the DiversityInc top fifty list for 2011. Its DiversityInc top fifty company profile attributes this to the health system's "strong values that are clearly articulated in its mission statement to 'put patients first' and to 'improve human life.' The hospital system does this by creating an inclusive workplace that results in culturally competent customer service." DiversityInc's profile of Henry Ford Health System highlights the health system's mandatory diversity training with associated metrics, fifteen employee-resource groups, and strong community ties among its notable initiatives. The profile cites Nancy Schlichting, president and CEO, and her commitment to diversity leadership. Schlichting chairs the diversity council, meets with the employee-resource groups, and signs off on the 7 percent of executive compensation linked to diversity goals. The profile quotes Schlichting as follows: "The current economic conditions make no difference in our continuing commitment to diversity at Henry Ford Health

Systems; it remains a social and moral responsibility for our company, regardless of the difficult times. Diversity remains a key component of our business strategy to achieve our goals of growth and service excellence." The health system's Institute on Multicultural Health works to ameliorate health disparities through research, education, and evidence-based programs.

University Hospitals, Cleveland, Ohio

Based in Cleveland, University Hospitals is an integrated network of hospitals, outpatient surgery centers, urgent care centers, cancer and pediatric specialty centers, rehabilitation, and mental health facilities throughout Ohio. Frankel (2011) of DiversityInc compliments University Hospitals on its strong CEO commitment, with CEO Thomas F. Zenty III appointing members of the diversity council and personally signing off on diversity goals and metrics as well as on executive compensation tied to diversity. Work and life benefits programs include telecommuting, flexible hours, adoption assistance, paternity leave, lactation programs, and religious accommodations (Frankel, 2010). University Hospitals' (2011) downloadable 2010–2011 *Report on Diversity* quotes CEO Zenty: "At University Hospitals, diversity and inclusion are woven into the fabric of our organization—they are a part of who we are and how we work" and provides a comprehensive overview of the health systems' diversity and cultural competence initiatives.

Cleveland Clinic

Also based in Cleveland, Ohio, Cleveland Clinic is a health system composed of nine regional hospitals and sixteen family health centers with about forty-three thousand employees. The Office of Diversity and Inclusion offers the following among key initiatives and programs:

- Mandated cultural competence education and training
- The diversity toolkit manual for employees
- Language acquisition programs such as Spanish for health care professionals, accent modification programs, and vocational English-as-a-second-language courses

- Diversity councils and employee resource groups
- Supplier diversity programs

Cleveland Clinic's website (http://my.clevelandclinic.org) prominently features its extensive complement of diversity and cultural competence initiatives, such as workforce development programs that include initiatives to increase diversity in the health professions and mentoring circles to build employees' leadership potential. The *Diversity & Inclusion Annual Report* is also downloadable from the website. DiversityInc (Frankel, 2011) compliments Cleveland Clinic on its strong CEO commitment; the CEO, Delos M. Cosgrove, chairs the executive diversity council and its supplier-diversity program.

Mayo Clinic

Although a new addition to the DiversityInc top five health systems list in 2012, the Mayo Clinic is certainly not new to the systems approach to diversity and cultural competence. Sharonne Hayes, MD, director, Office of Diversity and Inclusion (2012), provided the following overview of the Mayo Clinic and its approach to diversity and cultural competence:

> Mayo Clinic is the first and largest integrated, not-for-profit medical group practice in the world. Joined by common systems and a philosophy that the needs of the patient come first, doctors from every medical specialty work together to care for patients. Three thousand eight hundred physicians and scientists and 50,900 allied health staff work at Mayo, which has campuses in Rochester, Minnesota; Jacksonville, Florida; and Phoenix/Scottsdale, Arizona. Mayo Clinic also serves more than seventy communities in the upper Midwest through the Mayo Clinic Health System. Collectively, these locations care for more than one million people each year.
>
> Mayo Clinic ranked in the top five of DiversityInc's health systems list for 2012, and for a ninth year has made the *Fortune* 100 Best Places to Work.
>
> "This is acknowledgment that we're headed in the right direction," says John Noseworthy, MD, president and CEO, Mayo Clinic. "Greater diversity spurs innovation and understanding, and allows us to better serve the needs of all of our patients with a deeper level of compassion."

"The workplace environment we want to create reaches beyond diversity," says Sharonne Hayes, MD, director, Office of Diversity and Inclusion. "Inclusion is the ultimate goal. We are striving to create an environment where everyone can use their unique backgrounds and perspectives to contribute their best work. Mayo recognizes that successful diversity and inclusion efforts will lead to more creative innovation, better problem solving, increased productivity and quality, and, most important, enhance patient and employee satisfaction. We believe that if we do this, we'll be positioned to truly meet the needs of our increasingly diverse patients."

Mayo Clinic has long embraced diversity, and has a diversity roadmap that operationalizes its major priorities and initiatives, each of which is linked to its organizational operational plan. Recent initiatives include a clinical practice workgroup charged with examining health disparities and employee inclusion and engagement affecting GLBTI individuals, creation of a multicultural patient and family advisory group (One World), creation of an Office of Health Disparities, developing a veteran hiring program, and the transition of our employee networking groups to a new employee resource group model that aligns them to organizational strategic initiatives (personal communication, June 29, 2012).

Massachusetts General Hospital (Mass General)

Boston-based and affiliated with Partners Health Care and the Harvard Medical School, Massachusetts General Hospital admits forty-seven thousand inpatients and serves almost 1.5 million out-patients annually. Cultural competence training through patient care services and an array of employee groups, including the Association of Multicultural Members of Partners, the Multicultural Affairs Office, the Massachusetts General Hospital LGBT Employee Resource Group, and the Office for Women's Careers, are among the initiatives that reflect the systems approach to strategic diversity management and cultural competence at Mass General (http://www.massgeneral.org/careers/commitmenttodiversity.aspx). DiversityInc lauds Mass General's work and life benefits programs, including paid paternity leave, adoption assistance, job sharing, flexible hours, and on-site religious accommodations. Mass General's accomplishments are also discussed in the health care business case section.

Brigham and Women's Hospital (BWH)

Although not on the 2012 top five list, BWH ranked second in both 2010 and 2011. Also based in Boston, Massachusetts, Brigham and Women's Hospital employs more than thirteen thousand people. BWH and Massachusetts General Hospital founded Partners HealthCare in 1994. Partners HealthCare is a non-profit organization that includes community and specialty hospitals, a physician network, community health centers, home care, and other health-related entities and is a teaching affiliate of Harvard Medical School. DiversityInc cites the BWH's community philanthropy and the racial, ethnic, and gender diversity of its workforce among its distinguishing features. And, DiversityInc quotes BWH's former CEO Gary L. Gottlieb as saying, "An investment in our employees allows us to better serve those who depend on us to deliver the best care possible, even in the most challenging of economic times. Our workforce must reflect the richness of the populations we serve and the breadth of talents and strengths necessary to support our precious mission."

Conclusion

DiversityInc identifies the following as hallmarks of diversity leadership in the top five hospital systems:

- Supportive and involved administrators

- Deep community connections that include philanthropy

- Accountability, including executive performance reviews and compensation linked to diversity goals

- Talent development, including crosscultural mentoring programs with formal follow-up

ASSESSMENT AND THE SYSTEMS APPROACH

Virtually all discussions of diversity management and cultural competence in health care organizations emphasize the importance of beginning with a baseline assessment within the organization and using that assessment to move toward needed improvements. Because most designers of assessment models recognize that movement toward best practices in diversity management and cultural competence requires extensive organizational change, they urge periodic and ongoing assessment rather than a single snapshot. Assessment protocols generally reflect models such as the CLAS standards. Four assessment protocols, exemplary of cultural competence evaluation tools, are well regarded and easily accessible. The first, *Indicators of Cultural Competence in Health Care Delivery Organizations: An Organizational Assessment,* was developed by the Lewin Group (2002) under a contract with the Health Resources and Services Administration and is available on HRSA's website. The assessment is organized into several domains and is comprehensive in its reach:

- *Organizational values:* An organization's perspective and attitudes with respect to the worth and importance of cultural competence

- *Governance:* The goal-setting, policy-making, and other oversight mechanisms an organization uses to ensure the delivery of culturally competent care

- *Planning, monitoring, and evaluation:* The processes used to plan long- and short-term policy and operations and the procedures used to track the efficacy of the planned policies and operations

- *Communication:* The exchange of information between the organization and providers and the clients and communities, and internally, among staff, in ways that promote cultural competence

- *Staff development:* An organization's efforts to ensure that staff have the requisite knowledge, attitudes, and skills for delivering culturally competent care

- *Organizational infrastructure:* The organizational resources required to deliver culturally competent care

- *Services and interventions:* An organization's delivery of clinical, public health, and health-related services in a culturally competent manner

The HRSA website, *The Provider's Guide to Quality and Culture,* also offers a second assessment tool, *The Cultural-Competence Assessment Protocol for Health Care Organizations and Systems,* developed by Dennis Andrulis and his colleagues, which has a somewhat different emphasis: (1) a health care organization's relationship with its community, (2) the administration and management's relationship with staff, (3) interstaff relationships at all levels, and (4) the patient-provider encounter.

Another of the most thorough and comprehensive assessments was developed through the collaborative efforts of The California Endowment and the Joint Commission (Wilson-Stronks, Lee, Cordero, Kopp, & Galvez, 2008). As part of the Joint Commission's *Hospitals, Language and Culture* research program, the publication *One Size Does Not Fit All: Meeting the Health Care Needs of Diverse Populations* provides background and examples of various aspects of culturally competent care found in hospitals across the nation. There are specific illustrations of how and who should be involved in planning, how language-access services can be offered, how cultural competence staffing and training are accomplished, and specific instances of the use of cultural competence in direct patient care. The assessment instrument offered as part of the document covers cultural competence from every aspect, going from building a foundation to incorporating community input.

The fourth protocol, the Cultural Competency Assessment Tool for Hospitals (CCATH), was developed with funding from the Office of Minority Health and field tested with The Commonwealth Fund support. The CCATH, which measures adherence to the CLAS standards, assesses the extent to which the organization engages in best practices in each given area. The researchers (Weech-Maldonado et al., 2012) have also mapped the domains assessed by the CCATH to the National Quality Forum's (NQF) (2008) framework and preferred practices for diversity management and cultural competence.

In addition to these four assessment protocols, the National Center for Cultural Competence has a number of additional protocols on their website, and there are many more such assessments available on the Internet. Most of the good assessments such as the ones noted previously are broad enough to be applicable to small and large organizations: clinics, medical groups, hospitals, and health plans. There is considerable overlap in the items covered on different assessments but variation is usually only a matter of emphasis. These several assessment protocols are valuable not only for their thoroughness as evaluation instruments but, taken together, provide an excellent blueprint for actualizing cultural competence at the organizational level. Preassessment gives organizations the baseline data they need to take action to close the gap between current and best practices by developing the appropriate infrastructure and the processes of using that infrastructure to produce desired outcomes.

Broad-based assessments of overall performance should be followed by efforts to benchmark the organization's performance against best demonstrated practices and to directly define and assess success in achieving desired organization-specific outcomes so that the infrastructure and its processes can be fine-tuned and thus continually improved. The ultimate goal here is to apply standard quality improvement methods, including Six Sigma, to diversity initiatives. The next section discusses benchmarking and the following illustrates the application of Six Sigma and DMAIC to reducing racial and ethnic disparities in patient satisfaction.

BENCHMARKING

A benchmark is a norm or standard against which others are compared. Health care has yet to achieve consensus on a common set of benchmarks for best demonstrated practices in diversity management and cultural competence but the Institute for Diversity in Health Management and its partner organizations are working to change that. Using data from a biennial survey of US hospitals, first administered in 2008–2009, the institute hopes to develop national benchmarks against which health care organizations can assess their baseline performance to identify areas for targeted action.

The benchmarking survey was based on research included in *Strategies for Leadership* (AHA, 2004), a diversity and cultural competency assessment tool developed by the institute along with the American College of Healthcare Executives (ACHE), the American Hospital Association (AHA), and the National Center for Healthcare Leadership (NCHL). The checklist from this document is included in Chapter Three of this book. The survey instrument also drew from recent work in the areas of culturally competent patient care, health care disparities, and leadership conducted by the Joint Commission and the National Association of Public Hospitals and Health System's collaboration with the Institute for Healthcare Improvement and the Disparities Solutions Center at Massachusetts General Hospital.

The survey assesses performance on numerous specific diversity management and cultural competence practices in four areas:

- Expanding the diversity of the governance body and leadership team of the organization

- Strengthening a diverse workforce throughout the organization

- Effectively engaging the diverse communities that the organization serves

- Delivering culturally and linguistically competent patient care throughout the organization-quality patient care and effective language access

The survey was sent to 3,500 US hospitals and 182 responded during the October 2008 to February 2009 time frame. The 2011–2012 survey results are now being processed. With nine hundred respondents, participation has increased almost fivefold, demonstrating a growing interest among hospitals in assessing their performance and vying for national recognition in diversity management and cultural competence.

Although benchmarks for specific diversity management and cultural competence practices are not yet in place, the survey results have been used to identify best in class hospitals in each of the four areas assessed. Table 11.2 displays those hospitals identified as best in class on three or more of the assessed dimensions. Organizations that are best in class across all four dimensions and rank best in class overall most likely have linked their diversity and cultural competence initiatives through a systems approach, which is a hallmark of high-performing organizations.

ROLE OF METRICS IN THE SYSTEMS APPROACH

Every one of the organizations on the DiversityInc top fifty companies for diversity list collects and uses diversity metrics. Without metrics to guide and document the results achieved through engaging in best-demonstrated practices, the business case for diversity and cultural competence cannot be substantiated. In fact, the three-hundred-plus question survey described previously that DiversityInc uses to

---

Note: Certain content in the section "Role of Metrics in the Systems Approach" was adapted with permission from Dreachslin, J. L., & Lee, P. D. (2007). Applying Six Sigma and DMAIC to diversity initiatives. *Journal of Healthcare Management, 52*(6), 364–370.

TABLE 11.2 Institute for Diversity in Health Management Benchmarking Survey 2009: Best in Class Hospitals on Three or More Dimensions

Hospital	Leadership and Governance	Strengthening Workforce	Engaging Communities Served	Delivering Quality Care	Overall
Aurora Health Care, Wisconsin	X	X		X	X
Cambridge Health Alliance, Massachusetts	X		X	X	X
Cedars-Sinai Health Systems, California		X	X	X	X
Clarian Health, Indiana	X	X	X	X	X
UC Davis Medical Center, California	X	X	X	X	X
Veterans Affairs Medical Center, Washington, DC	X	X	X		X

select top performers and the Institute for Diversity in Health Management benchmarking survey are metrics driven. As is the case in other areas of business performance, collection and use of diversity and cultural competence metrics is a hallmark of best practices. This section describes how health care organizations can move to a focus on metrics and apply quality improvement approaches such as Six Sigma and DMAIC to their own diversity initiatives.

Metrics are central to gauging the success of any business endeavor—whether that endeavor is aimed at improving market share, creating efficiencies in the supply chain, or reducing infection rates. Metrics can also be used to assess the effectiveness of diversity and cultural competence initiatives, such as ameliorating racial and ethnic disparities in care or recruiting and retaining a diverse workforce. Unless we set goals and examine the activities for reaching those goals, we cannot be sure that we are achieving our targets.

Rohini Anand, senior vice president and global chief diversity officer of Sodexo, describes the centrality of metrics in Sodexo's nationally recognized success:

> At Sodexo the adage "what gets measured gets done" is a truism. In order to ensure that diversity and inclusion are imbedded in the organization, we established a sophisticated scorecard that measures both qualitative and quantitative progress, and more importantly measures the underlying processes and inclusive behaviors that impact the outcomes. Progress is measured and reported monthly and managers are held accountable by linking the metrics to incentive compensation, as we do with any other measures of organizational success. (personal communication, July 30, 2007)

Following are examples of performance metrics for each of three important diversity and cultural competence performance assessment foci for health care delivery organizations:

- Leadership, strategy, and climate:
  - Concordance between leadership team diversity and service area or workforce diversity
  - Employee satisfaction with the workplace by key dimensions of diversity, such as gender, race and ethnicity, generation, tenure, role, and department
  - Supplier diversity as measured by the proportion of procurement from women and minority-owned suppliers

- Human resource management:

  - Employee retention rates by key dimensions of diversity, such as gender, race and ethnicity, generation, tenure, role, and department

  - Compensation by key dimensions of diversity, controlling for human capital variables and performance

- Culturally competent care, interpreters, and translators:

  - Patient satisfaction with care across key dimensions of diversity, such as gender, race and ethnicity, generation, tenure, role, and department

  - Performance against Agency for Healthcare Research and Quality's (AHRQ) quality measures (http://www.ahrq.gov/qual/qrdr10/measurespec/)

These particular outcome metrics may not be the most appropriate first-tier choices for every organization because each organization must determine its own desired outcomes in light of its unique mission, vision, and strategy. However, these are key among the outcomes best practices health care delivery organizations strive to accomplish.

Application of Six Sigma and DMAIC

As discussed earlier in this text, demographic diversity presents challenges and opportunities. Research on diversity's impact such as that summarized in Chapter Ten reveals that its effect is heavily dependent on the organizational context, including business strategy, human resource practices, culture, climate, and leadership. As Kochan and his colleagues (2003) concluded from their comprehensive study, the business case for demographic diversity is nuanced. Responsible health care leaders ensure that their diversity dollars are well spent. They ensure not only that best demonstrated diversity and cultural competence infrastructure and practices are in place, but they also strive to improve results. Doing so requires using outcome-oriented metrics and committing to continual assessment of organizational performance.

Six Sigma and its five-step DMAIC (define, measure, analyze, improve, and control) process can be used to identify areas for improvement and measure progress against organization-specific diversity metrics. Originating in the manufacturing sector at Motorola, Six Sigma uses statistical analyses to measure and reveal opportunities for process improvement by uncovering **defects** (Lucas, 2002; Mader,

2007). For a service firm, a defect is any transaction, service encounter, action, or procedure that does not meet customer expectations. The five-step DMAIC technique is the most prevalent Six Sigma method used for **process improvement** (de Mast & Bisgaard, 2007). Its elements are as follows:

- *Define:* Select the process that needs improvement.

- *Measure:* Translate the process into quantifiable forms, collect data, and assess current performance.

- *Analyze:* Identify the root causes of defects and set goals for performance.

- *Improve:* Implement and evaluate changes (solutions) to the process to remove root causes of defects.

- *Control:* Standardize solutions and continually monitor improvement.

One important diversity and cultural competence metric is ensuring that patient satisfaction does not differ by race and ethnicity. DMAIC can help the health care provider organization identify and ameliorate disparities in satisfaction through identifying **root causes** and implementing solutions that minimize or remove those root causes. In this process improvement application, the DMAIC steps are as follows:

Define

Six Sigma processes selected for improvement are usually those that are critical to the success of the organization. At the define step, assume that customer satisfaction with care is critical to success. Any defect in that care process, as viewed by the customer, leads to dissatisfaction. Thus, the view of the customer is critical to success. Because the goal of Six Sigma and DMAIC is to remove defects, this method will focus on eliminating processes or factors in care that result in dissatisfaction. A patient satisfaction survey will reveal areas of dissatisfaction, which will define the process that needs to be improved using Six Sigma and DMAIC. One process or factor that could be improved in the diversity context is the lack of or minimal interpreter services.

Measure

Well-designed performance measurement systems use metrics that are quantitative, are easy to understand, encourage appropriate behavior, and are visible. In addition, performance measures must encompass outputs and inputs, which are defined and mutually understood by those who will use them. In short, performance measures should be multidimensional so that every member of the team has a clear understanding of what behavior patterns need to be changed.

A **Pareto chart** is the quality improvement tool most often used to display or array the data obtained in the measure step. A Pareto chart is a bar chart that graphically represents the frequency distribution of each performance metric. In the example we used in the define step—improving patient satisfaction with care—a Pareto chart can depict the availability of interpreter services by language. The chart can display the proportion of patients by primary language and the availability of interpreters for that language group. This way, availability versus need can be easily seen, allowing managers to uncover gaps in service and to determine which gap needs to be tackled first.

The measure step also involves setting goals for each metric. In the interpreter services example, a goal might be to increase the availability of Spanish language interpreters to meet the demand of the population whose primary language is Spanish.

Analyze

The analyze step involves determining the root causes of defective products and services. Data from patient satisfaction surveys and focus groups may be analyzed by race and ethnicity of respondents. If results indicate that patients of color are less satisfied than their white counterparts, the root causes of this finding should be explored. Determining root causes can be done through assessing the organization's conformity to best practices, as measured by assessment protocols such as those discussed previously, or the "Diversity Practices Checklist" included in Chapter Three of this text. Most important, the organization should also analyze its own processes.

A **cause-and-effect diagram** (also called a *fishbone diagram* or *Ishikawa diagram*, after its developer, Kauro Ishikawa) can be used to determine potential causes. Ideally, such a diagram is the product of participatory brainstorming or an assessment exercise in which potential causes of the identified defect are categorized into meaningful and manageable groupings. Figure 11.2 is a cause-and-effect diagram that displays the root causes of a gap in patient satisfaction by race and ethnicity. In this figure, four categories are used: policies, procedures, people, and plant and technology. Insights from assessment protocols such as

FIGURE 11.2 Fishbone Diagram: Root Causes of Racial and Ethnic Patient Satisfaction Gap

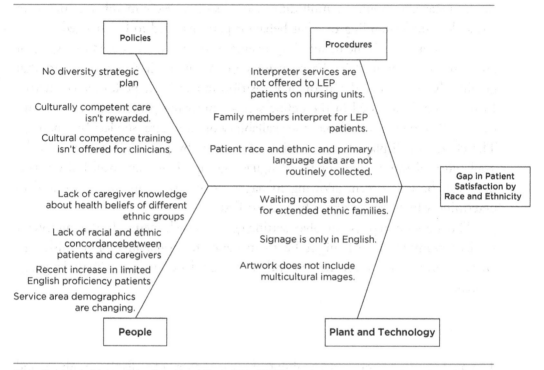

Source: Reprinted with permission from Dreachslin and Lee (2007).

those discussed previously or the assessment tool in Chapter Three are invaluable in identifying gaps through the brainstorming process.

Figure 11.2 displays the relationship among related causes on each of the four major categories. As shown in the figure, we performed only a first-level analysis. In an actual application of the diagram, the brainstorming group can jot down multiple levels of analysis, identifying causes behind causes. Once all possible causes have been entered, the group would then review the finished diagram, gain consensus on the top five or so root causes, and assign a priority ranking to each cause.

Improve

At the improve step, action is taken to address the previously identified root causes. For example, providing cultural competence training for clinicians would ameliorate the root cause "cultural competence training is not offered to clinicians."

Such training could improve the process of care and help close the racial and ethnic gap in patient satisfaction. In this step, solutions are identified and implemented for each of the root causes revealed in the analyze step and selected for improvement.

Control

The control step involves monitoring the status of the improvements to the process to ensure that goals are achieved and acceptable behavior patterns are maintained throughout the organization. When patient satisfaction metrics are monitored and made visible to everyone concerned, cultural competence becomes a critical success factor. At this stage, new possibilities for process improvement are revealed, enhancing the concept of continuous improvement inherent in the Six Sigma method. By beginning with satisfaction and expanding to other metrics, such as the AHRQ quality measures for patients, organizations can systematically improve their diversity performance.

Conclusion

Although Six Sigma and DMAIC are most often associated with the manufacturing sector, they can be used effectively to improve a health care delivery organization's diversity and cultural competence performance. By committing to the use of metrics and with continuous improvement, targets for high-quality care and goals of equitable treatment of all patients and employees can be reached. Health care organizations can emulate these best practices to realize the benefits of workforce diversity and meet the needs of diverse patients.

SUMMARY

Two landmark publications are widely credited with fueling the diversity movement in corporate America in the early 1990s that focused on the workforce and HRM: the Hudson Institute's report, *Workforce 2000: Work and Workers for the 21st Century* (Johnston & Packer, 1987) and Roosevelt Thomas's *Harvard Business Review* article, "From Affirmative Action to Affirming Diversity" (1990). Since that time, a growing number of organizations have arrived at the same conclusion: the systems approach to strategic diversity management and cultural competence is a business imperative not only for health care provider organizations but also for organizations in every sector of the US economy. A well-known and easily accessible source to identify exemplary performers and their strategic diversity management practices is the DiversityInc top fifty companies for diversity list and the associated specialty lists, including the DiversityInc top five hospital systems list. Many other valuable sources for best practices case examples within health care were also described.

The role of pre- and post-assessment, benchmarking, and metrics in the systems approach to diversity and cultural competence was also discussed. These are central to gauging the success of diversity and cultural competence goals such as reducing racial and ethnic disparities in care or recruiting and retaining a diverse health care workforce. Unless we set goals and measure performance from a baseline, we cannot be sure that we are achieving our targets. And unless we benchmark our organization's performance against best in class, we will not know that we are doing the best that can be done. In health care fields, measured outcomes make up an evidence base that is necessary for a practice or intervention to be widely adopted.

A business case must be made for health care because it is, in fact, one of the major industry sectors in the US economy. Health care organizations must market their services, be cost effective, and achieve their patient care goals, all while remaining financially viable. By looking at the hallmarks, activities, or distinguishing features of organizations outside of health care that are considered diversity leaders, we can identify diversity and cultural competence practices in health care organizations that can benefit from quality improvement. Additionally, nonprofit organizations that specialize in assessment of health care organizations and their practices, such as the Institute for Diversity in Health Management, the Joint Commission, the National Commission on Quality Assurance, and the National Quality Forum have identified the areas of diversity management and culturally competent service delivery as targets for improvement.

Organization-specific outcome metrics for each area targeted for improvement can be developed to assess performance. Health care organizations that strive to emulate best-demonstrated practices can do so by building and using a diversity infrastructure, comparing performance to best in class, defining outcome-based measures of impact, and using Six Sigma and DMAIC to assess and continuously improve organizational performance. By committing to the use of metrics and with continuous improvement, benchmarks for high-quality care and goals of equitable treatment of all patients and employees can be reached.

KEY TERMS

benchmarking

best demonstrated practices

cause-and-effect diagram

defects

distinctive competence

DiversityInc

DMAIC

metrics

Pareto chart

process improvement

root causes

Six Sigma

REVIEW QUESTIONS AND ACTIVITIES

1. In what way is health care a business? In what ways is it not? In what way is the business case in health care different from that of organizations in other sectors of the US economy? Do you believe the business case for diversity and cultural competence in health care is strong enough that leadership in US health care provider organizations should make strategic diversity management and cultural competence a high priority? Support your answers with logical argument and factual information.

2. CEO commitment is the highest weighted area of the four evaluated to select the DiversityInc top fifty companies for diversity. Leadership and governance is one of the four dimensions assessed in the Institute for Diversity in Health Management benchmarking survey. Using research findings, testimonies from experts, and logical argument, explain why leadership is key.

3. Choose one of the best practices organizations from this chapter and gather information about the organization's best practices and their effect on performance. Select one or two of those practices and describe how they would improve diversity management or cultural competence in a health care delivery organization in your community.

4. The terms *evidence-based* and *metrics* have been used several times in this chapter. Why do you think these concepts are so important in health care? Are there aspects of health care for which evidence-based proof can't be achieved through metrics? Why or why not?

5. Several organizations that specialize specifically in the assessment of health care were mentioned in this chapter, including the National Quality Forum (http://www.qualityforum.org/Home.aspx) and the National Commission on Quality Assurance (http://www.ncqa.org/). Go to their websites and download their protocols for assessing the cultural competence of health care organizations. In what ways are they similar? Different?

6. For each of the three quality improvement foci identified in this chapter—(1) leadership, strategy, and climate; (2) human resource management; and (3) culturally competent care, interpreters, and translators—develop two outcome metrics in addition to those already identified in the text. For each metric, explain its importance.

7. Imagine that you are an executive leader in a hospital that is having difficulty retaining male nurses. Describe how DMAIC could be applied to improve male nurse retention. Then, develop a hypothetical Ishikawa diagram (modeled on Figure 11.2) to identify root causes for the gap in nurse retention by gender.

REFERENCES

Agency for Healthcare Research and Quality (AHRQ). (2006). *National healthcare disparities report 2006. Appendix C: Measure specifications quality of health care.* Retrieved from www.ahrq.gov/qual/nhdr06/measurespec/index.html

Alliance of Community Health Plans Foundation. (2007). *Making the business case for culturally and linguistically appropriate services in health care: Case studies from the field.* Retrieved from www.minorityhealth.hhs.gov/Assets/pdf/Checked/CLAS.pdf

American College of Healthcare Executives, American Hospital Association, Institute for Diversity in Health Management, National Center for Healthcare Leadership. (2004). *Strategies for leadership: Does your hospital reflect the community it serves?* Chicago: American Hospital Association.

Beach, M. C., Price, E. G., Gary, T. L., Robinson, K. A., Gozu, A., Palacio, A., Smarth, C., Jenckes, M. W., Feurerstein, C., Bass, E. B., Powe, N. R., & Cooper, L. A. (2005). Cultural competency: A systematic review of health care provider educational interventions. *Medical Care, 43*(4), 356–373.

Betancourt, J. R., & Green, A. R. (2010). Commentary: Linking cultural competency training to improved health outcomes: Perspectives from the field. *Academic Medicine, 65*(4), 583–586.

Billington, M. G., & Billington, P. J. (2003). *Six Sigma: Quality performance.* Retrieved from http://clomedia.com/articles/view/six_sigma_quality_performance

Brach, C., & Fraser, I. (2002). Reducing disparities through culturally competent care: An analysis of the business case. *Quality Management in Health Care, 10*(4), 15–28.

de Mast, J., & Bisgaard, S. (2007). The science of Six Sigma. *Quality Progress, 40*(1). 25–29.

Dreachslin, J. L., & Lee, P. D. (2007). Applying Six Sigma and DMAIC to diversity initiatives. *Journal of Healthcare Management, 52*(6), 364–370.

Frankel, B. (2007, June). Domestic-partner benefits the top 50 litmus test. *DiversityInc Magazine*, p. 22.

Frankel, B. (2011). *The DiversityInc top 5 hospital systems*. Retrieved from http://www.diversityinc.com/article/8379/The-DiversityInc-Top-5-Hospital-Systems/.

Goode, T. D., Dunne, M. C., & Bronheim, S. M. (2006). *The evidence base for cultural and linguistic competence in health care*. Retrieved from http://www.commonwealthfund.org/Publications/Fund-Reports/2006/Oct/The-Evidence-Base-for-Cultural-and-Linguistic-Competency-in-Health-Care.aspx

Hampers, L. C., Cha, S., Gutglass, D. J., Binns, H. A., & Krug, S. E. (1999). Language barriers and resource utilization in a pediatric emergency department. *Pediatrics, 103*, 1253–1256.

Jacobs, E. A., Laurderdale, D. S., Meltzer, D., Shorey, J. M., Levinson, W., & Thisted, R. A. (2001). The impact of enhanced interpreter services on delivery of health care to limited-English proficiency patients. *Journal of General Internal Medicine, 16*(7), 468–474.

Jacobs, E. A., Sadowski, L. S., & Rathouz, P. J. (2007). The impact of an enhanced interpreter service intervention on hospital costs and patient satisfaction. *Journal of General Internal Medicine, 22*(suppl. 2), 306–311.

Johnston, W. R., & Packer, A. H. (1987). *Workforce 2000: Work and workers for the 21ˢᵗ century*. Indianapolis: Hudson Institute.

Kochan, T., Berukova, K., Ely, R., Jackson, S., Joshi, A., Jehn, K., Leonard, J., Levine, D., & Thomas, D. (2003). The effects of diversity on business performance: Report of the diversity research network. *Human Resource Management, 42*(1), 3–21.

LaVeist, T. A., Gaskin, D. J., & Patrick, R. (2009). *The economic burden of health inequalities in the United States*. Washington, DC: Joint Studies for Political and Economic Studies.

Lewin Group. (2002). *Indicators of cultural competence in health care delivery organizations: An organizational assessment*. Washington, DC: Health Resources and Services Administration.

Lie, D. A., Lee-Rey, E., Gomez, A., Bereknyei, S., & Braddock, C. H. (2011). Does cultural competency training of health care professionals improve patient outcomes? A systematic review and proposed algorithm for future research. *Journal of General Internal Medicine, 26*(3), 317–325.

Lucas, J. M. (2002). The essential Six Sigma. *Quality Progress, 35*(1), 27–31.

Mader, D. P. (2007). How to identify and select lean Six Sigma Projects. *Quality Progress, 40*(7), 58–60.

Millman, J. (2007, June). Why you need diversity to be competitive: Case studies from the 2007 DiversityInc top 50 companies for diversity. *DiversityInc*, pp. 24–44.

National Business Group on Health. (2003). *Why companies are making health disparities their business: The business case and practical strategies.* Prepared for the Office of Minority Health. Retrieved from http://minorityhealth.hhs.gov/assets/pdf/checked/business_case.pdf

National Business Group on Health. (2009a). *Eliminating racial and ethnic health disparities: A business case update for employers.* Retrieved from http://www.businessgrouphealth.org/pdfs/Final%20Draft%20508.pdf

National Business Group on Health. (2009b). *Addressing racial and ethnic disparities: Employer initiatives.* Retrieved from http://www.businessgrouphealth.org/pdfs/NBGH%20Webinar%20Slides.pdf

National Business Group on Health. (2011). *An employer's guide to reducing racial and ethnic disparities in the workplace.* Retrieved from http://www.businessgrouphealth.org/pdfs/DiversityReport_Final.pdf

National Committee on Quality Assurance. (2006). *Innovative practices in multicultural health care.* Retrieved from http://www.ncqa.org/Portals/0/HEDISQM/CLAS/CLAS_InnovativePrac06.pdf

National Committee on Quality Assurance. (2008). *Innovative practices in multicultural health care.* Retrieved from http://www.ncqa.org/Portals/0/HEDISQM/CLAS/CLASInnovativePrac_08.pdf

National Committee on Quality Assurance. (2009). *Innovative practices in multicultural health care.* Retrieved from http://www.ncqa.org/Portals/0/HEDISQM/CLAS/CLAS_InnovPrac_09.pdf

National Commission on Quality Assurance. (2011). *NCQA's multicultural health care distinction program.* Retrieved from http://www.ncqa.org/LinkClick.aspx?fileticket=_57ciAJz4xs%3D&tabid=61

National Quality Forum. (2008). *A comprehensive framework and preferred practices for measuring and reporting cultural competency.* Washington, DC: National Quality Forum.

National Quality Forum. (2011). *Promoting a common language for quality measures and electronic health records.* Retrieved from http://www.qualityforum.org/News_And_Resources/Press_Releases/2011/Promoting_a_%E2%80%98Common_Language%E2%80%99_for_Quality_Measures_and_Electronic_Health_Records.aspx

Pitturo, M., & Mahoney, S. S. (1991). Managing diversity. *Executive Female, 14*(3), 45–48.

Price, E., Beach, M. C., Gary, T. L., Robinson, K. A., Gozu, A., Palacio, A., Smarth, C., Jenckes, M., Feurstein, C., Bass, E. B., Powe, N., & Cooper, L. (2005). A systematic review of the methodological rigor of studies evaluations cultural competence training of health professionals. *Academic Medicine, 89*(6), 578–586.

Sodexo. (2011). *Diversity and inclusion annual report.* Gaithersburg, MD: Sodexo.

Solomon, C. M. (1989). The corporate response to work force diversity. *Personnel Journal, 68*(8), 43–53.

Thomas, D. A., & Creary S. J. (2011). *Shifting the diversity climate: The Sodexo solution.* Cambridge, MA: Harvard Business School.

Thomas, R. (1990). From affirmative action to affirming diversity. *Harvard Business Review on managing diversity* (pp. 1–32). Boston: Harvard Business School Publishing.

University Hospitals. (2011). *Report on diversity 2010–2011.* Retrieved from http://www.uhhospitals.org/portals/6/docs/about_uh/diversity/report-diversity2010.pdf

Weech-Maldonado, R., Dreachslin, J. L., Brown, J., Pradhan, R., Rubin, K. L., Schiller, C., & Hays, R. D. (2012). Cultural competency assessment tool for hospitals: Evaluating hospitals' adherence to the culturally and linguistically appropriate services standards. *Health Care Management Review, 37*(1), 54–66.

Wilson-Stronks, A., Lee, K. K., Cordero, C. L., Kopp, M. L., & Galvez, E. (2008). *One size does not fit all: Meeting the health care needs of diverse populations.* Oakbrook Terrace, IL: The Joint Commission.

THE FUTURE OF

DIVERSITY AND CULTURAL

COMPETENCE IN

HEALTH CARE

LEARNING OBJECTIVES

- To identify six trends that are expected to result in more widespread adoption of the systems approach to diversity and cultural competence in health care in the near future

- To explain how the sustainability movement supports the systems approach to diversity and cultural competence in health care

- To apply Kurt Lewin's change theory and force field analysis models to envision and shape the future of the systems approach to diversity and cultural competence in health care

In this final chapter, we identify and discuss the key trends that are expected to drive more widespread adoption of the systems approach to diversity and cultural competence in health care, not only in the United States but also in other countries. We describe how the sustainability movement and its focus on triple-bottom-line accounting will likely encourage the systems approach to diversity and cultural competence in health care. And we apply Kurt Lewin's widely used change management model along with his force field analysis method to not only identify but also to influence factors that will drive and factors that will restrain widespread adoption of the systems approach to diversity and cultural competence in health care in the future.

TRENDS THAT SUPPORT WIDESPREAD ADOPTION OF THE SYSTEMS APPROACH

It is clear that the diversity-associated disparities in health and health care and in career accomplishment and satisfaction discussed throughout this book will continue unless systematic action to ameliorate these disparities is taken by each and every health care organization. In this section, we discuss six trends that support the expectation that the systems approach to diversity and cultural competence in health care will become the norm rather than the exception in the future.

Trend One: The Demographic Imperative Is Well Established

As reported in Chapter One, by the middle of this century the United States will be a majority minority nation; less than half of the population will be non-Hispanic white. Figure 12.1 is a graphic representation of the percent of the total US population in each racial and ethnic group from the 2000 and 2010 censuses. The decline in the proportion of white non-Hispanics in the US population is apparent: 69 percent in 2000 and 64 percent in 2010.

This demographic sea change is especially evident in children; all of the increase in the population of children under age eighteen between 2000 and 2010 can be attributed to minority population growth. In fact, the number of non-Hispanic white children decreased 10 percent in that same time frame. See Figure 12.2 for the 2000 to 2010 percent change in the US population under age eighteen

FIGURE 12.1   Percent of the US Population in Each Racial and Ethnic Group, 2000 and 2010

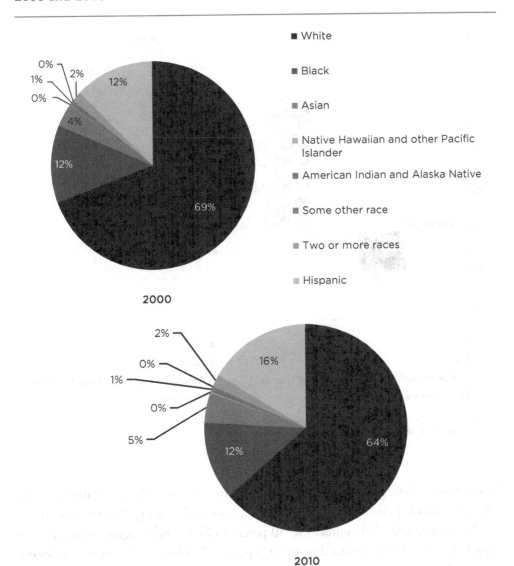

2000

2010

Legend:
- White
- Black
- Asian
- Native Hawaiian and other Pacific Islander
- American Indian and Alaska Native
- Some other race
- Two or more races
- Hispanic

Source: US Census Bureau (2011).

FIGURE 12.2 Percent Change in the US Population Under Age Eighteen, 2000–2010

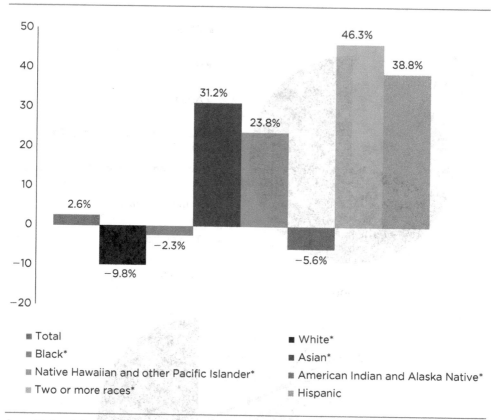

Legend:
- Total
- Black*
- Native Hawaiian and other Pacific Islander*
- Two or more races*
- White*
- Asian*
- American Indian and Alaska Native*
- Hispanic

Source: Mather, Pollard, and Jacobsen (2011). Reprinted with permission.

by racial and ethnic group and Figure 12.3 for the percent of the population in each racial and ethnic group for children compared to adults, using 2010 Census data.

Minorities will likely constitute 50 percent of the under-eighteen population even before the 2020 Census due, in large part, to US-born children of immigrant parents. In fact, children of immigrants account for 23 percent of the US population under age eighteen. And, because population growth in children is highest among families living in poverty with higher dropout rates and lower standardized test rates, the nation's ability to meet the needs of an increasingly diverse and aging population is of concern (Mather, Pollard, & Jacobsen, 2011).

FIGURE 12.3 Percent of the Population in Each Racial and Ethnic Group by Age, 2010

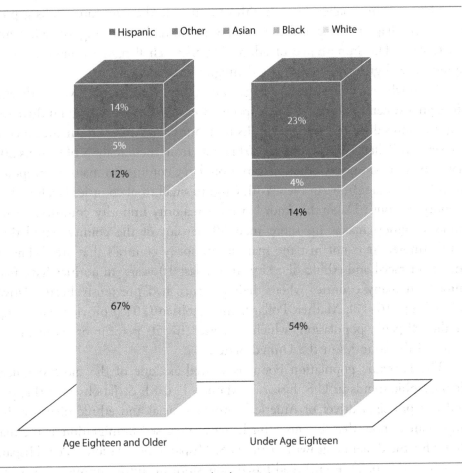

Source: Mather, Pollard, and Jacobsen (2011). Reprinted with permission.

The 2010 Census also reveals that California, Hawaii, New Mexico, and Texas are already majority minority states and, within ten years, Arizona, Florida, Georgia, Maryland, Mississippi, Nevada, New Jersey, and New York are projected to increase the number of majority minority states to twelve. Racial and ethnic demographics patterns differ significantly by state. For example, the 2010 US Census revealed that over 90 percent of the population in Maine,

New Hampshire, Vermont, and West Virginia is non-Hispanic white (Mather, Pollard, & Jacobsen, 2011).

Demographic challenges to health care include the workforce skills gap discussed in Chapter Three and the delivery of culturally and linguistically appropriate care. The importance of addressing these challenges through a systems approach will grow because of the demographic imperative.

Although every health care organization must be responsive to diversity through a systems approach, needs specific to each service area should drive each organization's diversity strategy and its resultant tactics and performance metrics. As Mather, Pollard, and Jacobsen (2011) note from their analysis of Census 2010 data, "majority-minority counties vary from large counties in major metropolitan areas (such as the Bronx in New York City) to small rural counties (such as Todd County in South Dakota)." And, "in most majority-minority counties, a single minority group makes up more than 50 percent of the county population." Furthermore, "it is not just the majority-minority counties that are feeling the impact of racial and ethnic diversity. In the last 10 years, minorities have made inroads in many counties where their presence had previously been relatively minor" (pp. 16–17). Mather, Pollard, and Jacobsen (2011) provide the example of the Hispanic population, which increased by 50 percent or more in two-thirds of the counties in the United States.

The Hispanic population boom is viewed as "one of the most significant demographic trends in U.S. history" (Mather, Pollard, & Jabobsen, 2011, p. 7) and is a principal driver of America's growing racial and ethnic diversity. It is important to note that, because "births have surpassed immigration as the main driver for the dynamic growth in the U.S. Hispanic population" (Pew Hispanic Center, 2011, p. 2), even broad-based opposition to future immigration would not significantly change the trends discussed in this section and the concomitant need for health care organizations to respond with a systems approach to diversity and cultural competence.

Trend Two: Diversity Is Increasingly Nuanced, Complex, and Multifaceted

As explained throughout this book, the broader culture; our own community, family, and other social networks; as well as our individual cognitive, emotional, and behavioral responses to our experiences shape the meaning of group identities and how we experience them. And group identities are increasingly nuanced, complex, and multifaceted.

In the 2000 US Census, which was the first to permit individuals to select more than one racial or ethnic identity group, about 2.1 percent of the population self-identified as bi-ethnic; this proportion increased to almost 3 percent in the 2010 Census. In fact, 5.6 percent of children under eighteen were identified with more than one racial or ethnic group in the 2010 Census, leading to the conclusion that "the children of these interracial unions are forming a new generation that is much more likely to identify with multiple racial/ethnic groups" (Mather, Pollard, & Jacobsen, 2011, p. 9).

Furthermore, individuals are juggling their own multiple group identities across diversity dimensions in different and more complex ways. For example, the Pew Research Center (2007) reports that "African Americans see a widening gulf between the values of middle class and poor blacks, and nearly four in ten say that because of the diversity within their community, blacks can no longer be thought of as a single race" (p. 1). Health care providers, as individuals and organizations, must be prepared to respond appropriately to the increasingly nuanced meanings that patients and their families attach to their group identities and test their own assumptions about who their patients and colleagues are, the groups they identify with, and what they believe about themselves, others, and health care itself.

And a growing number of people will experience the complexity of diversity in their personal lives, which, as discussed previously in this book, will influence how they deal with diversity's complex meaning in health care organizations. In 2008, 8 percent of married adults had a spouse of a different race or ethnicity compared to only 3.2 percent in 1980. The Pew Research Center reports that just over 14½ percent of new marriages in 2008 were between individuals of different races or ethnicities. The proportion of interracial and interethnic marriages in 2008 differed by racial and ethnic group as follows: 9 percent of whites, 16 percent of blacks, 26 percent of Hispanics, and 31 percent of Asians. US-born Hispanics and Asians were approximately three times more likely to be in an interethnic and interracial marriage than foreign-born members of their identity groups. Differences in gender were noted as well: whereas 22 percent of African American males married outside their race in 2008, only 9 percent of black women did. The gender pattern was just the opposite for Asians: 40 percent of Asian women and 20 percent of Asian male newlyweds married outside their own racial and ethnic group in 2008. For whites and Hispanics, there was no gender difference (Taylor et al., 2010).

Furthermore, another Pew Research Center report (Taylor, Funk, & Craighill, 2006) reveals that more than 20 percent of people in the United States have a relative in an interracial or interethnic marriage. A significant difference by age was also noted in the report. More than one-third of people between the ages of eighteen and twenty-nine said they had a relative in an interracial or interethnic marriage and only 14 percent of people over sixty-five did. The researchers conclude, "That degree of familiarity with—and proximity to—interracial marriage is the latest milestone in what has been a sweeping change in behaviors and attitudes concerning interracial relationships over the past several decades" (Taylor, Funk, & Craighill, 2006, p. 2).

Gender roles are changing as well, which will have an impact on the demographics of the health professions and will add to the complexity of gender dynamics in workplace interactions among health care professionals and with patients. For example, in 2009–2010 over 48 percent of medical school graduates were women as compared to about 27 percent in 1982–1983. Although not nearly as profound a change, a recent survey by the National League for Nursing (2010) found that approximately 13 percent of RN students across various types of nursing programs are men. That figure exceeds male RN current workforce representation.

Trends in religious identity, discussed in Chapter One, will also contribute to the growing complexity of diversity and cultural competence in health care. For example, the American Religious Identity Survey (ARIS) (Kosmin & Keysar, 2009) found that the percentage of US adults who self-identified as Christian declined from 86 percent in 1990 to 76 percent in 2008. ARIS attributed this decline to a growing proportion of Americans who either have no religious preference or self-identify as atheist or agnostic: 8.2 percent in 1990 and 15 percent in 2008. ARIS also saw growth in non-Christian faiths. Although still a rather small proportion of all US religious affiliations at just under 4 percent, the implications for health care are important and will affect areas from chaplaincy to food services to direct patient care by physicians, nurses, the allied health professions, and others.

This increasingly nuanced, complex, and multifaceted diversity calls for more widespread implementation of the systems approach because it is essentially through systematic efforts that health care organizations can deliver safe, effective, and high-quality care to each patient.

Trend Three: Support for Inclusion Is Broad Based and Growing, Especially Among the Young

Surveys reveal meaningful generational differences in explicit attitudes toward diversity, with younger generations more accepting of differences and more inclusive than their older counterparts. From interracial dating to gay marriage to gender roles in the family, attitude change is related to generation. For example, based on opinion survey data, the Pew Research Center (Taylor, Funk, & Craighill, 2006) concluded, "Acceptance of interracial dating is greatest among the young. In surveys conducted in 2002 and 2003, fully 91% of Gen Y respondents born after 1976 said that interracial dating is acceptable, compared with 50% of the oldest generation (those reaching adulthood during WWII) who expressed this view" (p. 2).

The Pew Research Center (Taylor et al., 2010) also found a similar age-related pattern regarding attitudes toward interracial and interethnic marriage. Survey data revealed no differences by race or ethnicity in acceptance of interracial and interethnic marriage by eighteen- to twenty-nine-year-olds, with over 80 percent expressing acceptance. However, those over fifty years old, and especially white respondents over sixty-five years old, are significantly less accepting of interracial and interethnic marriage, with only 36 percent expressing acceptance.

Similar age-related trends are seen in polls that assess explicit attitudes toward gay marriage. As with interracial and interethnic dating and marriage, overall acceptance is growing over time; only 27 percent supported gay marriage in 1996 when the question was first posed in Gallup's Values and Beliefs poll. The May 2011 poll was the first time that a majority (53 percent) in the United States expressed the belief that same-sex marriage should be legally recognized as are marriages between a man and a woman. Support for legal gay marriage is at 70 percent for eighteen- to thirty-four-year-olds and 39 percent among those fifty-five and older (Newport, 2011).

Attitudes toward gender roles and work-life balance also evidence a similar age-related trend. In its most recent survey, the Family and Work Institute (Galinsky, Aumann, & Bond, 2008) report the following among key findings:

- About two-thirds of men and women under twenty-nine years old want jobs with more responsibility; this represents a progressive closing of the gender gap since the first survey in 1992 when significantly more young men than women wanted more responsibility at work.

- Agreement with traditional gender roles has declined for all generations but only 35 percent of those under twenty-nine years old support traditional gender roles and 53 percent of those sixty-three and over do.

- Fathers under twenty-nine years old spend more time with their children than fathers who are twenty-nine to forty-two years old.

- As men take on more responsibility at home, their work-life conflict has increased from 37 percent reporting conflict in 1977 to 45 percent in 2008; the percentage of women reporting work-life conflict rose less steeply, from 34 percent in 1977 to 39 percent in 2008.

Age-related trends like these are harbingers of change that point to a future in which bias is less socially acceptable and inclusion is the norm, not the exception, in society at large and in health care organizations. In the future, inclusion in the workplace and personalized care will be expected and support for the systems approach to diversity and cultural competence in health care organizations more widespread.

Trend Four: Mandates Continue to Grow in Breadth and Depth

A growing number of professional associations and regulatory bodies are issuing regulations that recommend or require health care organizations to engage in training and adopt policies, practices, and procedures to ensure culturally and linguistically responsive care. This trend has been discussed in previous chapters and received special attention in Chapters Two, Six, and Eight.

The National Health Law Project reports that all fifty states have at least two laws that address language access in health care for LEP patients. These state requirements build on federal laws pertaining to LEP patients from Title VI of the Civil Rights Act of 1964 to the Hill Burton Act and others. State laws vary in breadth and depth, with California having the most laws and a more comprehensive approach to language access to health care for LEP patients than most other states. As noted earlier, there is a trend toward mandatory cultural competence training for health professionals as well as Medicaid funding for language services. New Jersey, California, and Washington all mandate such training. Some states such as California and Washington have extended language access mandates to commercial health plans and require access to interpreter and translation services as they pertain to accessing covered benefits. In a growing number of states, facility licensure is contingent on providing LAS to LEP patients. Some states, including Washington, Iowa, Indiana, and Oregon, now have certification requirements for medical interpreters or have passed laws that require development of interpreter standards. The researchers attribute the trend toward more state mandates to address changing demographics and the focus on quality and patient-centered care (Perkins & Youdelman, 2008). Although not mandatory, The Institute for Diversity in Health Care Management (IFD) recently began offering a certificate in diversity management program for diversity management professionals, which prepares participants to respond more effectively to the business case for diversity and cultural competence and to emerging regulations and mandates.

The Patient Protection and Affordable Care Act of 2010 also supports the trend toward more mandated policies and procedures to ensure culturally and linguistically appropriate care. Key relevant provisions include the following (Andrulis, Siddiqui, Purtle, & Duchon, 2010):

- Collect data on patient race and ethnicity and primary language and report and monitor health disparities in federally funded programs

- Collect and report data on workforce diversity and support initiatives to increase diversity in the health professions

- Support the development and implementation of cultural competence training curricula for health care professionals and organizations

- Support disparities research and prevention initiatives

- Address health insurance disparities

The report's conclusion is apropos here (Andrulis, Siddiqui, Purtle, & Duchon, 2010):

> The ACA and its provisions to improve access, affordability and quality of care—in supporting comprehensive action to improve health and health services for racially and ethnically diverse patients and communities—lays a strong foundation for eliminating the legacy of health disparities. In looking forward, this new law has the potential to seed, promote and guide diversity initiatives in this country for decades to come. Realizing its vision will do much to promote the longstanding promise of equality and equity for all. (p. 18)

Add to these initiatives the Joint Commission's (2010) standards for patient-centered communication, which were implemented in January 2011, The National Center for Quality Assurance's (2010) multicultural health care standards, the National Quality Forum's (2009) comprehensive framework and preferred practices for measuring and reporting cultural competence, and the CLAS standards enhancement initiative (www.thinkculturalhealth.hhs.gov), and the trajectory is clear. The demand for culturally and linguistically appropriate care as the norm not the exception will continue to grow, thus driving more health care organizations to implement a leadership-driven systems approach to ensure success.

Trend Five: The Business Case for Diversity Continues to Build

We reviewed the theory and research that undergird the systems approach to strategic diversity management and cultural competence in Chapter Ten and discussed the evolution of the business case in Chapter Eleven. Researchers and health care organizations are increasingly aware of the business case for diversity. And, because health care organizations are open systems and, therefore, interact with and are influenced by their environment, the previous four trends are principal drivers of this growing attention.

In a study of California hospital's diversity management practices, for example (Weech-Maldonado et al., 2012), hospitals performed better in patient-related cultural competence activities than in diversity management activities. This finding illustrates the power of mandates (trend four) in shaping the behavior of health care organizations. But, as Weech-Maldonado and his colleagues (2012) contend, "Organizations need a systems approach to cultural competency with strong leadership commitment and integration of cultural competency into management systems, such as human resources, information systems, and QI" (p. 9) as recommended by the NQF's comprehensive framework and preferred practices (National Quality Forum, 2009). And, as discussed in previous chapters, health care organizations that engage in a leadership-driven systems approach to diversity management and cultural competence have implemented more best practices than those who do not.

The growing recognition of the business case for the systems approach is also evidenced by DiversityInc's decision to add the top five hospital systems to its portfolio of specialty lists in 2010. And, in 2011, the American Hospital

Association's Health Research & Educational Trust (HRET) and IFD joined a growing list of professional associations and government agencies articulating the business case for cultural competence in health care and providing guidelines for health care organizations to help ensure effective implementation. HRET and IFD (2011) recommend that health care organizations make the following seven tasks an institutional priority and that they begin with a self-assessment of their current performance:

- Collect race, ethnicity, and language preference (REAL) data
- Identify and report disparities
- Provide culturally and linguistically competent care
- Develop culturally competent disease management programs
- Increase diversity and minority workforce pipelines
- Involve the community
- Make cultural competence an institutional priority

HRET and IFD (2011) also suggest that health care organizations address this central question: "Has your board set goals on improving organizational diversity, providing culturally competent care, and eliminating disparities in care as part of your strategic plan?" (p. 3). As the open systems perspective of organizations (Scott & Davis, 2007) articulates, adaptation and responsiveness to changes in the external environment are necessary to thrive and the systems approach is the best path forward.

Trend Six: Global Interest in Diversity and Cultural Competence in Health Care Is Growing

Interest in the systems approach to diversity and cultural competence in health care is growing in other countries as well. Australia's universal health insurance system, Medicare, for example, funds care that is provided by public health care organizations to a diverse patient base and employs a diverse workforce of health care professionals. Although the indigenous population of Aboriginal and Torres Strait Islander people constitutes only about 2½ percent of the total population, more than half of the population was either born overseas or has at least one parent born in more than two hundred countries from which they immigrated to Australia. An exploratory study that compared Philadelphia and Sydney hospitals on the extent to which they engaged in diversity and cultural competence best practices in six areas—planning, stakeholder satisfaction, diversity training, human resources, health care delivery, and organizational change—concluded that there is more similarity than difference between the two samples but also notes that "the discourse of diversity management has emerged out of the USA where scholars and practitioners are more comfortable in arguing the business case for greater market share and improved productivity in health care organizations, through diversity. In countries with a tradition of unionization and concern for social justice, such language may sit uneasily with values of collectivism" (Whelan, Weech-Maldonado, & Dreachslin, 2008, p. 135). So, although the same best practices in diversity and cultural competence are aimed for, the rationale for engagement may differ across countries.

The Council of Europe (COE), which is composed of forty-seven member states, was founded on May 5, 1949, and includes among its objectives "to promote awareness and encourage the development of Europe's cultural identity and diversity" (http://www.coe.int/aboutCoe/index.asp?page=nosObjectifs&l=en). In 2006, the COE's committee of ministers adopted a recommendation to member states on health services in a multicultural society, which noted that Europe is now a multicultural society because of migration; acknowledged ethnic disparities in health; advocated a broad definition of diversity that is not limited to race, ethnicity, or emigration status; and offered a series of recommendations for action that are consistent with the systems approach advocated throughout this book.

Recommendations put forth in a report from the COE's Committee of Experts on Health Services (2006) addressed the following:

- Provider bias

- Legal barriers

- Language access

- Cultural competence

- Workforce diversity

- Patient-centered care

- Multidisciplinary health care teams

Although the case for the systems approach may differ by country, it is clear that the commitment to leadership-driven strategic diversity management and culturally competent health care delivery is expanding across the globe.

THE SUSTAINABILITY MOVEMENT AND THE SYSTEMS APPROACH

As discussed in previous chapters, demographic diversity, whether in the work-force or the patient population, is more likely to do harm than good unless it is managed through the systems approach. Consequently, as Kochan (2003) aptly stated, "It may be that the business-case rhetoric has run its course . . . [D]iversity is both a labor-market imperative and social expectation or value" (p. 18). The emerging focus in the United States and globally on sustainability and the associated practice of triple-bottom-line accounting supports this perspective.

The sustainability movement, as applied to health care organizations, broadens the focus from short-term financial bottom-line performance to an emphasis on stewardship of the health care organization's human, financial, and environmental resources with the fundamental goal of contributing to the long-term well-being of the community. Triple-bottom-line accounting supports sustainability by expanding performance metrics that are solely financial to also including measures of social and environmental impact. The triple bottom line (TBL) is often referred to as people, planet, and profit. **Diversity dashboards**, which are graphical displays of performance metrics, should be designed in a way that is consistent with the philosophy of sustainability and TBL accounting by including goals and performance metrics that span people, planet, and profit.

Because the systems approach to diversity and cultural competence is grounded in the assumption that health care organizations that are not responsive to community needs and regulatory mandates will not endure, as the sustainability movement and TBL accounting gain traction, so will the systems approach to diversity and cultural competence. Sustainability and TBL may be especially apropos for nonprofit health care provider organizations, whose missions are grounded in social responsibility and the need to respond to stakeholders. In fact, Weech-Maldonado and his collaborators (2012) found that not-for-profit hospitals in California outperformed for-profit hospitals on a broad range of diversity and cultural competence practices. As evidence for the business case builds and the sustainability and TBL perspective is more widely adopted, the performance gap between for-profit and not-for-profit health care providers is likely to narrow.

CHANGE MANAGEMENT AND FORCE FIELD ANALYSIS: TOOLS TO ENVISION AND SHAPE THE FUTURE

Although the six trends discussed in the previous section strongly support widespread adoption of the systems approach to diversity and cultural competence in health care, this fundamental change to the status quo will not happen without the active involvement of change agents. **Change agents** are individuals who lead the process of organizational transformation from a reactive to a pro-active systems approach to diversity and cultural competence. Although, ultimately, buy-in from the health care organization's senior leadership, including the board, chief executive officer, chief financial officer, chief operating officer, chief nursing officer, and chief medical officer, is essential for enduring change, the process of transformation can begin anywhere and can be spearheaded by anyone.

Dreachslin's (1996) description of the origins of the Japanese community relations program at Good Samaritan Hospital and Health Center of Dayton, Ohio, is a case in point. Tomiko Cross, an employee at Good Samaritan for more than twenty years, had lived in the United States for more than thirty years but remained fluent in Japanese. A chance meeting in a Dayton park with a young Japanese woman who was treated at Good Samaritan after a miscarriage produced a flash of insight for Cross. The young woman, who spoke little English, told Cross that she wished she had known Cross while being treated at Good Samaritan because she would have found comfort in talking with someone in Japanese during her stay. It was then that Cross realized that she could serve as a bridge between the hospital and the growing community of Japanese nationals in the service area. Cross shared her insight with the Good Samaritan administrators and was appointed Japanese relations coordinator in 1990. Change agents such as Tomiko Cross are self-motivated catalysts for organizational transformation who literally show the way to a different way of doing things by acting on their vision and helping others to see what they see.

Two models from the renowned psychologist Kurt Lewin, who is commonly credited as the father of organizational development, are valuable additions to the toolkit of change agents in their quest to develop and transform the way health care organizations approach diversity and cultural competence. Lewin's (1947) widely used change theory model and his associated (1943) force field analysis model stress the importance of identifying and influencing driving and restraining forces that will affect the likelihood of a successful change process.

Lewin's change management model (1947) has three phases: unfreeze, transition, and freeze. In the first phase—unfreeze—the change agent's goal is to reduce forces that are serving to maintain the status quo and inspire others to recognize the need for change. In the second phase—transition—the change agent's goal is to introduce new ways of thinking and behaving that support the desired change. And in the third and last phase—freeze—the focus is on ensuring that the new ways of thinking and behaving are institutionalized and become the "new normal" so that the organization will not revert to its old ways of thinking and acting.

Lewin's **force field analysis** (1943) is widely used as a tool to identify driving forces that support the desired change and restraining forces that work against the desired change. Lewin (1943) himself explained that "field theory is probably best characterized as a method: namely a method of analyzing causal relations and of building scientific constructs" (p. 294). A force field is defined as the dynamic environmental context in which individuals and organizations respond to the status quo. Driving forces are factors in the force field that support a proposed change to the status quo, and restraining forces are factors that act against change. The goal of the change agent is to strengthen the driving forces and weaken the restraining forces, thus making successful implementation of the desired change more likely.

In the previous section we outlined six factors that are essentially driving forces for widespread adoption of the systems approach to diversity and cultural competence in health care:

- The demographic imperative is well established.
- Diversity is increasingly nuanced, complex, and multifaceted.
- Support for inclusion is broad based and growing, especially among the young.
- Mandates continue to grow in breadth and depth.
- The business case for diversity continues to build.
- Global interest in diversity and cultural competence in health care is growing.

But there are restraining forces as well, forces that make it less likely that we will see widespread adoption by health care organizations of the systems approach to diversity and cultural competence in the future:

- Recent Supreme Court decisions have weakened traditional affirmative action laws and regulations, which may discourage health care organizations from engaging in diversity-focused recruitment initiatives out of concern for legality.

- Public concern about illegal immigration may discourage health care organizations from language access or other programs for LEP patients beyond those that are required by regulation.

- Financial stress and regulatory mandates for change in other areas such as patient safety and information technology may draw attention away from diversity and cultural competence, especially if no more clear-cut evidence is forthcoming showing positive connections between cultural competence interventions and cost benefits and patient outcomes.

- Personal bias is hard to acknowledge or change and, even though younger people espouse more accepting explicit attitudes, their implicit attitudes are not significantly different than their elders.

- Concerns about the drawbacks of multiculturalism, an approach to diversity that emphasizes the coexistence of different subcultures in one society or organization, may discourage health care organizations from diversity initiatives out of concern that the shared culture will be lost in the process.

- The systems approach to diversity and cultural competence, especially its vision of partnership with the patient and its view of the relationship between diversity management and culturally competent care, shake the foundation of the traditional patient-provider relationship and the role of health care administration, which may engender strong resistance to calls for such fundamental change.

As Figure 12.4 illustrates, a change agent who advocates the systems approach to diversity and cultural competence can use the force field analysis method to first identify driving and restraining forces. Then, the relative strength of each force must be assessed, along with an evaluation of how malleable or resistant to change the force is. In some applications of force field analysis, change agents assign a qualitative numerical value to each driving and restraining factor. By

FIGURE 12.4 Force Field Analysis

Widespread Adoption of Systems Approach to Diversity and Cultural Competence in Health Care

Driving Forces	Restraining Forces
• The demographic imperative is well established.	• Weakened traditional affirmative action
• Diversity is increasingly nuanced, complex, and multi faceted.	• Public concern about illegal immigration
• Support for inclusion is broad based and growing, especially among the young.	• Pressure of financial stress and regulatory mandates in other areas
• Mandates continue to grow in breadth and depth.	• Personal bias is hard to acknowledge or change
• The business case for diversity continues to build.	• Concerns about the drawbacks of multiculturalism
• Global interest in diversity and cultural competence is growing.	• The systems approach requires fundamental change and can produce backlash to diversity and cultural competence.

adding up these numbers, the change agent can determine the likelihood of successful change. If the sum of the relative values associated with the driving forces exceed that of the restraining forces, change is more likely to succeed.

Of course, just identifying and assessing the relative power of driving and restraining forces is not enough. The final step in applying the force field analysis method is to identify and implement action to strengthen the driving forces and weaken the restraining forces. For example, interventions such as the following can serve to weaken the six restraining forces listed previously:

- Distinguish between diversity management and affirmative action and emphasize that diversity management is not dependent on affirmative action regulations but instead is driven by the business case.

- Acknowledge the impact of illegal immigration on the health care organization's bottom line and discuss appropriate action in the context of mission and sustainability.

- Demonstrate and build synergy among financial performance, mandates in areas such as information technology and patient safety, and the systems approach to diversity and cultural competence.

- Provide training in implicit bias to help participants identify, acknowledge, and learn how to change their own implicit biases to be more consistent with their explicit attitudes.

- Openly discuss the challenge and acknowledge the complexity of balancing the differences supported by multiculturalism and the need for a common culture within society and the health care organization.

- Allow stakeholders to express resistance to the systems approach and to mourn the loss of the old way of doing things.

Similarly, interventions such as the following can serve to strengthen the six driving forces discussed earlier in this chapter:

- Illustrate the diversity imperative using hard data specific to the health care organization's service area.

- Provide diversity training that encourages participants to acknowledge and respond appropriately to diversity's nuances, complexity, and multiple facets and dimensions.

- Reward support for inclusion but at the same time acknowledge, understand, and respect diversity in perspectives, especially regarding challenging social issues.

- Adhere to mandates through a comprehensive systems approach that identifies and capitalizes on their interrelationships.

- Develop a diversity dashboard, consistent with sustainability and TBL accounting, to support the business case specific to the health care organization.

- Participate in international forums to share challenges and successes in addressing diversity and cultural competence in health care.

What is the future of the systems approach to diversity and cultural competence in health care? Although no one knows for sure, we are convinced that more widespread adoption is on the horizon. And we can say with certainty that the hard work, dedication, and commitment of change agents will make a difference in our capacity to ameliorate disparities, capitalize on the power of diversity, and deliver personalized care that is culturally and linguistically appropriate.

SUMMARY

In this chapter we identified six forces that will drive more widespread adoption of the systems approach to diversity and cultural competence in health care in the future. We also emphasized the importance of change agents who advocate for the systems approach and influence the future of diversity and cultural competence with their personal commitment and deft use of tools such as Lewin's change model and force field analysis. For the systems approach to become more widespread, change agents must not only work to strengthen driving forces but also to counter restraining forces such as the six identified in this chapter.

In the end, people shape the future of the systems approach to diversity and cultural competence in health care and hold the keys to ameliorating disparities. Providers, patients, families, communities, payors, regulators, professional associations, and other stakeholders will determine our success or failure in meeting the health care needs of diverse communities. It is what we think, feel, and do about the systems approach to diversity and cultural competence that will mold our future. What role will you play?

KEY TERMS

change agents   force field analysis

diversity dashboards

REVIEW QUESTIONS AND ACTIVITIES

1. List the six trends that support widespread adoption of the systems approach to diversity and cultural competence in health care. Rank them from one to six, with one being the most important. Support your rankings with facts and logical argument.

2. What impact will the growing support for diversity and inclusion among younger people have on culturally and linguistically appropriate care? Discuss the impact of this trend from the patient as well as the provider perspectives.

3. Will health care organizations change more in response to the business case for diversity and cultural competence or in response to regulatory mandates? Explain your answer.

4. Use force field analysis to identify driving and restraining forces for one of the following organizational change initiatives or another of your choice: implementing a policy prohibiting the use of family members as interpreters, requiring mandatory diversity and cultural competence training for all employees, tying a percentage of administrators' compensation to diversity goal achievement, or hiring a chief diversity officer. What can you do as a change agent to strengthen the driving forces and counter the restraining forces?

5. Review the six restraining forces that work against widespread implementation of the systems approach to diversity and cultural competence. Rank them from one to six, with one being the most important. Support your rankings with facts and logical argument.

6. Do you believe that the systems approach to diversity and cultural competence in health care will be more widespread in the future? Support your answer with facts and logical argument.

7. What actions will you take to shape the future of the systems approach to diversity and cultural competence in health care?

REFERENCES

Andrulis, D., Siddiqui, N., Purtle, J., & Duchon, L. (2010). *Patient protection and affordable care act of 2010: Advancing health equity for racially and ethnically diverse populations.* Washington, DC: Joint Center for Political and Economic Studies.

Committee of Experts on Health Services in a Multicultural Society. (2006). *Adapting health care services to cultural diversity in multicultural Europe: Explanatory memorandum.* Strasburg, France: Council of Europe.

Dreachslin, J. L. (1996). *Diversity leadership.* Chicago: Health Administration Press.

Galinsky, E., Aumann, K., & Bond, J. T. (2008). *Times are changing: Gender and generation at work and at home.* New York: Families and Work Institute.

HRET (Health Research and Educational Trust) & IFD (Institute for Diversity in Health Management). (2011). *Building a culturally competent organization: The quest for equity in health care.* Chicago: Health Research and Educational Trust.

The Joint Commission. (2010). *Advancing effective communication, cultural competence, and patient- and family-centered care: A roadmap for hospitals.* Oakbrook Terrace, IL: Author.

Kochan, T., Bezrukova, K., Ely, R., Jackson, S., Joshi, A., & Jehn, K., et al. (2003). The effects of diversity on business performance: Report of the Diversity Research Network. *Human Resource Management, 42*(1), 3–21.

Kosmin, B. A., & Keysar, A. (2009). *American religious identification survey (ARIS 2008) summary report.* Hartford, CT: Trinity College.

Lewin, K. (1943). Defining the field at a given time. *Psychological Review, 50*(3), 293–310.

Lewin, K. (1947). Frontiers in group dynamics, concepts, methods, and reality in social science. *Human Relations,* 5–42.

Mather, M., Pollard, K., & Jacobsen, L. A. (2011). *First results from the 2010 census.* Washington, DC: Population Reference Bureau.

National Center for Quality Assurance. (2010). *Implementing multicultural health care standards: ideas and examples.* Retrieved from http://www.ncqa.org/Portals/0/Publications/Implementing %20MHC%20Standards%20Ideas%20and%20Examples%2004%2029%2010.pdf

National League for Nursing (NLN). (2010). *Executive Summary: Annual survey of schools of nursing, academic year 2009–2010.* Retrieved from http://www.nln.org/research/slides/index.htm

National Quality Forum. (2009). *Cultural competency: A comprehensive framework and preferred practices for measuring and reporting cultural competency: A consensus report.* Washington, DC: Author.

Perkins, J., & Youdelman, M. (2008). *Summary of state law requirements addressing language needs in health care.* National Health Law Program. Retrieved from http://www.lawhelp.org/ documents/383231nhelp.lep.state.law.chart.final.pdf

Pew Hispanic Center. (2011). *The Mexican-American boom: Births overtake immigration.* Washington, DC: Pew Hispanic Center.

Pew Research Center. (2007). *Blacks see growing values gap between poor and middle class.* Washington, DC: Pew Research Center.

Saad, L. (2012, May 14). *US acceptance of gay/lesbian relationships is the new normal.* Gallup Poll Social Series: Values and Beliefs. Retrieved from http://www.gallup.com/poll/154634/ Acceptance-Gay-Lesbian-Relations-New-Normal.aspx

Scott, W. R., & Davis, G. F. (2007). *Organizations and organizing: Rational, natural, and open systems perspectives.* Upper Saddle River, NJ: Pearson.

Taylor, P., Funk, C., & Craighill, P. (2006). *Guess who's coming to dinner: 22% of Americans have a relative in a mixed-race marriage.* Washington, DC: Pew Research Center.

Taylor, P., Passel, J., Wang, W., Kiley, J., Velasco, G., & Dockterman, D. (2010). *Marrying out: One-in-seven new U.S. marriages in interracial or interethnic.* Washington, DC: Pew Research Center.

US Census Bureau. (2011). *Overview of race and Hispanic origin: 2010. Table 1: Population by Hispanic or Latino origin and by race for the United States: 2000 and 2010 (p. 4).* Retrieved from http://www.census.gov/prod/cen2010/briefs/c2010br-02.pdf

Weech-Maldonado, R., Dreachslin, J. L., Brown, J., Pradhan, R., Rubin, K. L., Schiller, C., & Hays, R. D. (2012). Cultural competency assessment tool for hospitals: Evaluating hospitals' adherence to the culturally and linguistically appropriate services standards. *Health Care Management Review, 37*(1), 54–66.

Whelan, A. K., Weech-Maldonado, R., & Dreachslin, J. L. (2008). Diversity management in health: Cross national organizational study. *International Journal of Diversity in Organisations, Communities, and Nations, 8*(3), 125–137.

GLOSSARY

Accessible statuses: The group identity statuses that from time to time describe our reactions in situations where our group affiliation is salient. Differs from our dominant group identity status, which describes our usual or customary reactions in situations where our group affiliation is salient.

Acculturation: A process by which an individual coming in contact with a culture other than his or her own begins to internalize aspects of the new culture.

Ad hoc interpreters: Any bilingual family member, friend, health care worker, or passerby who is pressed into service as an interpreter.

Attitude: Favorable or unfavorable disposition or feeling toward a target such as an identity group or diversity dimension.

Benchmarking: Comparing performance to norms or standards.

Best demonstrated practices: A proven method or approach that leads to a reliable and desired outcome.

Bicultural: A personal identity formed by being socialized in two cultures with the resultant ability to function well in both.

Business case: Justification for a course of action in an organization based on the action's impact on organizational performance, including outcomes such as workforce and customer satisfaction, effective teamwork, market share, disparities reduction, and profitability.

Career pipeline: The flow of students or trainees into a specific profession.

Case studies: An in-depth analysis of a single example or a person, situation, or event for the purpose of exploring underlying principles or to develop contextual information.

Cause-and-effect diagram: A visual representation of the root causes of a defect, also known as a *fishbone diagram* or *Ishikawa diagram.*

Change agents: Individuals who lead the process of organizational transformation.

CLAS standards: An acronym widely used for the federal guidelines for cultural and linguistically appropriate services, which inform and direct the health care of diverse patient populations.

Cognitive reframing: A technique from cognitive psychology to reframe negative thoughts in order to produce more positive feelings and actions.

Community-based training: Learning that comes from community involvement in activities that bring the professional in contact with individuals and population groups in the context of their everyday lives.

Comparative effectiveness research: Research that assesses the efficacy of different treatments for the same disease or disorder.

Concordance: A match between the group identities of a patient and his or her caregiver, which research associates with patient preference and satisfaction.

Consensual validation: The process of determining whether the receiver in a communication exchange comprehended the intended message of the sender.

Contingency variables: Factors that mediate the relationship between dependent and independent variables.

Continuing education: Courses or activities that allow practicing professionals to stay up-to-date on new developments in their fields often required by licensing agencies in order to keep licenses current.

Crosscutting: A diversity dimension that can change during the life of an individual, including age, language, socioeconomic status, and religion.

Cultural awareness: Recognition of the strong effects of culture on self and others.

Cultural bias: Societal beliefs and customs that reinforce the assumption that majority culture—for example, dialect, traditions, and appearance—is superior and minority culture is inferior.

Cultural competence: The capacity of health care systems, organizations, and personnel to provide high-quality, culturally sensitive care to patients from diverse populations. Synonymous with cultural competency.

Cultural desire: A concept developed by Josepha Campinha-Bacote that refers to a provider's internal motivation toward self-development of cultural competence; the central affective construct in her *Process of Cultural Competence in the Delivery of Health Care Services* model (2008).

Cultural epidemiology: The study of how culture affects the onset, course, outcome, incidence, and prevalence of a disease or health condition.

Cultural humility: An attitude of lifelong self-reflection, self-critique, and respectful partnering with patients of all cultures.

Cultural identity: A multidimensional self-concept drawn from allegiance to and acceptance by an ethnic or cultural group.

Cultural relevancy: The act of making an idea, action, or behavior meaningful in the context of a cultural worldview.

Cultural responsiveness: The ability to respond to the needs of persons from cultures different from one's own.

Cultural sensitivity: Respect for the cultural concepts and needs of persons from cultures other than one's own.

Culture: Shared patterns of group thought and behavior acquired through intergenerational learning; worldview, knowledge, norms, values, and behavior shared by a group of people.

Data-driven strategies: Actions and plans that are informed by specific and relevant facts and information.

Decenter: The ability to take into account perspectives other than just one's own.

Defects: Any transaction, service encounter, action, or procedure that does not meet customer expectations.

Demographic data sets: Data programs used by health care organizations to record important characteristics of their patients, both individually and collectively.

Dependent variable: The outcome or effect a researcher wants to predict.

Developmental training: Training that occurs over time in several segments, each segment building on the prior segment.

Didactic: Contains a moral or political message.

Disparities: Differences in the incidence, prevalence, mortality, and burden of diseases and adverse health conditions that exist across population groups in the United States.

Distinctive competence: An area of expertise that differentiates an organization from others that deliver the same product or service and enhances the organization's reputation and performance.

Diversity: All of the similarities and differences that make each individual unique, including characteristics a person is born with and those determined by social factors.

Diversity dashboards: Graphic displays of performance metrics for diversity and cultural competence.

DiversityInc: A leading source of information on diversity management, founded in 1998, that publishes two websites and a magazine, sponsors events, and provides benchmarking data to organizations. DiversityInc's top fifty companies for diversity competition began in 2001 and is a highly regarded source of information on best demonstrated practices in diversity management.

Diversity sensitive orientation (DSO): A measure of the extent to which meeting the needs of a diverse population and recruiting and retaining a diverse workforce drive an organization's strategy.

DMAIC: An acronym for a systematic five-step quality improvement process: define, measure, analyze, improve, and control.

Dominant status: In terms of group identity status it best describes our customary and dominant reactions in situations when our group affiliation is salient.

Dual role interpreter: A bilingual person whose major job is not health care interpreting but is on call for interpreting if needed.

Enculturation: The socialization processes by which the cultural values, beliefs, and behaviors of an identity group are transmitted to its members.

Epidemiological transition: The process that occurs when the major causes of morbidity and mortality in a population change from parasitic and infectious diseases to chronic lifestyle diseases.

Epidemiology: The study of the onset, course, outcomes, incidence, and prevalence of diseases and disorders in populations.

Ethnic group: Groups whose members identify with each other through a common heritage, culture, and language.

Ethnicity: A shared, common ancestry or collective identity through a cultural heritage that generally includes a common language, family, values, norms, and religious traditions.

Ethnocentrism: The belief that the culture of one's identity group is superior to that of other cultures.

Ethnomedical syndromes: A collection of symptoms that are believed by a cultural group to signal a specific, culturally recognized disease or health condition.

Ethnopharmacology: A field of study that investigates responses to drugs that are related to genetic variation across ethnic or racial groups.

Etiology: The set of factors that are believed to contribute to or cause a disease or health condition.

Evidence-based medicine: Medical treatment that is based on scientifically and clinically proven efficacy.

Evidence-based strategies: Actions, plans, or structures that are based on specific and relevant facts and tests of efficacy.

Executive coaches: Professionals who provide one-on-one developmental support to a senior leader in order to build the leader's interpersonal awareness, knowledge, and skills so that the leader can transfer his or her learning into positive results for the organization.

Explanatory models: Patients' perspectives on the nature of their health problems, including etiology, likely course of development, and appropriate treatment.

Explicit biases: Consciously held attitudes toward a target such as an identity group or diversity dimension.

Face-to-face interpretation: A situation in which the interpreter is present in person during the interpreted encounter.

Force field analysis: A method to identify and influence driving forces that support a desired change and restraining forces that work against the change.

Genetic risk: Risk for disease or drug response that is based on inherited biological factors.

Group identity status: The constellation of attitudes and beliefs that shape how we experience and enact our group affiliation.

Hallmarks: Distinguishing characteristics.

Health care encounter: A planned or unplanned interaction between a provider of health care or related services and a recipient of care or information such as a patient, client, family member, or community member.

HEDIS: Commonly used acronym for the National Committee on Quality Assurance's Healthcare Effectiveness Data and Information Set, a tool used by more than 90 percent of public and private health plans to measure performance on many dimensions of care and service.

Human capital factors: Qualifications of individuals that affect career attainment, including education, experience, and technical and interpersonal competencies.

Identity groups: Socially relevant classifications of people such as gender, age, religion, race, or ethnicity.

Immutable: Personal characteristics that are biological in nature or that are highly resistant to change, including diversity dimensions such as gender, race, ethnicity, and sexual orientation.

Implicit biases: Unconsciously held attitudes toward a target such as an identity group or diversity dimension.

Inclusion: The outcome of effective diversity management; an organizational context that facilitates optimal performance, outcomes, and organizational commitment for diverse individuals.

Independent variables: Factors that predict change or variation in dependent variables.

Individual bias: Personally held attitudes, beliefs, and behaviors that reinforce the presumed superiority of the majority and inferiority of the minority.

Inequitable health care disparities: Differences in health access and status that are the result of discrimination, neglect, or socioeconomic variation.

Information value of diversity theory: The theory that heterogeneous groups will produce better outcomes than homogeneous groups because heterogeneous groups will generate a broader range of ideas.

In-group: A group of people united by a common identity and shared beliefs, attitudes, or interests, with the collective social power and influence to exclude outsiders.

Institutional bias: Policies, laws, and regulations that have the effect of systematically giving the advantage to one group and disadvantaging the other(s).

Internalize: The process of consolidating and embedding attitudes, values, and beliefs into one's personal worldview.

Interpretation: The verbal process of conveying the meaning of an utterance spoken in one language (the source language) into another language (the target language) by an interpreter.

Interprofessional or multidisciplinary teams: Synergistic teams made up of health care professionals with different areas of specialized expertise who collaborate to deliver patient care.

Job function: Discrete duties and responsibilities that accrue to a specific position in the workplace.

Language access services (LAS): The full spectrum of services available to provide meaningful access to persons with limited English proficiency.

Language barriers: The difficulties faced when two parties who have no language in common attempt to communicate by spoken or written means.

Language concordance: A circumstance in which both parties to a conversation or communication speak the same language.

Limited English proficiency (LEP): A limited English proficient person is someone who speaks a language other than English and has limited ability to speak, read, or understand English.

Locus of control: A theoretical construct in social psychology that refers to the extent to which individuals believe they can control events that affect their behavior. An internal locus indicates that a person feels in control and an external locus indicates that others are perceived to have that control.

Market share: The percentage or portion of sales controlled by a particular company or business enterprise.

Medical and healthcare interpreter certification: Certification indicating that a health care interpreter has been trained and meets the standards of the National Board of Certification of Medical Interpreters or the Certification Commission for Healthcare Interpreters.

Medical homes: A model of care in which each patient has an ongoing relationship with a personal physician who leads a team that takes collective responsibility for patient care over extended periods of time.

Metrics: A set of measures used to quantify results and evaluate performance.

Mnemonic: A short phrase, rhyme, word, or other mental technique for making information easier to memorize.

Model of developmental readiness: A conceptual model developed by Avolio and Hannah (2008) that defines five preconditions for self-development: learning goal orientation, developmental efficacy, self-concept clarity, self-complexity, and metacognitive ability.

National origin group: A group whose members are drawn from a specific nation state.

Nonverbal communication: Meaning conveyed from one person to another through body language, facial expression, or spatial distance.

Organizational behavior (OB): The study of the impact that individuals, teams, culture, climate, and infrastructure have on performance outcomes.

Organizational development (OD): The practical application of OB theory and research in organizations.

Organizational factors: Aspects of the organization that affect diversity management, including policies, procedures, plant and technology, and people.

Outcome measures: Tools that assess the results of preventive and curative health care strategies.

Out-group: A group of people united by a common identity and excluded from belonging to the in-group and, relative to the in-group, is seen as less powerful, less socially desirable, or contemptibly different.

Pareto chart: A bar chart that graphically represents the frequency distribution of a performance metric.

Patient-centered care: An approach to care that emphasizes that the specific characteristics of each patient such as gender, age, sexual orientation, ethnicity, and race as well as the patient's social environment are considered equally important as medical status or diagnosis.

Patient Protection and Affordable Care Act of 2010: The principal health care reform legislation of the 111th US Congress that expands health insurance to millions of Americans and contains specific measures to reduce disparities related to race and ethnicity, gender, and sexual orientation.

Personalized care: Medical care that is tailored to the individual and includes his or her genomic, social, and cultural contexts.

Power: The ability to change or influence the behavior and circumstances of others through influence, control, or coercion without having to change yourself.

Process improvement: An approach, fundamental to Six Sigma, to continuously improve performance by identifying and closing gaps between desired and actual performance. DMAIC is the most commonly used process improvement approach in Six Sigma.

Projected similarity: A phenomenon that occurs when individuals assume their own beliefs, values, and cultural behavioral patterns are universally shared and valued.

Proxemics: A field of study that focuses on the cultural meaning of interpersonal distance in communication.

Race: A term used by scientists and the general public to identify groups of people by physical characteristics such as skin color, hair texture, bone structure, and genetic markers.

Racial groups: Groups that share a common set of genetically transmitted physical traits.

Research: A systematic approach to testing theory that relies on rigorous methods to control for factors that could serve as alternative explanations for an observed relationship and replication of findings through multiple studies to build a strong evidence base to support or refute theory.

Root causes: The origin of a chain of problems that result in failure to achieve a desired metric.

Self-efficacy: The belief that one is capable of performing in a certain manner so as to achieve a specific goal or set of goals.

Self-monitor: The ability to identify how you are perceived by others and adapt your style to communicate more effectively with others.

Similarity-attraction theory: A proposition, consistent with social categorization theory, that people gravitate toward other people with whom they share salient commonalities and avoid people that they perceive as not sharing such commonalities.

Six Sigma: A customer-focused and data-driven approach to quality management, which improves organizational performance through setting high standards and reducing variation.

Skills gap: The difference between the education and competencies needed for the available jobs and the education and competencies actually possessed by available workers.

Social categorization theory: The proposition that people have a natural tendency to form in-groups with whom they share salient characteristics and associated out-groups that are perceived as not sharing such commonalities.

Social determinants of health: Contextual factors such as marginal living conditions, the environment, education, and literacy that affect health status.

Social diversity dimensions: Personal characteristics such as socioeconomic status, class, or religion that are defined by social classification and are subject to change by the individual.

Social factors: Aspects of society that can contribute to disparities in access and opportunities for diverse groups.

Social organization: The pattern of relationships among people in a group that is generally associated with ethnicity and is learned through the process of enculturation in the family and community.

Socialization: The lifelong process of learning one's culture from the teaching and modeling of others in that culture.

Stereotyping: The act of oversimplifying or overgeneralizing the characteristics of a group or of a member of a group.

Strategic diversity management: A leadership-driven systems approach in which organizational policies, practices, and the workforce promote inclusion and address the needs of diverse staff, patients, and communities through cultural and linguistic competence.

Subcultures: Groups of people with cultural traits that differentiate them from the larger culture to which they also belong.

Symptoms: Signs or indications of the existence of a disease or health problem.

System: A structure made up of interconnected people, policies, and practices designed to work in concert to achieve common goals and that provides feedback loops to inform and adjust the structure as needed to achieve the goals.

Systems approach: The process of considering how different parts of a whole influence and integrate with each other to achieve a goal and of viewing problems in a system as affecting the system overall.

Telephonic or video interpretation: Interpretation that takes place over the telephone or through a video hook-up.

Theory: A proposed explanation of a real-world phenomenon that requires testing and validation through research.

Therapeutic alliance: The interpersonal dynamic that takes place between a patient and doctor through their mutual interaction.

Trained health care and medical interpreters: Individuals who have received training in medical terminology and procedures as well as in techniques that facilitate interpreted encounters between care providers and patients.

Transcultural nursing: An area of nursing research and practice, founded by Madeline Leininger, that focuses on the impact of culture on patients' and providers' health values, beliefs, and behaviors and advocates provision of culturally appropriate care through providers' cultural awareness, sensitivity, and competence.

Transcultural self-efficacy: Confidence in one's own ability to develop and apply cognitive, practical, and affective transcultural nursing skills, a central construct in Jeffreys's Cultural Competence and Confidence Model.

Transforming experiences framework: A conceptual model developed by the Grubb Institute used to explore how professionals enact their roles by understanding the relationships among three constructs that affect how people experience their role in an organization and influence their actions: person, context, and system.

Translation: The process of transcribing a piece of written communication from a source language into a target language by a translator.

Value system: The hierarchy of beliefs and convictions that guide a person's conduct, choices, and goals.

Workforce diversity: Differences among employees in their identity groups, life experiences, cultures, and work-related and personal styles.

Worldview: A constellation of core beliefs that together define the overall perspective from which the world is seen and interpreted.

INDEX